AROMATHERAPY

AROMATH

REVISED AND UPDATED FROM
Aromatherapy for Vibrant Health and Beauty

ERAPY

ESSENTIAL
OILS FOR
VIBRANT
HEALTH
AND BEAUTY

ROBERTA WILSON

AVERY

A member of Penguin Putnam Inc.

New York

a member of
Penguin Putnam Inc.
375 Hudson Street
New York, NY 10014
www.penguinputnam.com

Copyright © 2002 by Roberta Wilson

Library of Congress Cataloging-in-Publication Data

Wilson, Roberta, date.
Aromatherapy : essential oils for vibrant health and beauty / Roberta Wilson.
p. cm.
Previous ed. published with title: Aromatherapy for vibrant health and beauty.
Includes bibliographical references and index.
ISBN 1-58333-130-1
1. Aromatherapy.   I. Wilson, Roberta, date. Aromatherapy for
vibrant health and beauty.   II. Title.
RM666.A68 W57   2002   2001056598
615'.321—dc21

Printed in the United States of America

9   10   8

Book design by Renato Stanisic

I dedicate this book
to my mother, Genie Stuart.

For all your generosity, goodness, help,
kindness, love, and support,
I thank you.

Acknowledgments

To my readers, *I offer my gratitude for your patronage over the years. Your curiosity, your quest for knowledge, your passion to improve your lives, your desire to take care of yourselves and others, and your support of aromatherapy and essential oils inspire and motivate me forward on this fragrant path that I chose to follow. I feel blessed that your needs and desires allow me to combine two of my great loves—writing and aromatherapy. I thank you for the opportunity to have an impact on your lives. You validate my endeavors to educate, to share, and to make the world a healthier and happier place. You help me keep the flames of hope and faith burning in my heart that someday, somehow, we will live once again in a paradise where peace and harmony prevail.*

The field of aromatherapy attracts many wonderful people who are willing to share their time, expertise, and experiences with others. I especially appreciate the gracious assistance and patience of Robert Gaffney and Nicole Syme at Omega Nutrition, and Kurt Schnaubelt and his staff at Pacific Institute of Aromatherapy. Your integrity and your commitment to quality and consumer education symbolize the aromatherapy experience for me.

I thank my family for always supporting me and for indulging me when necessary. Being a writer is challenging, but I suspect having a writer in the family is an even greater challenge. I especially am grateful to my mother and my sister for helping me prepare the revised manuscript for publication.

I am forever indebted to the many pioneers of modern aromatherapy, who revived the almost lost art of aromatherapy. Without their tireless efforts, none of us would reap the rewards of using essential oils. In my work, I strive to keep alive their life work and to fulfill their dreams of sharing with the world the value of true aromatherapy using essential oils.

Contents

Part Three:

WAYS TO USE AROMATHERAPY

Part Four:

COMMON CONDITIONS THAT CAN BE TREATED WITH AROMATHERAPY

Foreword

✳

Considering how *fast the world is moving today, one could almost say that modern aromatherapy has, to some degree, already come of age. In the early 1980s, modern aromatherapy became a popular phenomenon in Great Britain, then started to spread throughout the rest of the English-speaking world and beyond. Since then, many people have learned about the numerous ways in which aromatherapy and essential oils can improve their lives. The most obvious benefits of using essential oils are related to health conditions that are common in modern life. In the search for cures and remedies for afflictions ranging from herpes to stress-induced symptoms, many aromatherapy enthusiasts have found often unexpected healing through the use of these relatively simple and inexpensive essential oils.*

A rather brisk development of aromatherapy ensued, driven mostly by the idealism of those who wanted to make these safe and easy options available to consumers who did not yet know about aromatherapy. As is probably normal with such a wave of rapid development, the forces of commerce have made their imprint on aromatherapy. An avalanche of products that are "aromatherapy" in name only—not in substance—make it increasingly difficult for the layperson to distinguish true healing aromatherapy from superficial marketing gimmicks.

In light of this issue there could be no better timing for a book like *Aromatherapy: Essential Oils for Vibrant Health and Beauty*, which truly is a representation of what aromatherapy is all about in its pure essence. Roberta Wilson's book is of invaluable assistance to the reader who wants to get to the true substance of aromatherapy. On the one hand, it familiarizes the reader with the basic concepts of using essential oils for common ailments. Yet, on the other hand, it does so much more. It tells readers in equal depth about the many additional benefits of aromatherapy that they might not expect. When it comes to healing, most of us admittedly take our cues from our conditioning about conventional medicine. We focus on cause and effect, and on remedies that address specific pathologies. Indeed, investigating the effects of essential oils along those lines has presented us with many new applications for aromatherapy. This book gives a comprehensive overview of what readers can readily do with essential oils and the positive effects they can reasonably expect. We know through scientific studies that essential oils can be effective against bacteria and viruses. We know which components of essential oils are more likely than others to have such effects, even though we do not know the exact mechanisms by which their actions occur. In vitro experiments prove that essential oils can inhibit herpes and other viruses. In a fascinating alliance, our sometimes incomplete or fractionated scientific understanding of essential oils has been complemented by the popular practice of aromatherapy, which has added a large body of very real empirical knowledge. It is fair to say that the combined empirical knowledge of aromatherapy users bears out what the scientific data suggest. Essential oils work reliably when used with the right expectation and in the proper way.

Aromatherapy: Essential Oils for Vibrant Health and Beauty fills the reader in on the many ways and the many ailments for which essential oils present meaningful relief. While it is obvious that the understanding of the pharmacology of essential oils is valuable and has brought great benefits, Roberta's book also promotes an awareness that true healing—strengthening of the fabric of life— includes processes on other planes besides the purely pharmacological one. Essential oils speak to us because they are an expression of the evolution of life on planet earth. So rather than seeing essential oils as merely a mix of random natural chemicals, biologists today know that essential oils represent a finely tuned mélange of natural substances that must have benefited, in one way or another, the plants from which they originate. Essential oils can benefit the plants that produce them in many and diverse ways, ranging from fending off predators to actually providing benefits to other organisms—which, in a symbiotic exchange, then repay the emitter plants. While our understanding of the biological interactions that essential oils initiate is still very limited, this is where *Aromatherapy: Essential Oils for Vibrant Health and Beauty* especially shines. Readers are constantly reminded that in order to garner the full support that essential oils can provide, they must make sure that each essential oil they use is truly the product of a biological organism—that is, a once-living plant—rather than the product of a laboratory. Roberta makes it very clear that even slight alterations of essential oils with synthetics, or even with other natural substances, will diminish or eliminate their biological power.

Aromatherapy: Essential Oils for Vibrant Health and Beauty goes beyond simply listing the known applications of essential oils for a variety of conditions to also familiarize the readers with the subtle, but potentially very substantial, comfort that essential oils can provide. Given that many of us are submerged in modern urban civilization, we often suffer from our separation from nature or, even more significantly, separation from the goodness of creation in general. Essential oils put us back in touch with these primal aspects of our existence. They open our eyes to rediscover the rhythms of nature and the many ways in which physiological processes are interconnected with the mind and the soul. Essential oils, in the practice of aromatherapy, first surprise us with their unexpected efficacy in the realm of the physical. (Anyone who has treated a bruise or a hematoma with the oil of helichrysum will know that.) Yet essential oils go on to rebalance the autonomic nervous system, thus providing relief from the effects of ongoing stress factors. A gradual reintegration into healthy habits takes place as we mediate these stresses and take more time to just be and think clearly. We realize that essential oils not only relieve symptoms but also strengthen our instinctual and emotional processes. They strengthen our identities and, in so doing, ultimately strengthen our immune systems. As we realize that these gentle healing agents are right in front of us, practically as gifts from nature, we are filled with a sense of joyful humility, and our souls start to heal. By reaffirming our connection with nature, essential oils will ultimately support those of us embarking on the aromatherapy journey in doing whatever we do best on planet earth. If this sounds intriguing, *Aromatherapy:*

Essential Oils for Vibrant Health and Beauty is a perfect ticket to this journey. Readers will soon realize that true essential oils from once-living plants interact with the full spectrum of our consciousness, swiftly covering the realm of material remedies and integrating instinct, consciousness, and soul.

Kurt Schnaubelt, Ph.D.
Pacific Institute of Aromatherapy

Preface to the Second Edition

✳

When I returned *to the United States after living abroad for many years, I was stunned to see how aromatherapy had changed. Aromatherapy had entered the mainstream. Discount stores, supermarkets, drugstores, and even convenience stores were stocking their shelves with aromatherapy products. Prime-time television commercials promoted aromatherapy products. At first, I thought my dreams for educating the world about aromatherapy had been fulfilled. However, upon closer inspection, I sensed that something insidious was corrupting aromatherapy. Why was this happening? And, more important, what could I, one person alone, possibly do to educate the public about what was happening in the world of aromatherapy? People needed to know that their best efforts to buy therapeutic aromatherapy* products might be exploited by businesses willing to substitute inexpensive synthetic ingredients for pure essential oils.

When my editor at Penguin Putnam asked me if I would consider revising *Aromatherapy for Vibrant Health and Beauty,* I knew the time was right. At about the same time, I met an incredible woman, Mary Ellen Bowman, who had been using the formulas in my book to treat her friends, her family, and herself. She shared my belief in the powers of essential oils to help the human body heal itself. When she recounted her success stories with me, I asked her to help me develop an aromatherapy company. We are committed to being a valuable resource for people who want to engage in the healing experiences that essential oils offer. We want to provide the highest quality products and services such as the purest essential oils, blends, carrier oils, information, research, and education to encourage you to use your own abilities to take responsibility for your health and to encourage you to share your wisdom with others. We want to become a leading resource in your quest for vibrant health and beauty.

One of my greatest goals is to urge consumers to distinguish between true aromatherapy and commercial aromatherapy, and to understand the necessity of always choosing true aromatherapy for health and healing. Aromatherapy—the original and true aromatherapy—is in jeopardy of being corrupted and even disappearing. True aromatherapy requires the use of pure essential oils from once-living plants to prompt the body's own healing abilities to protect against or overcome illnesses. Conversely, commercial aromatherapy—or what I call *pseudo-aromatherapy*—employs synthetic scents that simply smell, yet lack therapeutic or medicinal benefits.

I am eager to share new knowledge with my readers and aromatherapy enthusiasts. To the original thirty-six essential oils featured in *Aromatherapy for Vibrant Health and Beauty,* I have added eight others that can expand your healing horizons. I have included some new conditions to offer more opportunities for people to take care of themselves. I have created almost all new formulas to reflect my view that using lower levels of essential oils brings equal or greater healing benefits than do higher levels. Essential oils are highly concentrated and so potent that less is plenty. In an expanded section on carrier oils, I stress the importance of using only the highest quality and freshest carrier oils in your blends to ensure the best aromatherapy experiences. I have changed my previous position on mixing pure essential oils with commercial cosmetics. I feel that doing so diminishes the effect of the essential oils and often can defeat your best intentions. Finally, I have included some information on hydrosols, or floral waters, for readers who wish to explore this avenue as an alternative or supplemental means of using aromatherapy.

On the surface, this book is about aromatherapy and health and beauty. Beneath the surface, I hope I convey deeper meanings. This book is also about responsibilities and choices. It is about attention and intention. It is about inner connections and outward connections. It is about human nature and mother nature. It is about caring and sharing. It is about love and life. It is about you and me, for together—and only together—we can make differences that acting alone we could not or would not make.

My greatest desire is to help others through education. I want to touch people's lives at the core, where they form the beliefs and make the choices that will determine the directions their lives and their health will take. I hope to empower people to assume responsibility for their health, lifestyles, and life choices. I invite every one of you to use the knowledge contained in this book to improve your health and your life.

Health is a reflection of the inner world you create with your thoughts, beliefs, and attitudes, as well as the energy you bestow upon your spirit or soul. Equally, health is a reflection of the outer world that you create with your actions, lifestyle choices, and priorities. Your attitudes and actions today determine the health of your mind and body tomorrow.

Modern lifestyles are harsh on health. Having vibrant health requires taking responsibility by playing an active role in caring for yourself. It requires remembering that you are your best doctor, for who can know your body and mind better? You have the power, within your body and your mind, to heal yourself. Healing demands that you look beyond symptoms to discover their sources, for silencing symptoms can heal neither body nor mind. Investigating underlying causes lets you look closely at your life and the lifestyle factors that cause or contribute to discomfort and disease. It brings awareness and offers opportunities to make change that can restore health and balance.

Balance promotes health, while imbalance brings illness. How can we find our way back to good health unless we address the various causes of poor health that lead to illness, pain, discomfort, and disease, which create imbalance? How can we address the causes of imbalance unless we investigate how our thoughts and actions contribute to or create illness? How can we take responsibility unless we reclaim the power to heal ourselves? How can we heal our bodies unless we heal our souls as well? And how can we heal our souls unless we heal our split with nature, with our fellow humans, and most of all within ourselves?

Humans are marvelous creatures and creators. With the magic of our thoughts and actions, you and I create the world around us. Your choices affect me; my choices affect you. If and when we assume responsibility for our powers of creation, we can create perfection and paradise on earth and in our bodies, and whatever else we desire. In a world out of balance, finding the way back to center and to balance sometimes seems impossible. Aromatherapy can guide us back to where we belong.

Humans are an integral and inseparable part of nature, and nature is a part of us. As the health of nature suffers, so too does human health. Nature is in serious trouble and so too are humans. It is no coincidence that the farther we stray from our natural relationships with plants and nature, the more out of balance we become, the more symptoms we suffer, and the more disease dominates our lives.

All of the plants that provide the precious essential oils that I treasure also are in jeopardy. Will we realize in time that we need plants more than we are willing to admit? Will we realize that we need plants more than they need us? Have we really forgotten one of the most basic principles of human life? We need oxygen to breathe, to live, to have healthy bodies, to energize our brains, and to survive as a species. Plants provide this oxygen. We fill our lungs with their oxygen, and their oxygen fills us with life. We also need plants to absorb our respiratory waste product, carbon dioxide. The quality and quantity of the oxygen that plants produce determine, to a large degree, the quality of our lives. The quality and the quantity of the plants on earth determine how much of our carbon dioxide waste can be absorbed. Yet we carelessly cut down plants, trees, and entire forests as though our lives don't depend on them.

We need a miracle to help us save ourselves. Rediscovering botanicals and integrating them into our lives may be the closest thing to a miracle that we can expect. In addition to practicing aromatherapy, growing, using, and appreciating fresh fruits and vegetables for foods, herbs for flavoring and medicinal properties, plants for natural-fiber clothing, forests for increased quality and quantity of fresh air to breathe, flowers and houseplants as a source of beauty all offer us viable solutions to many problems we face today. Embracing plants and nature may present us with a pleasant and practical chance to save ourselves, for we cannot do it without them.

Plants and botanicals seem to be the most likely sources for healing the human body. We are already doing a respiratory slow dance with plants, our intimate partners in life. Plants have the ability to automatically adapt to external and internal stressors by creating changes in their tissue that ensure their survival. Isn't it possible that, as they take in our carbon dioxide, they can interpret our state of health or illness? As plants adapt to survive ever-changing external conditions, such as the changing state of human health, could they possibly hold secrets that will help us survive too—if we will only use them?

One of the easiest ways to embrace nature is by practicing aromatherapy using pure essential oils. Essential oils are messengers from nature that offer us vital information about living in balance to heal ourselves. They offer us an ideal opportunity to reconnect with the whole of nature.

As we seek healing from botanicals, we learn to appreciate the delicate balance between the state of nature and the state of our bodies. We can feel the link between the health of nature and our own health. Essential oils can make us want to live a life based on reverence for the deep physical and spiritual connection of all things on earth.

Aromatherapy heals, but it also teaches. Essential oils encourage us to look inside ourselves for answers. Aromatherapy teaches us to look closely at the big picture and see our part in the whole. Aromatherapy can help us save ourselves. It makes us want to heal ourselves, heal our split within, and heal our split with all people and all things around us. Aromatherapy makes it clear that the farther we stray from the natural world, the more out of balance we become. The farther we stray from the spiritual pulse that runs through all life, the more we feel an insatiable need to fill the emptiness that persists within. Aromatherapy awakens us to the endless possibilities. Essential oils are the guides that can lead us forward on the path toward the future that we are creating today.

If I can help you to gain new respect for essential oils and true aromatherapy, I will feel genuinely rewarded for my efforts. I invite you to partake of aromatherapy as an effective and pleasurable means of restoring health, beauty, and balance to your body, mind, and soul, so that you will want to do your part to restore balance in the world.

With this book, I am rededicating my life's work to helping guide people on the healing path to vibrant health. Besides working to create a reliable source of accurate educational information and therapeutic-quality products, I will conduct research on essential oils and aromatherapy. I will continue to write other books on health, healing, and aromatherapy that will urge people to take responsibility for their health and their lives. Humans can accomplish great achievements in life when we embrace our potential, when we feel compassion toward ourselves and others, when we acknowledge that we are together in this life, when we aspire to harmony and peace with nature and one another, and when we commit ourselves to making the world a beautiful and safe place to live. We can do it by exploring, sharing, and playing together.

Preface

Since the day *in the early 1980s when I first discovered lavender oil, I have been fascinated by aromatherapy. I felt as if I had found a long-lost friend. Aromatherapy filled a gap in my life—both a personal and a professional one. I immediately incorporated essential oils into my skin-care practice, into my private life, and into my study of herbs, nutrition, and holistic healing. Using these concentrated plant extracts to improve physical and emotional health seemed like the perfect addition to my natural beauty treatments and lifestyle.*

Curious by nature, I became a sponge for knowledge about aromatherapy, soaking up every drop of information I could find on the subject, particularly on ways to use aromatherapy. Unfortunately, at the time, only a few books were available, and their highly technical approach was somewhat discouraging and confusing.

As a beginner, I was more interested in how essential oils could help me than I was in their chemical composition.

Through the years I've combed library and bookstore shelves, searching for books on the practical applications of aromatherapy. Today, although more than two dozen aromatherapy books are in print, simple and easy-to-understand books with explicit instructions for using essential oils are still scarce.

I have spent much of the past ten years researching aromatherapy and attending numerous aromatherapy classes. I have taken two certification programs, interviewed French physicians who use medical aromatherapy, and written more than two dozen articles on aromatherapy. I have become familiar with at least 110 different essential oils, and have mixed hundreds of blends for my friends, my clients, and myself. Everyone has responded with encouragement and enthusiasm.

Through the years I have also educated people—friends, neighbors, strangers, children, senior citizens, clients, skin-care professionals, cosmetic manufacturers, health-food store retailers, and the general public—about aromatherapy. I have come to realize that many people are simultaneously interested in and intimidated by aromatherapy. My primary objective in writing this book is to provide a complete, useful reference to help people learn how they can use aromatherapy to improve the quality of their lives. In the pages that follow, I will provide the important information you need so that you can use aromatherapy safely and effectively, without overwhelming you or inundating you with more information than you need or can use. At the same time, I have eliminated most of the guesswork by providing precise instructions for making aromatherapy blends to treat more than sixty common conditions. To keep it simple, I have omitted the chemistry and botany of essential oils. First of all, there are already many good books that address these subjects in detail (some of them are listed in Recommended Reading at the end of this book). Second, I believe that unless aromatherapy is presented in an easy, enjoyable manner, you probably won't use it. And only by using aromatherapy will you discover its many pleasures and benefits.

Though this book is simple and easy to follow, it is not intended only for beginners. Veteran aromatherapists, skin-care specialists, massage therapists, cosmetic manufacturers, and health-care professionals all will find plenty of practical information and useful formulas here that can complement the treatments they already use.

Aromatherapy plays a vital part in my life. From saving me from the stresses of hectic days to keeping my skin youthful and attractive; from soothing my sore throats to making my breathing easier; from freshening my home to fragrancing my bathwater; from providing me with delightful, emotionally soothing perfumes to furnishing me with great gifts for loved ones, essential oils have been my faithful friends and constant companions for the last decade.

My study of aromatherapy has awakened more than my sense of smell. I have become acutely aware of my other senses and my many abilities. Aromatherapy has also inspired in me a deep, abiding reverence for plants. These sometimes sturdy, sometimes fragile, but always amazing chlorophyll factories give us the gift of life. Without them, we would surely starve and suffocate. Beyond providing the basics of life, plants beautify our planet. In doing so, they sustain another aspect of human survival—the satisfaction of our senses. Their delightful perfumes seduce our sense of smell. Their rainbows of colors decorate our homes, offices, gardens, parks—the entire earth—and delight our sense of sight. They spice up our lives and our foods and satisfy our sense of taste. Their feathery leaves and silky petals tantalize our sense of touch. Without plants we could not live. And even if we could, would we want to? How dull life would be if we were deprived of the rich splashes of pastels and vibrant shades of flowers and greenery that color the earth!

I have written this book for several reasons. Writing is a true love of mine; it is something I must do. I especially love writing about essential oils and aromatherapy. I enjoy educating people about anything I've found valuable in my life, and essential oils head the list of tools that have helped me. Beyond my personal reasons, I saw the need for a book that would encourage people to incorporate aromatherapy into their daily lives by showing them exactly how to use it. I hope this book will spark your curiosity about aromatherapy, inspire you to experiment with essential oils, and make you want to continue seeking knowledge about aromatherapy. I am excited about sharing my discoveries with you. In writing this book, I have expanded my own knowledge about aromatherapy, and what I have learned has validated my work over the previous few years. As we embark on this adventurous journey of the senses, I hope aromatherapy will enhance your health and well-being and improve the quality of your life.

Thank you and bon voyage!

Roberta Wilson

Part One

THE BASIC PRINCIPLES
OF AROMATHERAPY

What Is Aromatherapy?

❋

Aromatherapy is *the practice of using naturally extracted essences of aromatic plants to promote the health and well-being of your body, mind, and emotions. These essences, called essential oils, contain the vital life force of fragrant botanical plants. Pure essential oils are the key to success with aromatherapy. They can restore balance and harmony to your body and mind, while adding depth, dimension, and definition to your life. The use of* pure essential oils *characterizes and distinguishes true aromatherapy, which always substantiates the work and supports the intentions of pioneers in aromatherapy.*

USES AND ACTIONS OF ESSENTIAL OILS

You can use essential oils in a variety of ways. Inhale them directly from the bottle. Use them for skin care, hair care, and body care, as well as for numerous other beauty purposes. Use them for personal hygiene and oral hygiene. Take aromatherapy baths. Soak your tired, aching feet in a foot bath fragranced with essential oils. Dangle your fingers in a delightful hand bath. Give and receive aromatherapy massages. Breathe in aromatherapy blends to relieve congestion, clear your head, and make your breathing easier. Make delightful fragrances with essential oils.

While essential oils are the primary tools of aromatherapy, other plant derivatives can benefit you as well. Smelling a fragrant flower or an aromatic herb is aromatherapy, simple and honest. Crushing peppermint leaves between your fingers releases some of its essential oil. As you breathe in its exhilarating essence, you experience healing qualities of the herb. Spraying rose water or lavender water on your face freshens your skin as it disperses the soothing properties of the plant onto your skin. Floating a sprig of rosemary or a handful of orange blossoms in your bath releases skin-softening and emotion-balancing properties into the warm water. Burning dried herbs such as sage smudge sticks or using fresh herbs in homemade potpourri allows their aroma to waft through your home. Pouring boiled water over herbs for a facial steam bath releases aromatic essences that you can smell and feel immediately. When you squeeze a lemon or lime wedge into a glass of water, its aromatic molecules escape into the air. Eating fresh basil or fennel seeds in your food releases their healing attributes into your body.

Aromatherapy can help prevent or ease an assortment of ailments. Essential oils can boost your immune system and help you stay well. You can treat aches, pains, and injuries with essential oils. Essential oils can also help you reduce stress, lift depression, and restore or enhance emotional well-being. You can even disperse essential oils in the air throughout your home or office to help improve your productivity, alter the atmosphere, or modify your moods.

In this book, you will discover hundreds of aromatherapy blends, each designed for a specific purpose, as well as many different ways you can incorporate aromatherapy into your life. You will also learn how to choose and experiment with essential oils on your own. You can learn how to listen to your body and trust your innate instincts to take care of your body, mind, and spirit. Aromatherapy offers a natural approach to wellness that can infuse your life with a new sense of vitality, vibrancy, and pleasure.

WHAT IS *NOT* AROMATHERAPY?

The practice of using essences that did not originate from an aromatic plant that was once alive is *not* aromatherapy. No regulations restrict the use of the word *aromatherapy*. Anyone can sell anything and call it aromatherapy, and plenty of companies are doing exactly that. The result is that about 95 percent of the products sold as aromatherapy are counterfeits—pseudo-aromatherapy. Their aromas derive from synthetic scents, and they offer no therapeutic value whatsoever. True aromatherapy *never* uses synthetic aromatic substances.

Pseudo-aromatherapy relies on synthetic petrochemicals that merely smell but have no healing qualities. Simply having an aroma doesn't make something aromatherapy; fragrant man-made chemicals can never qualify as true aromatherapy.

Every day, thousands of consumers unknowingly purchase pseudo-aromatherapy products as mass marketers strive to gain a greater market share of the aromatherapy "trend." In fact, aromatherapy is not a trend. For more than 5,000 years, people have been practicing aromatherapy as a sincere healing practice. Many mass-market merchandisers have corrupted the category and robbed the word *aromatherapy* of its original meaning and its authenticity.

In their confusion, and through misplaced trust, millions of people mistakenly purchase "aromatherapy" products they believe will improve their health and well-being. If deceit was the only offense, it would be bad enough, but these petrochemical impostors possess the potential to seriously harm the health of the people who seek healing from them. Another sinister side effect is that these potent petrochemicals numb the senses to the subtle aromas of nature.

Below are some considerations to help you detect pseudo-aromatherapy products and petrochemical impostors:

• *Place of purchase.* Don't expect to buy quality products containing pure essential oils at department stores, discount stores, drugstores, national or international chain stores, or supermarkets. Rarely, if ever, do these products contain pure essential oils. Likewise, your chances are slim of finding pure essential oils or true aromatherapy products in the bath and body boutiques in shopping malls or at most beauty salons. Nowadays, even few health-food stores offer products that contain pure essential oils.

• *Type of product.* The following are frequently sold as aromatherapy products but almost always are impostors: aerosol air fresheners, bath oils, bath salts, bubble baths, candles, electric oil burners or plug-ins, facial sprays and toners, feminine hygiene products, hair dyes and perms, nail polishes and nail polish removers, potpourri and simmer herbs, scratch-and-sniff products, sexual lubricants, shampoos and hair conditioners, and most skin-care products. These products rarely contain pure essential oils. Even if they did, the amounts of essential oils in them would be so minute as to be useless.

• *Other ingredients.* Always consider the other ingredients in the product. Essential oils can accelerate the absorption of these ingredients into your body. Read the list of ingredients of any product you are considering and think about whether you want them entering your body. What therapeutic value are essential oils if they are swimming in synthetic chemicals such as emulsifiers, stabilizers, surfactants, propellants, petroleum waxes, and preservatives? Often, these ingredients are petrochemical derivatives that compromise the integrity and negate the effects of the essential oils.

• *Price of the product.* Price can often indicate whether or not a product is true aromatherapy. Think about whether "rose" aerosol spray selling for $4.00 or a "jasmine" candle priced at $6.00 could possibly contain pure essential oil, when even one drop of pure rose or jasmine oil can cost several dollars.

Do your arithmetic. Consider the price of an "aromatherapy" body lotion that sells for $20.00. Subtract the retailer's typical 100-percent markup, about $10.00. Next, subtract the cost of packaging, advertising, and freight, about $5.00. Estimate the manufacturer's profit, about $3.00. That means the manufacturer likely spent a total of about $2.00 on *all* the ingredients. At that price, the lotion cannot contain any therapeutic levels of pure essential oils.

Before buying, always ask yourself: How likely is this product to be true aromatherapy? You are wiser to invest your money in pure essential oils and make your own cosmetics. Don't just trust labels or clever advertising. Use your common sense.

WHAT AROMATHERAPY CAN DO FOR YOU

Through essential oils, nature provides us with a network of therapeutic plant essences that have valuable healing properties. These highly concentrated essential oils are ideal for treating an array of physical, mental, and emotional problems. People around the world are searching for safe, effective, and environmentally responsible alternatives to conventional medicines and cosmetics. Those who have discovered aromatherapy have found exactly what they need to help maintain and improve their health and take care of their skin, hair, and bodies. Women, men, and children are all benefiting from the use of aromatherapy.

Aromatherapy works with your body in a very natural, holistic way. By gently activating your body's own healing energies, aromatherapy helps to restore balance to your body, mind, and spirit. Aromatherapy complements almost any other type of therapy or healing practice, whether conventional or alternative.

Aromatherapy offers you easy ways to enhance the quality of your life and improve your health. Aromatherapy can prompt your body and mind to function more efficiently. It can help boost your immune system. Often, you can prevent common ailments or illnesses with aromatherapy. If you do get sick, you can use aromatherapy to minimize the discomforts and speed up your recovery. Aromatherapy can help you get back on your feet after an illness. It also makes a safe and effective first-aid treatment.

Aromatherapy can help you reduce and manage stress. Since none of us seems to be spared from modern-day stress, any reduction in stress will certainly improve or enhance the quality of our lives and restore balance to our lives. Stress plays a major role in almost all illnesses, both physical and mental. The regular use of essential oils can help you control stress, alleviate anxiety and tension, and minimize the physical aches and pains they cause. You can use aromatherapy to relax and unwind after a stressful day at work, at home, or on the road. Or you can use it to refresh and recharge yourself so that you can keep up the pace of your busy life.

Aromatherapy has a positive influence on the emotions. Many essential oils can help you regulate your moods. Some are uplifting and energizing; others are calming and sedating. Some work to restore balance. In Part Two of this book, you will learn about essential oils that can elevate your mood, soothe your emotions, clear your mind, quiet your anger, and even inspire your creativity.

You can make aromatherapy treatments for your skin, hair, and body that will add a new dimension to your beauty or personal hygiene routine. These creations can be among the most natural and effective types of beauty treatments. Aromatherapy can give a healthier appearance to any skin, especially troubled or problem skin. Essential oils can revitalize dry or prematurely aging skin, regulate oily skin, clear problem skin, and add a healthy glow to all complexions. Men as well as women will enjoy using essential oils in skin-care products and for hair care. Men also can employ essential oils in skin-softening and protective aftershave preparations.

In addition to offering a natural, holistic approach to enhancing health and well-being, the practice of aromatherapy supports the environment. Growing plants—lots of them—for the production of essential oils helps the planet and helps us. Too many people, in their race to turn the world into a concrete jungle, forget that without plants, humans could not exist. Plants provide us with a most vital element for life—oxygen. They manufacture and circulate this life-sustaining gas so that we may breathe. In doing this, they utilize the carbon dioxide we exhale—a waste that otherwise contributes to the greenhouse effect. Besides beautifying its surroundings, every plant that flourishes makes the air a little cleaner, reduces some of the effect of greenhouse gases, and diminishes global warming.

Cultivating crops for the production of essential oils has other environmental advantages. By avoiding chemical fertilizers and pesticides, farmers who grow botanicals using organic methods help to counter soil erosion and reduce the toxic wastes that contaminate waterways and ground water. In developing countries, growing botanical crops can provide farmers with a greater economic return than other, more harmful industries, such as logging, cattle grazing, and growing crops for illegal drugs. People thus have an opportunity to make a better living in ways that are not as destructive to the land or to society.

Growing botanicals can help protect the world's diminishing forests instead of demolishing them. Farmers need not clear-cut huge tracts of forest for grazing a few head of cattle. They can also restore lands depleted from grazing by growing botanicals for essential oil production. By reducing greenhouse gases, plants may also help preserve the fragile ozone layer. Each time you purchase pure essential oils, you cast a vote for natural botanicals that can have immediate and long-term effects on your health, well-being, and longevity, as well as on the health, well-being, and future of the planet. You send the message to manufacturers that you want to buy products that are good for the planet, that help sustain agriculture around the world, that preserve precious and valuable plant species, and that support life on earth.

You can use your purchasing power to make a significant statement and have a positive influence on the environment. Plants can help us solve some of the problems we face, if we will only let them do what they instinctively want to do—grow. By using botanicals in your everyday life, you can help guarantee plants' survival. Their survival has a crucial impact on humanity. We need plants. We cannot live on earth without them.

Using pure essential oils has another far-reaching effect: It provides a perfect opportunity to connect with nature. In these stress-filled times, we often forget about nature and fail to appreciate the many advantages that the earth offers. In fact, the neglect of nature is largely responsible for the current global environmental crisis. Could there also be a connection between our irreverence for nature and the rising rates of disease?

Opening a bottle of an essential oil, which possesses the vital life force of a once-living plant, and breathing in its fragrant and therapeutic aroma can subtly yet powerfully remind you that you too are an integral part of nature whether you live on a farm in the rural Midwest or in a penthouse 100 floors above a modern metropolis.

Aromatherapy can make a big difference in your life. In this book, you will learn exactly how you can use aromatherapy for body, hair, and skin care; for creating personal perfumes and fragrancing your environment; for first-aid treatments; for relaxation; for maintaining or improving health; for boosting immunity; for reducing stress; and for enhancing or restoring emotional equilibrium. You will learn how to make many different cosmetics, skin oils, massage oils, fragrances, diffuser blends, inhalants, and therapeutic blends for treating a variety of conditions. You will find out about essential oils—what they are, what they do, and how to select them. You will discover how you can easily use aromatics in your everyday life. In short, you will come to appreciate essential oils for the value they can add to your daily life. In fact, once you begin using them and realize what a difference they can make, you will probably wonder how you ever managed without aromatherapy.

The History of Aromatherapy

✳

Aromatherapy is *nothing new. Virtually every ancient culture recognized the value of botanicals and aromatic plants and practiced primitive forms of aromatherapy. Ancient people used botanicals to adorn their bodies, to maintain physical health, and for religious purposes. The ancient Egyptians were among the first practitioners of aromatherapy. Fragrance was a dominant aspect of their lives, particularly for pharaohs and priests. Priests often doubled as physicians and perfumers; they guarded the secrets of their craft closely. Royalty and the rich lavished on themselves such botanicals as cedarwood, coriander, cypress, elemi, frankincense, juniper, myrrh, and rose, often anointing each part of the body with a different essence.*

THE ANCIENT WORLD

The first perfumes were incense. The word *perfume* derives from the Latin *per,* meaning "through," and *fume,* meaning "smoke." Religious rituals celebrated a connection between physical matter and the spirit. Many ancient peoples believed that any disrespect or irreverence for the laws of nature could create illness or disease. They burned plants to invoke an atmosphere of reverence and to transcend the mundane world into the realm of the divine. They used botanicals to ward off evil spirits, purify their thoughts, and invoke meditation.

Incense burned day and night in early Egyptian temples. The Egyptians also used botanical gums; ointments; perfumed powders; and scented oils, waters, and wines. During elaborate religious rituals, Egyptians anointed their bodies with aromatic oils and burned elemi, frankincense, myrrh, and sandalwood incense to glorify their gods. Incense helped them to heighten their spiritual experiences by deepening meditation, inspiring inner transformation, and purifying the spirit. Benzoin, cedarwood, juniper, and thyme incense freshened the air and expelled evil spirits in homes and temples. What ancient Egyptians considered evil spirits, we today might equate with psychological or emotional problems.

The Egyptians were famous for embalming their dead. Embalmers would hollow out the body cavities of the dead and fill them with aromatic plants and oint-ments. If the deceased came from a wealthy family, myrrh and cedarwood would be used. Less costly plants, such as cinnamon, elemi, sandalwood, and thyme, were used to preserve the bodies of commoners. Beauty and cosmetics were of prime importance to Egyptians, both in daily life and in preparing for the afterlife. Perhaps the world's first cosmetic chemists were Egyptian embalmers who transferred their knowledge of preserving the flesh of the dead to treating the skin of the living.

Aromatic oils were the key ingredients in the earliest cosmetics. The ancient Egyptians believed in bathing frequently and anointing their bodies with botanicals to keep their skin healthy and youthful, as well as to protect against the harshness of the desert climate and the sun. Ancient Egyptians believed that perfuming their bodies made them more attractive and alluring. Indeed, Cleopatra supposedly seduced Mark Antony with her extravagant use of roses and other aromatics. Many of their perfumed oils and ointments also had healing properties and served as medicines.

At around the same time, Ayurvedic medicine, the oldest known form of medicine, was developing in India. The Vedic texts mention the healing properties of such aromatic plants as coriander, ginger, myrrh, sandalwood, and rose. The *Kamasutra* suggested using sandalwood for lovemaking and for beauty purposes. Sandalwood was also an integral part of early Indian religious and spiritual rites. The practice of perfumery was described in early Sanskrit literature, and ancient Indians took full advantage of the abundant aromatic plants of their country. Perfumery lore was intertwined with Indian legends and spiritual beliefs. Indians especially enjoyed the sweet scents of sandalwood, rose, and jasmine.

Hindu worshippers anointed themselves with perfumed oils to purge themselves of spiritual impurities and wash away their sins. In the temples, priests burned incense made of benzoin, sandalwood, and patchouli to banish evil spirits. At weddings, fires burning sandalwood and other scented woods, aromatic oils, and incense emitted lovely aromas into the air. The bride's feet were anointed with sacred, scented oil. At the end of the wedding ceremony, the guests would toss scented rice at the newlyweds to validate their marriage vows.

Following their exodus from Egypt, the ancient Hebrew people traveled to what is now Israel, bringing with them their knowledge of incense and perfumery. Frankincense soon burned in their temples. Moses made a special holy oil from olive oil, myrrh, calamus, cassia, and cinnamon, and anointed priests with it. During their captivity in Egypt, the Hebrews had adopted the Egyptian custom of scenting their bodies with aromatic oils and their homes with incense. However, Hebrew law forbade the private use of certain aromatics that were designated as sacred: Only con-

secrated priests could use them in the temples.

Hebrew law required that maidens, before being presented at the royal court, undergo a yearlong purification process with myrrh and many other fragrant oils. When a heavily perfumed Jewish bride arrived at her wedding, guests joined in the celebration, and all were anointed with sweet-scented oils.

The Bible mentions the use of numerous aromatic essences, including cedarwood, cinnamon, coriander, cypress, frankincense, juniper, mint, myrrh, myrtle, pine, rose, and spikenard. Well known is the tale of the Magi presenting gifts of gold, frankincense, and myrrh—three of the most valuable commodities of that time—to the baby Jesus.

The Babylonian empire was the main source of fragrant botanicals during ancient times. Babylonians themselves consumed vast quantities of such scents as cedarwood, cypress, fir, juniper, myrtle, pine, and rose. While in Egypt only the wealthy enjoyed perfumes, Babylonian law compelled all citizens to douse themselves with fragrance, probably to subdue offensive body odors. On festive occasions, Babylonians burned immense amounts of aromatic woods and incense and saturated their entire bodies with scented oils.

Other ancient cultures made use of aromatic botanicals as well. The Assyrians burned tons of frankincense in religious rituals and drenched their bodies with botanical perfumes made from frankincense. They used cedar, cypress, and myrrh in cosmetics and for medicinal purposes. During the regal gatherings of King Antiochus Epiphanes of Syria, thousands of people were anointed with precious perfumes while aromatic incense burned all around. Every guest left these feasts with a garland of frankincense and myrrh.

The ancient Chinese and Japanese used perfumes in religious rituals. In both cultures, aromatic woods and herbs were burned at funerals. The Chinese used jasmine to venerate their ancestors; mourners would carry burning jasmine incense along the funeral procession. Both the Chinese and Japanese used botanicals for personal hygiene and beauty purposes, which they considered essential. Chinese women massaged fragrant jasmine oil into their bodies after bathing. The Chinese used some botanicals, such as cinnamon, ginger, and jasmine, to help restore health and balance to the ill.

Some ancient Africans also anointed their bodies with botanicals, primarily to soften their skin and protect it from the searing effects of the sun. In preparation for their wedding ceremony, a bride and groom would coat their bodies with scented oils and unguents, both to beautify their bodies and to deter evil on their wedding day. Many ancient Africans bathed their bodies with oils that were sweetly scented with aromatic roots and woods. The regular application of these oils helped their skin maintain its suppleness and elasticity while preventing skin problems.

The ancient Greeks learned about the art of aromatics and botanicals from the Egyptians. They respected the healing power of fragrant botanicals and perfumes, which they embraced as holy and healing medicines. Perfumes played a major role in Greek mythology. Aphrodite, the Greek goddess of love, supposedly delivered perfume to earth from the heavens. The Greeks believed that plants derived from divine origin, and that plant extracts therefore possessed spiritual and godlike qualities. They honored their gods and goddesses at elaborate feasts and squandered vast quantities of aromatics during these celebrations. Wishing to partake of the good fortune of their deities and receive their blessing, the Greeks enthusiastically adorned their bodies with an abundance of personal fragrances in hopes of gratifying the gods.

The ancient Greeks figured that these therapeutic and medicinal perfumes would also have favorable effects on their minds, especially in treating ailments of an emotional or nervous nature. Healing the mind, they assumed, would restore physical health. During their daily routines, they anointed each part of their bodies with different aromatic oils. Wealthy Greeks built altars in their homes at which they held daily rituals involving the burning of incense. Perfumes played an essential part in funerals, and the dead were buried with bottles of their favorite fragrances.

Hippocrates, the "father of medicine," studied the healing properties of herbs. In the fourth century B.C.E., he suggested that imbalances in food, occupation, and environment could create sickness and disease. He prompted people to take responsibility for their own health as he taught them to heal themselves with plants and diet.

Theophrastus, who is known as the "father of botany," suggested common fourth-century B.C.E. botanicals: all-heal (St. John's wort), cassia, cinnamon, cardamom, dill, ginger grass, iris, lily, marjoram, myrrh, myrtle, rose, saffron, spikenard, and storax. He recommended infusing most plants in olive oil to ensure that their fragrances would endure, although he preferred using sesame oil to make rose perfume.

Besides being praised for their fine fragrances, perfumes were valued for their medicinal properties, such as the ability to relieve the inflammation of wounds and to reduce or eliminate tumors. Healing properties attributed to perfumes increased their popularity among Greeks. Dioscorides, a Greek physician and author of *De Materia Medica,* one of the earliest and most influential herbal-medicine references, praised rose for relieving headache and toothache, and for fighting bacteria and tuberculosis. People from all classes of society congregated at perfume shops in Athens. Artists and craftsmen, statesmen and philosophers, and wealthy men and poor peasants met to share gossip, ideas, and political views while whiffing thought-provoking fragrances.

Greeks loved the sweet scents of botanicals and crowned their heads and those of guests with garlands of laurel and rosemary. Garlands of roses were used to relieve headaches and provide relief from drinking too much wine.

The ancient Romans gained their knowledge of both medicine and perfumery from the Greeks. They enjoyed using aromatics for cosmetics, hygiene, massage, and medical treatments. Bathing was an important ritual for the Romans; public baths became centers for cultural activities. The ancient Romans added aromatic oils to steam baths and hot tubs. Massage with scented oils followed their baths. Besides scenting their bodies and hair, the Romans fragranced their clothing and homes with botanicals. Aromatics and perfumes also figured in civic ceremonies. Following each conquest of the Roman Empire, the Romans introduced botanicals to their new domain.

Since time immemorial, indigenous tribes throughout the Americas have revered plants and have used them in rituals of cleansing, purification, and healing. Native Americans prepared ointments and salves from cedarwood, pine, and spruce. They burned smudge sticks—bound bunches of dried herbs such as cedarwood, cypress, and sage—to produce smoke that could purify the spirit, heal the sick, and induce spiritual and meditative states. They sought relief from respiratory problems, rheumatism, headaches, skin ailments, and various other complaints with botanicals such as cedarwood, pine, sage, and spruce.

THE MEDIEVAL PERIOD

With the collapse of the Roman Empire in the fifth century, the influence of Roman civilization in Europe waned, and the use of expensive and rare botanicals for beauty, bathing, and perfumery declined dramatically. Much ancient knowledge of perfumery disappeared forever. With the spread of Christianity, the popularity of botanical medicine waned, although commercial caravans and ships continued bringing supplies, such as cinnamon bark for heart, liver, and digestive tonics; nutmeg for pain relief; and rosewater for a soothing eyewash.

As Europeans allowed aromatic fragrances and medicines to vanish into obscurity for centuries, Arabs continued to explore perfumes' myriad applications. Although archeologists have recently unearthed primitive stills dating back to 2000 and 3000 B.C.E., Avicenna, a tenth-century Arab physician, regularly receives credit for originally discovering the means of extracting the aromatic essences of flowers by distillation. His first creation was rose oil. Soon, he easily obtained many other essential oils. The popularity of perfume spread rapidly among the Arabs, Moors, and Spaniards. By the thirteenth century, as trade resumed between Europe and the East, the use of essential oils for beauty, health, hygiene, and medicinal purposes became popular throughout Europe.

THE RENAISSANCE AND BEYOND

By the middle of the sixteenth century, perfumers had become prominent and prevalent throughout Europe. They created essential-oil blends, some with claims bordering on the miraculous or magical. Many Europeans believed that bathing was unhealthy and preferred to perfume their bodies to conceal offensive body odors. The popularity of essential oils rose with this practice. During the reign of Henry III of France (1551–1589), perfuming became so extravagant that it was actually wasteful. The French fragranced everything—public fountains, leather goods, stationery, wines, and drinking water, as well as their homes, their bodies, their hair, and all of their clothing. Throughout the medieval period in Europe, great quantities of such herbs and essential oils as juniper, laurel, neroli, pine, and thyme were used to help combat and prevent the spread of illness, particularly epidemics and plagues.

In the sixteenth and seventeenth centuries, the moral and philosophical climate of Europe shifted to emphasize stern religious discipline and lifestyle. In England, Puritanism prospered. The Roman Catholic Church adopted austere attitudes. This religious atmosphere exerted a mighty influence on people's every action. Many members of the clergy frowned on any personal use of aromatics, partially because pagans and witches had incorporated them in their rites, and partially because religious leaders of the time felt that any display of vanity or adornment detracted from religious devotion.

As late as the eighteenth century, puritanically minded people discouraged women from using perfumes and fragranced cosmetics. Some British lawmakers felt that perfume possessed special powers that gave women an unfair advantage over men, so they proposed a law to prohibit women from wearing scents. Perfumes and cosmetics, according to these men, were forms of witchcraft that allowed women to seduce men and lure them into marriage while the men were not in full command of their senses. The law failed to pass, however, and the sale of perfumes, cosmetics, and medicines continued.

Essential oils remained the most powerful antiseptics available until modern chemicals appeared. Yellow fever responded to sandalwood and thyme oils, cinnamon combated typhoid fever, and lavender treated tuberculosis. After the middle of the nineteenth century, however, as modern chemistry and science evolved, perfumes shifted from the category of medicines into cosmetics. In 1869, scientists created the first synthetic fragrance, coumarin. The list of man-made perfumes unacceptable for medicinal purposes grew quickly. Essential oils fell from favor as other synthetic chemicals replaced botanical ingredients in medicines, perfumes, and beauty products. By the early twentieth century, modern perfumers were using more synthetic fragrances than essential oils in their scents. The natural beauty and health benefits of essential oils and aromatics were all but forgotten as scientists and perfumers switched to cheaper, consistent, and readily available man-made chemicals. Today, only the most costly commercial fragrances contain even the tiniest amounts of pure essential oils.

AROMATHERAPY IN THE TWENTIETH CENTURY

The modern revival of essential oils began during the 1920s, with the work of René-Maurice Gattefossé, a French chemist and perfumer who coined the term *aromatherapy*. While experimenting in his laboratory, Gattefossé severely burned his hand. He immediately plunged it into the nearest liquid, which happened to be a bowl of lavender oil. He noticed that his hand healed very rapidly and without scarring. After his speedy recovery, Gattefossé dedicated the rest of his life to researching the therapeutic aspects of essential oils. His studies helped to revive an ancient, almost-forgotten art.

In the past several decades, with the emerging trends toward holistic health and natural skin care, interest in aromatherapy is reviving. Concern about the environment and the desire of many people to be closer to nature are probably partially responsible for this. In addition, the escalating costs of conventional medicine, the lack of personal attention provided by modern health-care facilities, and alarm over the numerous adverse side effects of many modern drugs and synthetic chemicals in cosmetics, plus the growing awareness of the advantages of preventive health care, contribute to aromatherapy's popularity. As people take increasing responsibility for their own physical and emotional health, they warmly welcome aromatherapy into their lives. Today, aromatherapy is experiencing its greatest popularity in centuries, as people are becoming aware of its potential for enhancing the quality of their lives.

AROMATHERAPY FOR THE FUTURE

Today, aromatherapy stands at a crossroads. Mass-market pseudo-aromatherapy contradicts true aromatherapy as a tradition that healers have practiced for thousands of years. This misuse and mockery of aromatherapy violate the intentions of the pioneers who recognized its value in preserving health and life on this planet.

In the late nineteenth century, chemists began transforming the healing practice of perfumery into a petrochemical industry that today generates billions of dollars. Likewise, modern chemists are transforming the therapeutic and medicinal nature of true aromatherapy into another multibillion-dollar outlet for their petrochemical scents.

Will aromatherapy go the way of per-fumery, or will it remain a healing practice? To a large degree, the future of true aromatherapy depends upon the demands of consumers. It also depends on their awareness and education about true aromatherapy. Most important, true aromatherapy depends upon the availability of pure essential oils, which require tons and tons of plants to produce. As we bulldoze forests to make farmland for the expanding purposes of "progress," less land is available for growing plants. Beyond aromatherapy, we must remember that we require plants for our very breath of life. Those of us who care about the future of aromatherapy must be willing to share our wisdom and knowledge to educate people who have forgotten about our special alliance with plants. We hold the power to keep plants alive on earth; plants can keep us alive and breathing and can contribute to our health. No amount of money, drugs, or technology will keep us alive without plenty of plants to produce ample oxygen for us.

Beyond scent, we need to decide what aromatherapy means. We can choose aromatherapy, with pure essential oils that can heal and transform our lives with their therapeutic powers, or we can shop at the local mass merchandisers for pseudo-aromatherapy, with synthetic scents that merely smell and may actually harm us.

Essential Oils

✻

Essential oils *are essences that are extracted from the bark, leaves, petals, resins, rinds, roots, seeds, stalks, and stems of certain aromatic plants. Essential oils are what give plants their characteristic smells. Pure essential oils are extremely concentrated. Many pounds, even tons, of plant material may be required to produce a relatively small amount of essential oil. For example, more than 150 pounds of lavender flowers will yield only 1 pound of lavender oil; approximately 5,000 pounds of rose petals produce but 1 pound of rose oil.*

Essential oils are not oils in the same sense as vegetable oils like almond, olive, or sunflower oils. Essential oils are usually very liquid and do not feel greasy at all. Most will not leave an oily stain on clothing or paper. Essential oils are sometimes called volatile oils because they evaporate readily when exposed to air. They are soluble in vegetable oil and partially soluble in alcohol. However, they do not readily dissolve in water.

Sometimes essential oils are referred to as *plant essences*. The word *essence* can mean "heart," "soul," or "spirit." Indeed, essential oils are the heart, soul, and spirit of aromatic plants. They contain the vital energy and the life force of the plants. Aromatic plants store essential oils in tiny pockets between their cell walls. As the plant releases the essential oils, they circulate throughout the plant and send messages that help it function efficiently, much as hormones do in humans. Many botanists believe that essential oils activate and regulate such activities as cellular metabolism, photosynthesis, and cellular respiration. Some scientists speculate that essential oils may trigger immune responses that assist plants in coping with stressful changes in climate and environment. Some plants release essential oils that protect them by repelling harmful insects and diseases, while others emit essential oils to attract insects or animals that aid in the plants' pollination and propagation. Essential oils thus play an important part in the daily life and survival of plants.

Of the thousands of plants that populate the plant kingdom, relatively few produce essential oils. Even among those that do produce essential oils, many yield such a minute amount that it is not financially feasible to extract them. Other plants produce essential oils, yet the oils smell nothing like the plants; often, this is due to chemical reactions that occur during the extraction process.

Ironically, some of nature's most fragrant flowers—gardenia, lilac, lily of the valley, magnolia, violet, and wisteria—yield no essential oils through steam distillation. Some flowers, such as carnation, honeysuckle, and narcissus, yield absolutes through solvent extraction (see page 23), but they are quite costly and smell little like the original flowers. Most fruits, with the exception of some citrus fruits, do not produce essential oils. Scents such as apple, banana, cherry, coconut, mango, papaya, peach, pear, pineapple, raspberry, strawberry, and watermelon are not essential oils. Scientists in chemistry labs synthesize these fragrances from petrochemicals or fossil fuels. They are inappropriate for inhalation or therapeutic purposes. Frequently, synthetic scents can aggravate the problems or symptoms that the pure essential oils could ease or relieve.

HOW ESSENTIAL OILS WORK

Essential oils work on several different levels. The first way they affect most people is through the sense of smell. The sense of smell is the most complex and most sensitive of the five senses. Smell is also the least understood and least appreciated sense. Whenever you open a bottle of an essential oil, its volatile aromatic molecules permeate the air. As you inhale the aroma, odor molecules enter your nostrils and drift upward into the olfactory receptors—the structures in the nose where smell originates. The olfactory nerves are the only sensory pathways that open directly into the brain. They are also the only nerves in the body that can normally replace themselves.

A single odor molecule can excite olfactory receptors. When odor molecules reach the mucous membranes in your olfactory apparatus, they are greeted by about 10 million olfactory receptors on two small patches of tissue at the end of each nostril. Atop these receptors are cilia, tiny hairlike projections that wave rhythmically back and forth, waiting to detect scents and transmit information about them. The olfactory nerves terminate in the olfactory bulb, in the front portion of the cerebrum. Odor molecules then travel across nerve synapses to the olfactory tract, which sends sensory impulses into the olfactory area of the cerebral cortex, or the smell cortex, of the brain. Here the brain recognizes odors that initiate the sensation of smell.

Scientists theorize that each olfactory receptor acts like a key that fits a certain odor, allowing it to unlock, or identify, an aroma. The human olfactory system needs as few as forty odor molecules to recognize a specific smell. Some people can differentiate over a thousand different odors, while others have difficulty distinguishing even a few.

Once receptors identify an odor, nerve cells relay this information directly to the limbic system of the brain, or the "smell brain," even before the odor molecules themselves actually arrive. The limbic system is a group of deep brain structures that are involved in the sense of smell and the experience of emotions, among other things. Here odors can trigger memories and influence behavior. In addition, the limbic system works in coordination with the pituitary gland and the hypothalamus area of the brain to regulate the hormonal activities of the endocrine system. Odors can thus trigger the production of hormones that govern appetite, bodily functions, insulin production, overall metabolism, stress levels, sex drive, and temperature. The limbic system also influences immunity. Through their action on the limbic system, essential oils can have a positive impact on all of these functions by bringing balance to the body. In addition, the limbic system interacts with the neocortex area of the brain, and odors can affect conscious thoughts and reactions.

The limbic system affects the nervous system as well. Desires, motivation, moods, intuition, and creativity all originate within the limbic system. Because they act on the limbic system, smells can improve your psychological disposition, in addition to enhancing your physical health. Research shows that people who surround themselves with pleasant scents enjoy higher self-esteem and an increased sense of well-being. Smells prompt both physical and psychological reactions by stimulating the release of neurotransmitters and endorphins in your brain. These hormonelike chemicals produce gratifying sensations, even feelings of euphoria, and generate an overall sense of well-being. Neurotransmitters can arouse sexual feelings, assist motor control, reduce stress, regulate alertness and sleepiness, relieve pain, and restore emotional equilibrium.

Smells can gain direct access to your emotions and work on a subconscious level to modify emotional imbalances or change behavior. Odors also can trigger long-forgotten memories and alter your attitude. Inhaling certain essential oils can enhance your emotional equilibrium, either calming and relaxing you or stimulating and energizing you. Calming floral fragrances such as neroli, rose, or ylang ylang oil will relax you, while the stimulating scents of black pepper, ginger, or peppermint oil will energize you. Some essential oils, such as geranium and lavender, work to restore equilibrium, according to what your body needs.

When you inhale essential oils, they also enter into your respiratory system. In your lungs, minute molecules of essential oils attach themselves to oxygen molecules. These oxygen molecules then carry the essential oil molecules into your bloodstream and circulate them, in much the same way that blood delivers nutrients, to cells in your body. Within the cells, essential oils can activate the body's ability to heal itself and improve health.

Essential oils work through the skin, too. They can stimulate circulation to surface skin cells and encourage cell regeneration, the formation of new skin cells. They can calm inflamed or irritated skin. Some oils can release muscle spasms, soothe sore muscles, and relieve muscular tension.

Your skin can absorb the tiny molecules of essential oils. They can penetrate through the pores of the sebaceous (oil-secreting) glands. Once they enter the skin, essential oils travel through the intercellular fluid surrounding the skin cells. They then pass into your bloodstream where blood transports them to your internal organs and your lymphatic system. Throughout their journey, essential oils can benefit your immune system. Scientists suspect that essential oils stimulate the body's own natural defense systems. Certain oils can encourage the production of white blood cells, thereby boosting your body's immune response. Many essential oils fight harmful bacteria, fungi, viruses, and other foreign invaders within the body. Others boost immunity by reducing physical and emotional stress.

When taken internally, essential oils are absorbed directly into the bloodstream through the digestive system. However, the internal use of essential oils for medicinal purposes is beyond the scope of this book. (There are several books available that focus on the internal use of aromatherapy for medical purposes; see Recommended Reading in the Appendix.) A health-care professional trained in medical aromatherapy should supervise any internal use of essential oils. Essential oils are the most highly concentrated form of botanical, and it is important to respect their power and potency.

Essential oils can improve your health and well-being in many different ways. Open a bottle of an essential oil and inhale it. Apply aromatherapy cosmetics to your face. Massage aromatherapy skin oils over your body. Take aromatherapy baths. Blend your own perfumes with essential oils. Disperse essential oils throughout your home or office with a diffuser. Whatever form you choose to use, aromatherapy offers you a wealth of opportunities to discover new levels of health. Essential oils can become your allies in caring for your body, mind, and spirit.

THE EXTRACTION OF ESSENTIAL OILS

During certain hours of the day in certain months of the year, farmworkers harvest crops that have been cultivated especially for essential oil production. By gathering the plants at these specific times, they can produce greater quantities of higher quality essential oils. To further ensure the freshness and quality of essential oils, extraction often takes place in or near the fields in portable stills.

Steam Distillation

Steam distillation is the most common method of extracting essential oils. Many old-time distillers favor this method for most oils, and say that none of the newer methods produces better quality oils.

Steam distillation is done in a still. Distillers place fresh, or sometimes dried, botanical material in the plant chamber of the still. A separate chamber generates pressurized steam, which enters the plant chamber and circulates throughout the plant material. The heat of the steam forces the tiny intercellular pockets that hold the essential oils to open and release the essential oils. The temperature of the steam must be high enough to open the pouches, yet not so high that it destroys the plants or fractures or burns the essential oils.

As they are released, the tiny droplets of essential oil evaporate and, together with the steam molecules, travel through a tube into the still's condensation chamber. As the steam cools, it condenses into water. The essential oil forms a film on the surface of the water. To separate the essential oil from the water, the film is then decanted, or skimmed off the top.

The remaining water, a byproduct of distillation, is called *floral water, distillate,* or *hydrosol.* It retains many of the therapeutic properties of the plant, as well as water-soluble properties that the essential oils do not contain. Hydrosols are valuable in skin care for facial mists or toners, as well as for many other conditions and ailments. Floral water may be preferable to pure essential oil in certain situations, such as when treating a sensitive individual or a child, or when a

more diluted treatment is required. (*See* HY-
DROSOLS in Part One.)

Cold Pressing

Cold-pressed expression, or scarification,
obtains citrus fruit oils such as bergamot,
grapefruit, lemon, lime, mandarin, orange,
and tangerine. In this process, fruit rolls
over a trough with sharp projections that
penetrate the peel and pierce the tiny
pouches containing the essential oil. Then
the whole fruit is pressed to squeeze the
juice from the pulp and to release the essential oil from the pouches. The essential oil
rises to the surface of the juice, and cen-
trifugation separates the juice from the essential oil.

Enfleurage

Some flowers, such as jasmine or tuberose,
have such low contents of essential oil or
are so delicate that heating them would destroy the blossoms before releasing the essential oils. In such cases, an expensive and
lengthy process called *enfleurage* can remove
the essential oils. Flower petals are placed
on trays of odorless vegetable oil or animal
fat, which absorbs the flowers' essential oils.
Every day or every few hours, after the vegetable oil or fat has absorbed as much of the
essential oil as possible, the depleted petals
are removed and replaced with fresh ones.
This procedure continues until the fat or oil
becomes saturated with the essential oil.
Adding alcohol to this enfleurage mixture

separates the essential oil from the fatty substance. Afterward, the alcohol evaporates,
and only the essential oil remains.

Solvent Extraction

Another method of extraction used on delicate plants is solvent extraction, which
yields a higher amount of essential oil at a
lower cost. In this process, a chemical solvent such as hexane is used to saturate the
plant material and pull out the aromatic
compounds. This renders a substance called
a *concrete*. The concrete can then be dissolved in alcohol to remove the solvent.
When the alcohol evaporates, a substance
called an *absolute* remains.

Although more cost-efficient than enfleurage, solvent extraction has disadvan-
tages. Residues of the solvent may remain
in the absolute and can cause side effects.
While absolutes or concretes may be fine
for fragrances or perfumes, they are not especially desirable for skin care or therapeutic applications.

Some trees, such as benzoin, frankincense, and myrrh, exude aromatic tears, or
sap that is too thick to use easily in aromatherapy. In these cases, alcohol or a solvent such as hexane can extract a resin or
essential oil from the tears. This renders a
resin or an essential oil that is easier to use.
However, only those oils or resins extracted
with alcohol should be used for therapeutic
purposes.

Several modern methods of extraction

are becoming popular alternatives to traditional steam distillation. They include carbon dioxide extraction, hydrodiffusion extraction, and turbodistillation extraction.

Carbon Dioxide Extraction

Supercritical carbon dioxide extraction employs carbon dioxide under extremely high pressure to extract essential oils. Plants are placed in a stainless steel tank, and as carbon dioxide enters the tank, pressure inside the tank builds. Under high pressure, the carbon dioxide turns into a liquid and acts as a solvent to extract the essential oils from the plants. As the pressure decreases, the carbon dioxide returns to a gaseous state, leaving no residues behind.

Many carbon dioxide extractions have fresher, cleaner, and crisper aromas than steam-distilled essential oils, and they smell more like living plants. Scientific studies show that carbon dioxide extraction produces essential oils that are very potent and have great therapeutic benefits. This extraction method uses lower temperatures than steam distillation, making it gentler on the plants. It produces higher yields and makes some materials, especially gums and resins, easier to handle. Many essential oils that are impossible to extract by steam distillation are obtainable with carbon dioxide extraction. In the future, many botanicals that are now unavailable may be extracted by this method.

Hydrodiffusion Extraction

In the hydrodiffusion process, steam at atmospheric pressure disperses throughout the plant material from the top of the plant chamber. In this way, the steam can saturate the plants more evenly and in less time than with steam distillation. This method is also less harsh than steam distillation, and the resulting essential oils smell much more like the original plant.

Turbodistillation Extraction

Turbodistillation is suitable for hard-to-extract or coarse plant material, such as bark, roots, and seeds. In this process, the plants soak in water, and steam circulates through this plant-and-water mixture. Throughout the entire process, the same water continually recycles throughout the plant material. This method allows faster extraction of essential oils from hard-to-extract plant materials.

THE PURITY AND QUALITY OF ESSENTIAL OILS

Selecting high-quality essential oils is more of a challenge today than ever before. When you first begin buying essential oils, you must rely almost entirely on the reputation of the supplier to guarantee the purity and quality of the oil you purchase (see Aromatherapy Resource Guide in the Appendix). Over time, as you smell different grades of essential oils and compare pure oils to synthetic ones, you will gain experience in recognizing the difference between high-quality essential oils and lower quality oils or synthetics. You'll learn to trust your nose as time goes by.

Whenever possible, smell the real plants in their natural environment. Compare the essential oils to the plants. What is similar? What is different? Many oils smell identical to but stronger than the plant. Others smell different. Through smelling the plants, you will begin to understand what their essential oils should smell like. Surrounding yourself with the plants from which these essential oils derive increases your experience of aromatherapy. Touch the leaves. Enjoy the beautiful shapes of the blossoms. See the vibrant colors. Hear the plants' movements in the wind. Feel the emanations of their vital energies. Breathe in their living essence. Being close to plants can make you aware of their subtle qualities and aromatic nuances that no chemist can copy. When you form a connection with them, you can remember them as you use their essential oils. This recollection can make your treatments more meaningful and more effective.

Pure Essential Oils Versus Synthetic Substitutes

The key factor in selecting essential oils is to understand the difference between pure essential oils and synthetic products. The practice of aromatherapy requires essences extracted from plants, not synthetic scents made from petroleum byproducts in laboratories. In aromatherapy, as with any other type of treatment, results are the goal. Synthetic oils can never produce the same desirable results that pure essential oils can, even if advancements in technology allow the production of synthetic scents almost identical in smell to pure essential oils.

Pure essential oils produce their effects by the relationships and synergy of their chemical components. Often the components that create their actions or prevent side effects are imperceptible to the most advanced scientific equipment. Even if these components are detected, scientists may deem them inactive when they are isolating important ingredients. Omitting any component completely changes the chemistry and physiology, thereby altering its action. This is one reason that so many synthetic scents and pharmaceutical drugs produce side effects, even if they are synthesized from botanical sources.

Whole essential oils work best for aromatherapy; they contain all the elements of the plants' essential oils, just as nature created them. Therefore, they have greater therapeutic benefits than do the isolated components, which lack many of the important properties of the plants. All of the components of essential oils work in a synergistic manner, and all are necessary to achieve the best results.

Quality and Price

The highest quality essential oils are extracted from plants that have been cultivated under optimum conditions—they were planted at the right time, in balanced soil, and grown using organic farming methods; they flourished in an ideal climate with the right amount of water and sun; and they were harvested at the most opportune time of day during the most suitable season. Ideally, workers cultivating and caring for the plants nurture them with love and view them as a valuable asset beyond the mere financial gain they bring.

Distillation also determines the quality of essential oils. The type of equipment used, its age, the size of the still, the capacity of the plant chamber, the size and length of the coil in the condenser, and the pressure and temperature of the water in the condenser all affect the finished product. Another consideration is the distillation time. The time required to produce the highest quality oil varies from plant to plant. Most plants will release up to 85 percent of their essential oils within one hour. Some distillers hurry distillation to minimize labor costs or to increase profits by distilling more batches during the day. Rushing distillation may produce weak or inferior oils, whereas patience and a willingness to accept lower profits can produce superior oils with remarkable therapeutic properties that are released later during the distillation process. Other producers may add solvents to the water, increase the water pressure, or raise the temperature to produce more oil. Any of these measures compromises the quality of the oil.

Quality affects the price of essential oils.

Growing plants and distilling essential oils are labor-intensive activities. This is why high-quality, pure essential oils are not inexpensive. Some plants are easier to grow and more readily available than others; some oils are easier to extract than others. The price of essential oils depends on the availability of the botanicals, the amount of essential oils contained within the plants, the ease of obtaining the essential oils, the location of the fields, harvest conditions, cultivation methods, local labor costs, seasonal and regional growing conditions, soil conditions, transportation and shipping costs, types of fertilizers used and their costs, weather, and world economics. In addition, the color, smell, and consistency of essential oils can differ from season to season and year to year. This also affects price. As a rule, the higher the quality of the essential oil, the higher the price.

Unfortunately, many suppliers of essential oils have researched the market and know what prices good essential oils can bring. They prey on the public's lack of knowledge, inexperience, or gullibility. They pass off inferior oils or synthetic substitutes as pure essential oils by charging the prices consumers would expect to pay for higher quality essential oils. The only recourse is to know and trust your suppliers.

Adulterated and "Nature-Identical" Oils

When purchasing essential oils, you should be aware of a number of warning signs that may indicate that you are not getting the purest product available. *Adulteration* is the addition of other substances—either synthetic or natural—to extend or to alter the appearance, the chemical composition, or the smell of an essential oil. Some suppliers magically transform 1 pound of pure essential oil into 10 pounds of adulterated oil. Many manufacturers engage in this practice to expand their profits. For example, it's common knowledge that the demand for French lavender oil is so high that each year France sells far more "lavender oil" than it produces. Sometimes companies, knowingly or unknowingly, sell products labeled as pure essential oils that are in fact synthetic or adulterated oils.

Adulterating essential oils with vegetable or carrier oils is perfectly acceptable if the label reflects this addition. For example, a facial oil that contains essential oils diluted in jojoba oil is fine, as long as the label doesn't imply that the product is pure, undiluted essential oil. Unfortunately, some companies don't disclose all the ingredients in their products. One way to detect if a product contains carrier oils along with pure essential oils is to place a drop of the product on a piece of paper. Pure essential oils will evaporate, usually leaving no trace, whereas those in carrier oils will leave an oily spot.

Adulterating one essential oil with a different essential oil is a frequent and fraudulent practice. For example, melissa oil often contains lemongrass oil to increase both the quantity of oil the company can sell and the profits the company can earn. Even more dishonest and dangerous is the adulteration of pure essential oils with synthetic scents. The most despicable and by far the most hazardous form of adulteration occurs when a supplier sells 100-percent petrochemical scents as pure essential oils. Not only do consumers who purchase such products fail to experience the therapeutic benefits of pure essential oils, but the synthetic substitutes can, in some cases, pose a danger to their health.

With aromatherapy's growing popularity, and with the entrance of mass-market merchandisers into the aromatherapy arena, more and more businesses are selling aromatherapy products. The owners may know little or nothing about aromatherapy except that, if manipulated properly, it can produce great profits. This manipulation usually includes substituting synthetics for pure essential oils. Sadly, some companies that honestly want to offer pure essential oils and true aromatherapy don't know enough to buy pure essential oils. They believe they are selling the real thing, yet their suppliers are deceiving them; they unknowingly pass the deceit on to the consumer.

Some signs may alert you to adulterated oil or synthetics. If a company sells all of its essential oils for the same price, chances are they aren't pure. Essential oil prices vary dramatically. While one-half ounce of orange oil may sell for several dollars, the same amount of rose oil costs several hundred dollars. Any "rose oil" selling for several dollars an ounce is surely synthetic. However, many shrewd business owners now realize that consumers judge the quality of essential oils by price and, therefore, charge the current price for high-quality pure essential oils while providing buyers with poor-quality essential oils or, sometimes, synthetic substitutes.

If the label on a product doesn't specify "essential oil" or "pure essential oil," the product probably is not an essential oil. Unfortunately, even the words *essential oil* or *pure essential oil* on the label are no guarantee of purity. Some companies sell synthetic oils mislabeled as essential oils. Companies also often sell products called perfume oils. These are rarely made with pure essential oils. While the label may read "Oil of Neroli," "Oil of Rose," "Rose Oil Perfume," or "Jasmine Perfume Oil," the product is likely to be a blend of synthetic oils that attempts to simulate the smell of real flowers. Price may be an indication. If a very expensive essential oil is selling for several dollars as a perfume oil, it cannot be a pure essential oil. The few companies that make natural perfumes with pure essential oils and other botanicals usually specify on the label that their ingredients are essential oils in a base of alcohol or jojoba oil. These natural fragrances provide excellent alternatives to commercial colognes and perfumes.

Sometimes people confuse infused oils with essential oils. Infused oils are prepared by soaking or simmering botanicals in vegetable oils to impart some of the properties of the plant into the oil. These infused oils are greasy and are different from pure essential oils. Most infused preparations are natural and possess many therapeutic properties. I mention them to distinguish them from pure essential oils and to alert you to their existence. Common infused oils are aloe vera, arnica, calendula, chamomile, comfrey, mullein, and St. John's wort. Calendula, chamomile, and St. John's wort are also available as essential oils.

Nature-identical is a very misleading term that you should understand. So-called nature-identical oils are actually man-made petrochemical-based products that have been scientifically reconstructed to closely mimic the smell and, sometimes, the chemical composition of pure essential oils. There's really nothing about them that is identical to nature. They do not derive from nature (except, perhaps, their fossil-fuel components), and they certainly are not identical to pure essential oils. The scientists who make these synthetics strive primarily to duplicate the smell. While only a dozen or so chemical components may be responsible for the smell of an essential oil, essential oils contain literally hundreds of components that combine to create their unique therapeutic properties. Many of these components are present in such minute amounts that even advanced laboratory equipment cannot detect their presence, yet these unidentified parts can contribute significantly to the synergistic and therapeutic effect of the essential oil. In addition, so-called nature-identicals lack the vital energy that essential oils have as a result of coming from plants that once reached their roots into the earth, felt the nourishing fire of the sun, bathed their flowers in the life-sustaining rainfalls, and fluttered their leaves in the caresses of the winds.

The action of an essential oil depends upon the delicate balance and synergy of all its components. With all the marvels of modern science, chemists still cannot duplicate essential oils in their laboratories. Some synthetic oils may smell very much like the real thing, but because they lack all of the genuine oil's many components, they cannot produce the desired therapeutic results. Synthetic substitutes also lack the balance and synergy of pure essential oils.

Finally, when selecting your essential oils, question the products of any company that sells animal extracts, such as musk or civet oil, as essential oils. All pure essential oils come from plants, not from animals. Moreover, almost all of the so-called musk and civet oils sold are synthetic; the smell of real musk or civet oil is so offensive that most people would never consider wearing it. Be suspicious if a company offers essential oils that don't exist or sells animal extracts as essential oils. All or some of their other oils may also be synthetic.

STORING AND HANDLING ESSENTIAL OILS

Storing your essential oils properly will protect their freshness and effectiveness, while extending their shelf life. Exposure to sunlight and heat can alter the properties of essential oils. Always keep your essential oils in dark bottles in a cool, dry place, away from sunlight or heat. Avoid leaving them in a moist or damp place, such as the bathroom.

Essential oils are very volatile and evaporate rapidly if exposed to air. In addition, oxygen can compromise their quality or change their chemical compositions. Always keep the bottles tightly capped when not in use. When using essential oils, never leave the bottles uncapped for more than a few seconds. To prevent contamination of your oils, avoid touching the dropper or the opening of the container to your skin or to anything else. Instead, allow the oils to drop from the bottle or dropper into the palm of your hand or into the bottle you are using for blending. Most essential oils will remain fresh for one year or longer with proper care and storage. The quality and aroma of some essential oils, such as patchouli, valerian, and vetiver actually improve with age.

Pure essential oils are the tools of aromatherapy. Choosing the highest quality pure essential oils available will ensure that your aromatherapy experiences are as therapeutic and pleasurable as possible. As you become more and more familiar with essential oils, your appreciation of essential oils, their purity, and their potency will surely increase.

As you read on, you will learn about the specific applications of individual essential oils. You will also learn how to make the blends in this book and how to create some of your own. You are embarking on an aromatherapy adventure that can improve the quality of your life and your health.

Hydrosols

✳

Hydrosols are *byproducts of the steam distillation of essential oils. They come from the same parts of the plants that essential oils do; the same procedure produces both essential oils and hydrosols. In essence, hydrosols are the "waste" product of steam distillation. When the steam that has coaxed the essential oils out of the plant material turns back to water, it contains therapeutic water-soluble molecules released by the plant.*

Hydrosols may possess properties similar to the essential oils, or they can have different ones. The term hydrosol *derives from the Latin word* hydro, *meaning "water," and* sol, *meaning "solution." Other names for hydrosols include aromatic waters, floral waters, hydrolates, hydrolats, and plant waters.*

Hydrosols offer a gentle, safe, and effective way to use low dilutions of botanicals for healing and health. The plant waters are much milder than the essential oils. You can splash them on your skin as a skin toner or aftershave. Smelling hydrosols, like smelling essential oils, can evoke emotions and memories and change your mood. You can spritz your face with floral waters to freshen your skin. You can mist hydrosols into the air to alter the atmosphere, prevent the spread of infection, and impart a delightful aroma to any room. You can also use them as a base for some of your aromatherapy blends by adding a few drops to several ounces of hydrosol. You can even take hydrosols internally for a variety of conditions. Some hydrosols can provide a delicious addition to your culinary creations in beverages, dressings, sauces, soups, and stews.

In this book, I offer such formulas as facial toners, skin sprays, and oral hygiene products that suggest adding essential oils to distilled water. These are not the same as hydrosols, nor are they intended to replace them. These waters have different properties than hydrosols.

Hydrosols lack the stability of essential oils. Since hydrosols can spoil easily, distillers often put preservatives in them before shipping. This practice renders them unsuitable for aromatherapy purposes. Unpreserved hydrosols require storage in a cool, dark place with a constant temperature of around 50°F (10°C). Variations in temperature can cause condensation that can promote the formation of mold. Light and heat can degrade the hydrosol and contribute to spoilage.

There is not a corresponding hydrosol available for every essential oil. The high costs of shipping "water" from overseas distillation sites and the risks of shipping "waters" without preservatives deter many distillers from making the effort of exporting hydrosols. In Part Two, at the end of each section on an essential oil, I include suggestions for ways to use hydrosols if they are available.

Carrier Oils

✳

In aromatherapy, *a carrier oil is any vegetable oil that dilutes pure essential oils for safe application on the skin. Carrier oils are extracted from nuts, kernels, seeds, and other parts of plants. Although any vegetable oil will work, some are preferable due to their specific properties, therapeutic qualities, and valuable nutrients that make them beneficial for treating certain conditions. Pure essential oils are so concentrated and so potent that if you apply them directly to your skin without diluting them, they may irritate or burn your skin. You also might develop sensitivity to them. When diluted in carrier oils, essential oils are safer to use, spread more evenly, can cover a greater area of skin, and are more economical to use in aromatherapy treatments.*

Your skin is the largest organ of your body, providing protection from and a barrier against the outside world. The tiny openings of sweat and oil glands in your skin provide passageways for various substances from the surface of your skin into your body. Topically applied products can penetrate through the layers of the skin, enter the bloodstream, and travel throughout your body. Your skin, your body, and your health all can benefit by choosing the highest quality carrier oils to blend with your pure essential oils.

Unfortunately, carrier oils have not received the attention they deserve. As a result, consumers, particularly aromatherapists, have not received the education they need about choosing and using carrier oils wisely. Some people feel that the freshness or the quality of the products they put on their skin doesn't matter. They generally give little or no thought to how carrier oils will affect their aromatherapy treatments. Frequently, people buy commercial-grade oils straight off the shelves of supermarkets. Others mistakenly believe that all the oils available at health-food stores are pure, safe, and of high quality.

People then disperse their expensive essential oils into suspicious carrier oils that can sabotage any therapeutic benefits because of the presence of chemical solvents, bleaching agents, preservatives, and other additives. Commercial carrier oils are almost always rancid by the time they reach store shelves. The very nature of the commercial oil extraction process robs carrier oils of nutrients and renders them lifeless,

colorless, and flavorless, while encouraging the formation of age-inducing free radicals.

HOW TO DETERMINE HIGH-QUALITY CARRIER OILS

Since not all carrier oils are equal, selecting therapeutic-grade carrier oils requires careful attention. Important factors in choosing carrier oils are the origin of the nuts and seeds, growing methods, the process of extraction, any added ingredients, the quality and freshness of the finished product, the shelf life or longevity, the safety and protective capabilities of the packaging, the best methods for use and storage, and the therapeutic properties.

The highest quality carrier oils are organic and unrefined food-grade oils that are suitable for human consumption. They are extracted from organically grown seeds and plants that have not been genetically modified. People who are committed to producing healthful products nurture the plants in a natural environment. The producers use sustainable agriculture methods, without the use of petrochemical herbicides, pesticides, or fertilizers. They harvest the plants at the optimal time, often by hand. Soon after harvest, they ship the nuts or seeds to the extraction facility. During the process of extracting the oil, heat never exceeds 110°F. High heat destroys the nutrients inherent in the oil. During processing, no hydrogenation occurs, since hydrogenation requires high temperatures to solidify the oil. Nor is the oil deodorized, since this requires high heat, which can distort the structure of the fatty-acid molecules. Structural changes can impair the oil's ability to perform its functions, invite further chemical breakdown or transformation, and promote free-radical formation. These chemical changes within the oil can cause or contribute to many health problems. During production, the purest carrier oils are exposed to neither light nor oxygen—two chief causes of chemical degradation and rancidity.

Quality carrier oils are free of preservatives, chemical additives such as solvents used for extraction, bleaching agents, deodorizing chemicals, hexane, heptane, or other harmful chemicals commonly used to make an oil clear, odorless, free of bacterial contaminants, and to extend shelf life. At the end of the extraction process, high-quality carrier oils retain their nutrients. They contain no traces of harmful substances that can sabotage your essential oils, your aromatherapy treatments, or your health.

By contrast, most commercial producers of vegetable oils select the cheapest seeds or nuts. Often, these are infested with worms, insects, or fungi. Many growers use genetically engineered seeds, genetically modified organisms (GMO), or hybridized plants to increase their harvests. Conventional cultivation methods rely heavily on petrochemical pesticides, herbicides, and fertilizers. Residues of these chemicals often remain on the seeds and nuts. After harvest, seeds and nuts may sit in silos or warehouses for months or years before undergoing oil extraction. To maximize yields during processing, expellers force out oils with friction heat, then solvents such as hexane or heptane leech out the residual oils. During extraction, workers may introduce other chemicals such as bleaching agents, deodorizing agents, toxic metals, additives, and preservatives. In addition, they may subject the oils to temperatures up to 520°F. Heat above 320°F distorts the molecular structure of the fatty acids within the oils. These changes can present threats to health—on the skin and in the body. Heat also promotes the formation of free radicals, atoms, or molecules that can attack healthy tissue on the skin and inside the body. Free-radical damage can contribute to aging, deterioration of health, weakened immunity, and disease.

Commercial producers generally have little regard for limiting the interaction of light and oxygen with the oil during processing. Light initiates the process of photo-oxidation, whereby light rays attack the molecules within the oil, changing the molecular structure, degrading the oil, and producing rancidity. The attack also creates free radicals, which can continue damaging the oil even after light is no longer present. Light is one of the greatest contributors to rancidity. Commercial oils are usually already rancid even before they leave the warehouse. The finished products of commercial extraction are highly refined oils that are devoid of any nutritional or therapeutic properties and have virtually no value in aromatherapy. In fact, they can damage your treatments by contaminating your essential oils and promoting free-radical damage to your skin and in your body.

WHAT IS RANCIDITY, AND WHAT CAUSES IT?

Some synonyms for *rancid* are *bad, foul-smelling, gamy, malodorous, putrid, rank, rotten, sour, stale,* and *stinking.* Rancid oils are not something you would want to mix with high-quality pure essential oils for use on your body. Yet most available carrier oils and many commercial aromatherapy preparations are already rancid when they are sold.

A major concern when choosing carrier oils is how long they will remain fresh. All triglyceride oils turn rancid eventually, but some do so more quickly than others. Of all the carrier oils mentioned in this book, only jojoba oil is not a triglyceride oil. Instead, it is a type of compound known as a wax ester, and for all practical purposes, it does not go rancid. For this reason, you may prefer jojoba oil for fragrance blends or for blends containing precious or expensive oils such as jasmine, melissa, neroli, and rose. You can also add some jojoba oil to help lengthen the life of other carrier oils.

Smell is the most frequent indication of rancidity. If the oil smells sour, spoiled, or "off," it is rancid. Other indications are a change in color, a change in texture, or the formation of a film or crusty particles around the rim of the bottle. The feel of the oil can change from its natural slippery quality, becoming sticky to the touch.

Unrefined oils may look cloudy after refrigeration; this is a normal occurrence and does not interfere with their therapeutic benefits.

INTERACTION OF OILS ON AND IN THE BODY

The human body can absorb varying amounts of almost anything placed on the skin. These ingredients can affect surface skin cells. Because the molecules of essential oils are especially small, they can easily penetrate the skin. Via the essential oils, the molecules of the carrier system (oils, creams, lotions, shampoos, conditioners, or any other cosmetic that contains essential oils) may also gain more immediate access into the body through the skin. This is the best reason to use only the freshest, unadulterated carrier oils or systems available for your aromatherapy blends. It is also the best reason to make your own aromatherapy preparations so that you will know the quality of all the ingredients.

Fatty acids are the main components of all fats and oils. The human body can produce all but two fatty acids—linoleic acid and linolenic acid. These are known as essential fatty acids, or EFAs, because they are essential nutrients that we must obtain through the diet. They function more efficiently in the body when they are present in the right ratio of 1:1 of omega-6, or linoleic acid, to omega-3, linolenic acid. The average American diet, however, has a ratio of 20:1. That imbalance may be one factor responsible for the decline in overall health and weakened immunity.

EFAs assist the body in building cell membranes, producing new cells, and regenerating damaged cells. They improve the quality of the skin and hair. They can reduce blood pressure, lower cholesterol, and minimize the risk of developing heart disease. They may prevent arthritis. They can benefit many disorders such as skin problems, heart conditions, and candida. They also produce hormonelike substances called prostaglandin precursors that contribute to metabolism, circulation, healthy skin, and immune function. Brain and nerve tissues consist of more than 50 percent EFAs. They aid in learning, retaining facts, and recalling information. EFA deficiencies and imbalances may contribute to other disorders such as attention deficit disorder (ADD) or hyperactivity, cancer, depression, eye problems, and heart disease. Proper balance provides opportunities for immune boosting. Through the skin's ability to absorb varying amounts of anything applied topically, the use of nutritious carrier oils for skin applications of aromatherapy may help enhance the body's ability to absorb and utilize EFAs.

High heat, chemical solvents, bleaches, and preservatives can destroy or chemically alter the properties of EFAs, leaving the refined vegetable oils inert and lacking in therapeutic properties. In addition, chemically altered carrier oils can create reactions on the skin, such as free-radical ravages that promote skin disorders, lines and wrinkles, and weakened immunity.

CHOOSING CARRIER OILS

The carrier oils employed most frequently in aromatherapy are almond, coconut, flaxseed, hazelnut, hemp, jojoba, olive, safflower, sesame, and sunflower oils. In addition, borage, calophyllum inophyllum, evening primrose, rose hip seed, and wheat germ oils are often added in small percentages to enhance aromatherapy blends. Since canola and soy crops are now prime targets for genetic engineering and modification, I no longer recommend them as carrier oils for aromatherapy blends. Nor do I include peanut oil, due to the presence of a fungus that grows on the peanuts and of aflatoxins, which are its carcinogenic byproducts. I don't recommend using mineral oil in aromatherapy. This petroleum derivative is made up of very large molecules that sit on the surface of the skin and prevent the penetration of essential oils. Besides, petroleum products are contrary to the whole purpose of aromatherapy since they may alter the therapeutic properties of essential oils.

USE AND STORAGE

Light presents an ever-present threat to carrier oils; packaging becomes a crucial consideration to prevent light from entering to do its free-radical damage. Vegetable oils can turn rancid quickly. To keep your carrier oils as fresh as possible, always refrigerate them until you are ready to use them. The ideal containers for storing oils are black opaque bottles that permit no light to enter. Clear bottles allow light to do its damage, constantly creating more free radicals and degrading the quality of the oils. You may freeze oils to increase their longevity. Frozen unrefined carrier oils can retain their freshness, when unopened, for up to two years. Before blending, allow time for the oil to defrost.

Agitating or vigorously shaking oils excites their molecules and initiates free-radical chain reactions. These actions can compromise the quality of the oil, and free radicals can be transferred to your skin when you apply the oil. Therefore, when you blend essential oils with carrier oil, do so by gently turning the bottle up and down or back and forth in your hand, until the oils are combined.

Essential oils act as mild antioxidants and can extend the shelf life of some carrier oils. Your blends will stay fresher if you mix small amounts and use them quickly. Be sure the bottle in which you blend them is clean and dry. Dirty bottles with residues of rancid oils, deposits from commercial cosmetics, or droplets of water can instantly alter and damage your formula.

AN INTRODUCTION TO THE CARRIER OILS

All carrier oils have lubricating properties. You may choose to work with certain oils because of their specific characteristics and therapeutic properties. Some possess protective properties. Recent research indicates that sesame oil can block about 30 percent of the burning rays of the sun, while coconut and olive may reduce them by about 20 percent. In addition, vitamin E, present in large amounts in wheat germ oil, can reduce sun damage to skin cells by reducing burning and by decreasing oxidation. Another study suggests that topical application of some oils may protect against certain types of skin cancer. Vegetable oils with a high content of linoleic acid may inhibit the growth of malignancies in melanocytes, the cells partially responsible for producing skin pigmentation. Some of the oils with the highest percentages of linoleic acid include safflower (78 percent), sunflower (71 percent), hemp (58 percent), and sesame (45 percent).

Following are brief descriptions of some of the best carrier oils for aromatherapy, along with their nutritional benefits. Since the skin can absorb particles of the carrier oils along with the essential oils and transport them into the body, the nutritional aspects of oils become more meaningful and validate the practice of using healthy carrier oils in your aromatherapy blends.

Almond Oil (*Prunus amygdalis,* var. *dulcis*)

Unrefined sweet almond oil is good for all skin types, especially for people with dermatitis and eczema. It has a mild nutty aroma and is golden yellow. It helps to relieve itching, irritation, and inflammation, and it also softens, soothes, and smoothes dry skin. Almond oil is very lubricating and lingers on the skin, making it good for massage and for protecting the surface of the skin. Shelf life is about one year if the oil is refrigerated after opening.

Borage Oil (*Borago officinalis*)

Borage oil stimulates skin cell activity and encourages skin regeneration. It contains high levels of gamma-linolenic acid (GLA), making it useful in treating all skin disorders, particularly allergies, dermatitis, inflammation, and irritation. GLA is helpful in treating the hormonal imbalances of menstrual difficulties, menopause, and premenstrual syndrome (PMS). Borage penetrates the skin easily and benefits all types of skin, particularly dry, dehydrated, mature, or prematurely aging skin. Add borage oil to other carrier oils to promote healthy skin and hair and for added protection. Historically, physicians and herbalists recommended borage oil as a blood purifier and tonic, a heart strengthener, and a cure for depression. Other conditions that borage may help include arthritis, circulatory problems, diabetes, hyperactivity, liver and intestinal complaints, obesity, and weakened immunity. Borage oil lasts about six months after opening if it is refrigerated.

Calophyllum Inophyllum Oil (*Calophyllum inophyllum*)

Calophyllum inophyllum oil is rich, thick, and dark, with a delicate nutty or spicy smell. It boosts immunity and stimulates cell regeneration. It has anti-inflammatory and pain-relieving properties, making it suitable for use in the treatment of arthritis, back pain, carpal tunnel syndrome, rheumatism, and sciatica. It nourishes fragile or broken capillaries. It helps heal wounds and soothe eczema and skin irritations such as burns, chapped skin, rashes, and insect bites. Calophyllum inophyllum remains stable for a year or longer without refrigeration.

Coconut Oil (*Cocus nucifera*)

Coconut oil is a saturated fat and is solid at room temperature. It may have little aroma, or it may have a mild aroma of coconut. Liquid coconut oil has usually been refined and may also have fragrance added. Coconut oil stays fresh longer than other oils, about one year even without refrigeration. Women and men in the tropics treasure coconut oil as a treatment for luxurious hair, for silky skin, and for protection against the harsh rays of the sun. It improves immune function and can protect your skin and body against microbes such as bacteria, fungi, parasites, and viruses. It can improve the absorption, digestion, and metabolism of nutrients within the body. Coconut oil doesn't promote the formation of free radicals within the oil, on your skin, or in your body. Aromatherapy blends made with coconut oil will last longer with less risk of going rancid. Before blending it with essential oils, you may need to melt the coconut oil. Heat does not harm it. You can set a container of coconut oil in a bowl or pan of hot water to melt it. Allow the coconut oil to cool slightly before adding essential oils.

Evening Primrose Oil (Oenothera biennis)

Evening primrose oil has a high GLA content that promotes healthy skin and skin repair. It is usually yellow in color. It soothes skin problems and inflammation, making it a good choice for people with eczema, psoriasis, or any type of dermatitis. Evening primrose oil discourages dry skin and premature aging of the skin. It is a useful treatment for female hormonal imbalances and menopause. It also serves as a treatment for hyperactivity. It shares many properties with borage oil, including its short shelf life of about three months. When purchasing evening primrose oil, choose a reputable source, since many manufacturers extract it using chemical solvents.

Flaxseed Oil (Linum usitatussimun)

Flaxseed oil is one of the richest sources of essential fatty acids, particularly linolenic and linoleic acids, making it one of the most therapeutic and nutritious oils. Because of its high omega-3 oil and vitamin-E content, it can prevent scarring and stretch marks. This rich, golden oil smells similar to melted butter. It nourishes the skin, especially dry skin, and promotes cell regeneration. It boosts immunity on the skin and in the body. Flaxseed oil is useful for treating any skin irritation or inflammation, including burns, dermatitis, eczema, psoriasis, and seborrhea. Its anti-inflammatory properties can also reduce the pain and swelling of joints and muscles associated with arthritis, backache, carpal tunnel syndrome, rheumatism, and sciatica. Flaxseed oil helps overcome depression. It lowers blood cholesterol and helps maintain healthy arteries. Flaxseed oil contains lignins, compounds that fight microbes and cancer. Historically, many ancient cultures prized flax for uses such as nourishing pregnant and nursing mothers, soothing skin disorders, overcoming malnutrition, and increasing men's virility. If refrigerated after opening, flaxseed oil retains its freshness for up to two months. Freezing can increase its longevity up to two years.

Hazelnut Oil (Corylus avellana)

Hazelnut oil is golden and has a hint of nuttiness in its aroma. It lubricates and nourishes all types of skin. It tones and tightens the skin and helps to maintain firmness and elasticity. It also helps to strengthen capillaries. Add hazelnut oil to facial oils to encourage cell regeneration. Skin disorders such as dermatitis, eczema, and psoriasis benefit from topical application. Historically, hazelnut oil has been used to treat intestinal problems such as colitis and parasites, cystitis and other urinary-tract conditions, diabetes, and tuberculosis. When refrigerated, it stays fresh for one year after opening.

Hemp Oil (*Cannabis sativa*)

Hemp oil is green and rich, with an earthy, nutty scent. Although it comes from the same plant as marijuana, this oil contains no tetrahydrocannabinol (THC), the psychoactive component. You will not hallucinate or get high from using it. Hemp has high levels of both EFAs and some GLA, making it a very balanced vegetable oil. Because of its anti-inflammatory actions, it is excellent for treating a variety of skin complaints, such as dermatitis, eczema, itching, psoriasis, redness, and swelling. It also can relieve the discomfort and swelling of arthritis, backaches, bursitis, carpal tunnel syndrome, joint problems, rheumatism, and sciatica. Hemp oil retains its freshness for about two months if refrigerated after opening. Frozen hemp oil lasts for several years.

Jojoba Oil (*Simmondsia chinesis*)

Jojoba oil is very similar in composition to sebum—the oil your body secretes. Color can range from clear from highly refined oil to golden yellow from unrefined oil. It penetrates the skin rapidly to nourish it. It softens and moisturizes mature and dry skin.

Jojoba oil helps to heal inflamed skin conditions such as eczema, psoriasis, and dermatitis; it also helps control acne, oily skin, and an oily scalp. Jojoba has regenerative value for both skin and hair because of its ability to balance oil production. Many people report that it has the ability to stimulate hair growth. Jojoba has antioxidant properties and can keep other oils from going rancid as quickly as they otherwise would. Use jojoba oil in fragrances and facial oils, and add it to massage oils, body oils, and hair treatments. Jojoba oil has an indefinite shelf life, even stored at room temperature.

Olive Oil (*Olea europaea*)

Olive oil has very therapeutic properties that benefit both skin and hair. It soothes, heals, and lubricates the skin. Olive oil has a distinctive odor and is golden in color. A green color indicates that the oil was extracted too soon from unripe olives. The term *extra virgin*, which signifies that it is unrefined and came from the first pressing of the olives, designates the olive oil of choice for aromatherapy. Neither high heat nor chemical additives have destroyed its nutrients. Even extra virgin and virgin olive oil from the supermarket are unrefined and, if packaged in light-protected containers, are suitable for aromatherapy purposes. Olive oil makes a nice facial oil for all skin types. It retains its freshness for one year after opening, when refrigerated.

Rose Hip Seed Oil
(Rosa mosqueta)

Rose hip seed oil reduces scarring, heals burns, and softens scars and keloids. It is reputed to reduce fine lines and retard premature aging by promoting the regeneration of skin cells. It can help diminish the appearance of broken capillaries. However, rose hip seed oil may aggravate acne or blemished skin. Because it goes rancid quickly, refrigerate it and use it within several months.

Sesame Oil *(Sesamum indicum)*

Sesame oil is a rich golden oil with a nutty aroma. Unrefined sesame oil has a much milder odor than refined, toasted sesame oil commonly sold in supermarkets. It makes a fine facial oil that doesn't normally cause the skin to break out. Sesame oil is good for all skin types and especially benefits eczema, psoriasis, and prematurely aging skin. Some people claim that it helps arthritis. One study suggests that topical application of sesame oil that is high in linoleic acid may inhibit the growth of some malignant melanocytes, or skin-cancer cells. Another study confirms that sesame oil acts to screen out about 30 percent of the burning rays of the sun. The U.S. Food and Drug Administration (FDA) recognizes sesame oil as an approved sunscreen ingredient. Sesame oil is highly valued in Ayurvedic medicine for treating depression, nervous disorders, poor circulation, and stress. In massage, it soothes and relaxes the body and

mind. Its high levels of lecithin help support and strengthen the entire nervous system. Unrefined sesame oil lasts one year after opening, if refrigerated.

Sunflower Oil *(Helianthus annus)*

Sunflower oil is a light, golden oil that is easily absorbed. It contains about 71 percent linoleic acid. It is suitable for all skin types. Its high vitamin-E content makes it especially helpful for delicate and dry skin. Traditionally, people used sunflower oil to treat circulatory problems, endocrine imbalances, and nervous disorders, as well as to heal wounds. Sunflower oil stays fresh, if refrigerated, for one year after opening.

Wheat Germ Oil *(Triticum vulgare)*

Wheat germ oil is a thick, sticky, and dark golden oil with a high content of vitamin E. It nourishes dry or cracked skin and soothes skin problems such as dermatitis, eczema, and psoriasis. It helps to prevent or reduce scarring and may prevent stretch marks. All skin types benefit from wheat germ oil, particularly mature skin. When refrigerated after opening, it may remain fresh for one year.

OTHER CARRIER SYSTEMS FOR ESSENTIAL OILS

While carrier oils provide the easiest means to dilute essential oils safely and economically for use on the skin, they may not always be the most suitable or desirable means of doing so. Alcohol and apple cider vinegar are two alternative systems. They offer a wide range of possibilities for making your own aromatherapy creations. You can treat numerous ailments and conditions by blending them with your choice of essential oils.

Alcohol

Essential oils usually combine nicely with alcohol. If local laws permit, you can purchase pure grain alcohol, also called ethyl alcohol, or ethanol. If not, vodka makes a suitable substitute for blending aftershaves, colognes, facial toners, hair tonics, and perfumes. Brandy might appeal to you for making gargles, mouthwashes, tonics, and even fragrances. Do not inhale directly from the bottle. Apply it to your skin and allow the alcohol to evaporate for thirty to sixty seconds. Never use isopropyl alcohol, or rubbing alcohol, for aromatherapy purposes.

Apple Cider Vinegar

Organic apple cider vinegar made from whole food-grade apples provides a good base for many aromatherapy formulas. Because it is acidic by nature, it can maintain or restore the skin's natural acid balance, which is an essential factor in immunity. It is antiseptic and cleansing, both internally and externally. Its many therapeutic topical uses include minimizing age spots, blemishes, fine lines, and wrinkles. It soothes burns, including sunburn, and rashes. It can relieve the discomfort of skin disorders, such as dermatitis, eczema, psoriasis, and seborrhea. It calms itching and redness of insect bites, poison ivy, and poison oak.

Essential oils disperse fairly well in apple cider vinegar. You can use it to create facial toners, soaks for athlete's foot, splashes for skin disorders, sunburn relief treatments, and tonics to banish blemishes. You can make soothing treatments for almost any skin disorder, such as dermatitis, eczema, psoriasis, red or inflamed skin, or seborrhea. You can also create hair tonics to stimulate growth or prevent hair loss, to diminish dandruff, to soothe seborrhea, or to minimize oiliness. Generally, add 2 to 8 drops of an essential oil or a combination of essential oils to 1 ounce of apple cider vinegar. Avoid using white vinegar or commercial apple cider vinegar in aromatherapy.

Part Two

AN INTRODUCTION TO FORTY-FOUR ESSENTIAL OILS

Introduction

*

Of the estimated *350,000 species of plants on earth, relatively few produce essential oils. Only between 150 and 300 essential oils are currently available with the existing methods of extraction. Many of these essential oils are readily available and easily affordable. Others are harder to obtain, but with patience—and for the right price—you can purchase them. Some are extremely rare and quite costly. Still others I have only heard or read about, and I have yet to see or smell them.*

This section features discussions of forty-four different essential oils. Selecting these oils was not an easy task. I have enjoyed every essential oil I have ever used and have profited from each one. I feel, however, that those in this selection are among the most useful and valuable essential oils, which will bring the greatest benefits to the most people. These essential oils have a broad range of activities for health, beauty, and emotional well-being. They are fairly common and easy enough to obtain. Most are relatively affordable. Some of the oils discussed, including jasmine, melissa, neroli, and rose, are rather expensive, but I include them because they are among the best essences for treating emotional problems. They also have tremendous value in skin care and the treatment of skin disorders. When you consider the value that just one drop of these oils can bring, their worth far exceeds their price. Besides, these possess four of the most delightful smells on earth.

Each of the sections in this part of the book is devoted to a single essential oil. The section begins with an introduction that describes the plant that is the source of the essential oil and tells you its botanical name, its botanical family, its native habitat, and the countries that cultivate it. I include information about the physical characteristics, the aroma, and the extraction of the essential oil. Each section is then subdivided into four parts: Folklore and Herbal Heritage, Medicinal Uses, Beauty Benefits, and Emotional Effects. When appropriate, I include a fifth and/or sixth part: Hydrosol Uses and Precautions.

Folklore and Herbal Heritage traces the plant's colorful history and tells about some of the ways people have used it in the past. Since the beginning of recorded history, people have trusted plants to feed them, clothe them, provide shelter, and help them maintain or regain their health. Botanicals have protected and preserved the human race. In many cases, you will see how you can treat modern ailments with the same faithful botanicals as your ancestors did hundreds or even thousands of years ago.

Medicinal Uses focuses on the role of the essential oil today in maintaining health and treating physical problems. Much of the information in this part comes from medical evidence of European physicians, who have greater success with botanical medicine than with allopathic drugs for their patients. Some data come from patient studies conducted by practicing aromatherapists. I complement these findings with my extensive research, my personal experiences in healing myself, and my experiments in caring for other people around the world.

Beauty Benefits explains how to use a particular essential oil to improve your appearance through skin, body, and hair-care treatments. Aromatherapy skin care offers one of the most natural and effective forms of skin care. Skin and hair-care specialists across America and abroad are using essential oils to achieve results that satisfy their clients.

Emotional Effects discusses the impact that the essential oil can have on the emotions. Many psychotherapists in Europe treat their patients with essential oils and report satisfaction with their results.

Hydrosol Uses lists conditions and suggested treatments for using the hydrosols, or plant water, of the essential oil. Hydrosols are the water byproduct from steam distillation. Though their properties are often similar to the essential oils, they are much less potent than essential oils and are safer to use. However, hydrosols are not available for all essential oils.

Precautions indicates warnings that might restrict the use of an essential oil. Not all essential oils require precautions.

This segment of the book will provide you with enough background information on each essential oil to help you decide which oils you want to use, and to help you feel comfortable and confident in using them. Essential oils can make a great difference in your daily life, as well as being enjoyable to use. They are a great gift from nature that can open a gateway to healing and guide you on a path toward improved health.

BASIL

Sweet basil is a tender annual herb with dark-green pointed oval leaves that may be fuzzy. It bears whorls of green, white, or pink flowers. The entire basil plant, *Ocimum basilicum,* emits a fresh, sweet, herbaceous scent. Steam distilling the flowering herb produces oil that is colorless, pale yellow, or pale green. Basil oil has a light, spicy smell with a balsamic or camphorlike undertone.

Native to tropical Asia and Africa, this member of the *Lamiaceae* family is cultivated throughout Europe, the Mediter-ranean, on islands in the Pacific, and in North and South America. Brazil, Bulgaria, Egypt, France, Hungary, Indonesia, Italy, Morocco, South Africa, and the United States all produce basil oil.

FOLKLORE AND HERBAL HERITAGE

The word *basil* stems from the Greek words *basilokos,* meaning "royal," and *basileus,* meaning "king." The ancient Greeks considered basil the "king of plants." It was an important ingredient in a regal oil for anointing kings. The Greeks also prized the herb for its medicinal and culinary properties.

Hindus believed basil to be sacred to the deities Vishnu and Krishna. They placed sprigs of basil on the chests of deceased loved ones to protect them from evil and provide safe passage into the next life. Ayurvedic doctors prescribed basil to relieve respiratory problems such as asthma, bronchitis, colds, coughs, and emphysema.

Ancient Chinese doctors treated digestive and kidney ailments with basil. They also used it to cure epilepsy. Basil was a popular antidote for poisonous insect or snake bites. People fought fevers, epidemics, and malaria with it. Herbalists have recommended basil to alleviate headaches and to comfort colds. Basil soothed irritated skin conditions, nervous disorders, and the pain of rheumatism as well. Many people have considered basil an aphrodisiac, and it has been closely linked to love. Italian women placed basil plants on their balconies to alert suitors to their availability; a man would give a woman a sprig of basil in the hope that she would fall in love with him and remain forever faithful.

MEDICINAL USES

Today, European physicians treat a variety of respiratory ailments with basil oil. It can restore a lost sense of smell, relieve sinus congestion, and avert attacks of asthma, bronchitis, and emphysema. Basil can ward off colds and the flu and relieve whooping cough. Digestive disorders respond to its stomach-soothing properties. It aids digestion and stimulates appetite; dispels gas and prevents constipation; and relieves nausea, stomach cramps, and vomiting.

Basil oil opens and clears the head and can ease headaches, including migraines. It helps overcome the nasal stuffiness of colds and the flu, while at the same time fighting infection. It stimulates circulation and reduces muscle spasms and cramping. It can revive someone who has fainted. It reduces the pain of menstrual cramps and promotes menstrual flow. Basil oil helps relieve the pain of arthritis, rheumatism, muscular aches and pains, injuries, and physical overexertion. Basil oil also eases the discomfort of earaches, soothes mouth ulcers, and fights gum infections. It acts as an insect repellent and can soothe the sting of mosquito bites and wasp stings. It also provides relief for many of the symptoms of chronic fatigue syndrome and stress.

BEAUTY BENEFITS

Because basil oil has the ability to stimulate circulation, it enlivens dull-looking skin, improves skin tone, and gives the complexion a rosy glow. It can reduce cellulite. It helps to control acne. It also adds luster to dull hair and can stimulate circulation to the scalp.

EMOTIONAL EFFECTS

Basil oil possesses both sedating and stimulating qualities. Its sedative action wards off anxiety attacks and nervous tension and helps to vanquish insomnia; its stimulating action fights mental fatigue and strengthens mental functions, including memory. Basil oil increases concentration, sharpens the senses, clarifies thoughts, and clears the head. As a nerve tonic, basil oil can calm nervousness. In Europe, psychologists and physicians use it to treat melancholy and depression. It produces a sense of joy and happiness. Basil oil can minimize fear and sadness while overcoming indecision and indifference. It fortifies weak nerves and strengthens the entire nervous system.

HYDROSOL USES

Basil hydrosol can be used as a digestive aid for bloating, gas, and constipation. It is calming, balances emotions, and reduces stress. It is also beneficial for headaches and muscle spasms, and can be used in cooking.

PRECAUTIONS

Basil oil stimulates menstrual flow; avoid it during pregnancy. It may trigger epileptic seizures in susceptible individuals. If you suffer from a seizure disorder, avoid it. The overuse of basil oil may have a sedative or stupefying effect. Basil oil may irritate sensitive skin.

BENZOIN

Fragrant clusters of silky white blossoms adorn the benzoin tree, *Styrax benzoin,* which can attain an imposing height of up to 115 feet. When workers slash triangular cuts into the bark of benzoin trees that are over seven years old, the trees secrete a thick sap. The sap flows forth in tears, or lumps, that harden into a yellow to reddish-brown resinous mass. During an average productivity cycle of one decade, each tree yields about 30 pounds of benzoin resin.

Native to Java, Sumatra, Thailand, and other tropical areas of Asia, this member of the *Styraceae* family produces a thick, exotic-smelling resin. The resin of the Siam benzoin tree *(Styrax tonkinensis),* which comes from Cambodia, Laos, Thailand, and Vietnam, is yellowish red; that of benzoin Sumatra *(Styrax paralleloneurus),* which comes from Java, Malaysia, and Sumatra, is reddish or grayish brown. Both resins are thick and viscous, with a vanillalike aroma, although benzoin Sumatra has an undertone suggestive of cinnamon. Benzoin is also called gum benzoin, gum benjamin, and styrax

benzoin. Because these gums or crude tears are so thick, they are either melted by heat or extracted with alcohol or a chemical solvent such as hexane before they can be used.

For aromatherapy purposes, use only solid benzoin tears or benzoin dissolved in alcohol. Also, while for the sake of simplicity benzoin is often considered together with the essential oils, it is more accurate to refer to it as benzoin resin.

FOLKLORE AND HERBAL HERITAGE

Ancient peoples incorporated benzoin into incense for its sweet, soothing smell. They believed it could drive away evil spirits. For centuries Buddhist and Hindu priests have burned benzoin in temples to invite divine inspiration and heighten spiritual awareness. Ayurvedic doctors treated shingles, ringworm, and other skin disorders with benzoin. Southern Asians used it to heal sores on their feet.

Benzoin was often added to cosmetics to keep skin clear and youthful. People in many different cultures have appreciated its ability to soothe and stimulate the skin. By adding benzoin to the animal fats used in making jasmine and tuberose enfleurage, perfumers protected those precious oils from turning rancid. Benzoin was also an important fragrance component in pomanders, potpourris, sachets, and soaps.

Tincture of benzoin, also known as friar's balsam, was used to help warm chills, fight the flu, and soothe sore throats, coughs, and laryngitis. By encouraging the movement of fluids through the body, it improved circulation, promoted urination, relieved congestion, and dispelled gas. Ballerinas applied friar's balsam to heal their battered feet.

MEDICINAL USES

Physicians in Europe still use benzoin resin for respiratory ailments such as asthma, bronchitis, colds, coughs, laryngitis, sinusitis, sore throats, and tonsillitis. Its soothing action tones the lungs, while its expectorant qualities reduce congestion and help the body expel phlegm. Benzoin resin helps improve physical strength, endurance, and energy, and is especially helpful during convalescence. Benzoin resin increases circulation, eases the aches and pains of arthritis and rheumatism, and relieves sore muscles and stiff joints due to overexertion or physical activity. It improves digestion, calms the digestive tract, and alleviates flatulence. As a diuretic, benzoin resin increases urination, which can relieve the discomfort of urinary tract infections or prostate problems where urination is difficult or scant. Because of its antibacterial activity, it can fight leukorrhea and yeast infections. Benzoin resin can also relieve some of the symptoms of premenstrual syndrome (PMS).

Benzoin resin soothes rashes and speeds the healing of wounds and sores. It calms inflamed and irritated skin and relieves the redness and itching of psoriasis, as well as eczema and other forms of dermatitis.

BEAUTY BENEFITS

Cosmetic chemists often add benzoin to protective skin-care products because it helps chapped or blistered skin to heal. Its rejuvenating action repairs dry, cracked skin, especially on the hands and heels. Benzoin resin helps to maintain skin's elasticity and preserve its suppleness. Regular application can soften scar tissue over time.

EMOTIONAL EFFECTS

Benzoin has warming and soothing qualities that extend to the emotions. It relaxes and pacifies a worrisome mind. By calming the central nervous system, it eases nervous tension, stress, and anxiety. When you are feeling drained or emotionally exhausted, benzoin can soothe your frazzled nerves. It offers comfort in times of sadness or loneliness, and its uplifting effect helps to overcome depression and restore confidence and esteem. Benzoin encourages meditation and spiritual growth by providing focus and direction. Benzoin resin dispels anger, diminishes irritability and hyperactivity, and reduces worrying. It promotes feelings of love and sensuality. Its sweet scent is slightly sensuous, exotic, and euphoria-inducing. Some people say that it helps overcome sexual problems, especially impotence and premature ejaculation.

PRECAUTIONS

For aromatherapy, use only solid benzoin tears or benzoin resin that has been dissolved in alcohol. If benzoin has been diluted with solvents, their residues remain and can penetrate the skin and enter the bloodstream.

BERGAMOT

Lush green leaves and tiny white star-shaped flowers cover the branches of the bergamot tree, which can attain a height of sixteen feet. It bears a pear-shaped yellow fruit that is smaller than an orange and was once called the bergamot pear. The bergamot tree is the result of the crossbreeding of the lemon tree and the bitter orange tree, which created the bergamot hybrids *Citrus bergamia* and *Citrus aurantium*, subspecies *bergamia*.

A member of the *Rutaceae* family, bergamot originated in tropical Asia. Farmers in most countries have had little or no success in cultivating the tree commercially. Today, bergamot grows in the Ivory Coast in Africa, in the Calabria region of Italy, and in Sicily.

A simple pressing or expression of the rinds of the sour green fruit renders a pale emerald-green oil. It has a flowery lemon-orange smell with a slightly sweet, balsamic undertone. The best quality oil is hand pressed. Peels from 1,000 bergamot fruits yield about 30 ounces of oil.

FOLKLORE AND HERBAL HERITAGE

Some controversy exists about the origin of the word *bergamot*. According to one story, the name originates from the Turkish word *beg-armudu*, meaning "prince's pear." Another account claims that it comes from the name of the small town of Bergamo in northern Italy, supposedly the site of the original distribution of bergamot oil in Italy. Early tales credit Christopher Columbus with transporting bergamot from the Canary Islands to Italy, where it has been cultivated ever since. Bergamot was virtually unknown to the rest of the world until relatively recently, and therefore most of the folklore concerning bergamot comes to us from Italy. Italians used it to cool and relieve fevers and protect against malaria. They took it internally to expel intestinal worms. Italians valued bergamot for its antiseptic actions. French perfumers enlivened fragrances, particularly eau de cologne, with the sweet citrus notes of bergamot. It imparts a delightful flavor and distinctive aroma to Earl Grey and Constant Comment teas.

MEDICINAL USES

Bergamot oil possesses strong antiseptic properties, making it useful against urinary tract infections such as cystitis and urethritis. Using it in sitz baths helps to prevent bacterial infections from spreading from the urethra to the bladder. Bergamot oil's antiseptic properties also alleviate respiratory ailments. It cools fevers, subdues the symptoms of colds and flu, and soothes sore throats, tonsillitis, and laryngitis. As a digestive aid, bergamot oil calms stomach cramps and regulates the appetite, either stimulating or suppressing it as needed.

Applied topically, bergamot oil can minimize the discomfort and hasten the healing of cold sores and other herpes infections, as well as mouth ulcers. It alleviates the pain of shingles and chickenpox, which are also caused by a herpes virus, varicella zoster. It can heal dry, chapped, and irritated skin, making it an excellent choice for relieving symptoms of eczema and psoriasis.

Bergamot is useful in treating chronic fatigue syndrome. When used as an inhalant or in a lamp or diffuser, bergamot oil can help people who wish to break the smoking habit. Bergamot oil fights fatigue from stress, helps restore physical and emotional strength, and is useful for restoring immunity in a person convalescing from a long illness.

BEAUTY BENEFITS

Bergamot oil's antiseptic action makes it useful for the treatment of acne and skin infections. Its astringent quality helps regulate excessive oiliness of the skin or scalp. Its deodorizing action can freshen your body, your home, or your office. Bergamot oil compresses help draw out the inflammation of blemishes or boils and promote rapid healing. Bergamot also repels insects and soothes insect bites. Along with neroli, orange, and rosemary, bergamot was a component of the original eau de cologne. Modern perfumers prize it for the fruity-floral bouquet it imparts to their creations.

EMOTIONAL EFFECTS

Bergamot oil is refreshing and uplifting. It acts as a stimulant and tonic to balance the emotions and nerves. Research conducted in Italy indicates that bergamot oil relieves feelings of fear, anxiety, and panic. It diminishes depression and sadness. It can calm aggression and anger. Its soothing nature encourages release of resentment and forgiveness through the beneficial expression of repressed emotions that distort perception and interfere with health. Studies show that it equalizes emotions and moods by balancing the activity of the hypothalamus. It regulates trapped or misdirected energy and redirects it toward healthy pursuits. Smelling bergamot oil can stabilize a person in a shaky emotional state. It evokes feelings of happiness and joy and can restore self-confidence and self-esteem. Bergamot's balancing properties help minimize the tendency toward compulsive or obsessive behavior. During times of sadness or grief, bergamot oil helps to heal emotional wounds and can inspire or restore loving feelings.

PRECAUTIONS

Bergamot oil promotes sensitivity to the sun. Avoid wearing it outdoors in sunlight to prevent sunburn or uneven darkening of the skin.

BLACK PEPPER

A woody perennial crawling vine, the black pepper plant has heart-shaped leaves, small white flowers, and red berries that turn black when mature. The plant can climb up to twenty feet. The dried, crushed berries—or peppercorns—of *Piper nigrum* produce a clear to pale-green oil when steam-distilled. Its fragrance is fresh, dry, and warm, with woody, spicy, and sweet notes.

Native to southwest India, this member of the *Piperaceae* family is now cultivated and distilled in many tropical areas, primarily China, India, Indonesia, Madagascar, and Malaysia. Europe and America also produce some black pepper oil from imported peppercorns.

FOLKLORE AND HERBAL HERITAGE

Ayurvedic and Chinese doctors have used pepper for thousands of years to treat malaria and cholera and to relieve digestive difficulties such as dysentery and diarrhea. Indian monks ate black pepper every day to sustain their endurance and increase their energy.

MEDICINAL USES

Black pepper oil stimulates circulation and improves muscle tone, offering relief for the discomfort of arthritis, backache, muscular aches, rheumatism, sports injuries, and sprains. When massaged onto muscles before exercising, it prevents stiffness and soreness. Black pepper oil also relieves pain and stiffness following strenuous physical activity. Black pepper oil helps to ward off and speed recovery from colds and the flu. It warms chills, clears congestion, and fights infection. As a digestive aid, black pepper oil increases the appetite and stimulates sluggish digestion. It soothes stomach cramps, reduces intestinal gas, and can help reduce colic, diarrhea, heartburn, and nausea. It can fight feelings of faintness. It also boosts red blood cell production in the spleen and may help overcome anemia.

BEAUTY BENEFITS

Applied to the skin, black pepper oil can be extremely stimulating and even potentially irritating. As a result, it is not usually used for skin-care purposes unless very diluted. However, some women use it to eliminate cellulite because it stimulates circulation.

EMOTIONAL EFFECTS

Black pepper oil increases alertness and improves concentration. It stimulates mental energy, especially blocked energy. Black pepper oil can motivate people into action when they feel stuck. It helps resolve past emotional issues so you can move forward. It encourages feelings of courage and bravery, particularly about speaking in public. It is a very settling and stabilizing oil, especially during change. It provides a sense of protection for vulnerable people. Some people use black pepper oil as an aphrodisiac.

PRECAUTIONS

Black pepper oil may irritate the skin.

CEDARWOOD

Three types of cedar trees produce essential oils for aromatherapy purposes. The most common is red cedar, or *Juniperus virginiana*. Native to North America, this slow-growing tree attains a regal height of up to 100 feet. It grows primarily in the mountainous regions east of the Rocky Mountains. Distillation of its reddish heartwood and seed-bearing cones renders a yellow to orange oil with a sweet, balsamic scent.

Texas cedarwood, or *Juniperus mexicana*, is a smaller tree that grows up to twenty-one feet tall. It is native to the southwestern United States, Mexico, and Central America. Its viscous dark-orange or brown oil has a sweet, smoky, and woody aroma and is distilled from the tree's stiff green needles and twisted branches.

The Atlas cedar, *Cedrus atlanticus,* grows atop the Atlas Mountains of North Africa. This member of the *Pinaceae* family can reach a height of 100 feet. Steam distillation of wood chips and sawdust from the Atlas cedar yields a thick yellow- to honey-colored oil with a soft and sweet, warm and woody, pinelike odor.

About 29 pounds of plant material can produce 1 pound of cedarwood oil. To obtain the oil of the red cedar, the tree must be felled; the other two cedar trees remain intact during the harvesting of their plant material. Some cedars can live for 1,000 to 2,000 years.

FOLKLORE AND HERBAL HERITAGE

During Biblical times, the famed cedars of Lebanon *(Cedrus libani)* provided one of the world's earliest perfumes. Visitors sought solitude in this holy forest, praying and seeking spiritual guidance. Although the oldest surviving cedar tree is 2,500 years old, most *Cedrus libani* trees were destroyed long ago.

Noah purportedly burned an offering of cedarwood and myrtle incense to show his gratitude for surviving the great flood. Tibetans likewise burned cedarwood incense in their temples; they also used it as a medicinal remedy. The temple of King Solomon was built of cedarwood to symbolize strength, nobility, and dignity. In Greek mythology, Artemis was given the surname *Cedreatis* because images of her were hung high atop the cedar trees.

Cedarwood oil was an important ancient antidote for poisoning. The ancient Egyptians included cedarwood oil in their embalming preparations, and they also constructed sarcophagi from cedarwood. Many of these 3,000-year-old coffins are still in good condition. Egyptian incense, perfumes, and cosmetics often contained cedarwood. When they discovered that the reddish-brown wood repelled insects, the Egyptians built ships and furniture from cedarwood. Each pharaoh owned his own ceremonial cedarwood barge. A coating of cedarwood oil protected papyri.

Native Americans in what is now New Mexico treated skin rashes, arthritis, and rheumatism with Texas cedarwood. Other Native Americans burned cedar leaves as incense and used red cedarwood to fight respiratory ailments, tuberculosis, kidney infections, skin disorders, gonorrhea, venereal warts, and delayed menstruation. They also repelled insects and vermin with it. For centuries, people have lined closets and chests with cedarwood to protect valuable clothing and personal belongings from moths and other insects. At one time, a popular commercial insecticide contained cedarwood and citronella oils as active ingredients. Sachets and potpourris commonly contained cedar chips to release a fresh, clean aroma into the atmosphere and to combat insects.

MEDICINAL USES

Like the oils from other coniferous trees, cedarwood oil makes an excellent choice for treating respiratory problems. It eases coughs and decreases the discomforts of colds and the flu. As an expectorant, it helps expel mucus from the lungs; it also decreases the congestion common with bronchitis and sinusitis. Cedarwood oil promotes urination and is useful against urinary tract infections and prostate problems. It tones the urinary tract and may help control incontinence. Its antiseptic action assists in combating infection, particularly cystitis and urethritis. It helps to reduce the pain and swelling of arthritis, backache, carpal tunnel syndrome, rheumatism, and sciatica. Cedarwood oil heals skin rashes, soothes the discomfort and irritation of dermatitis and psoriasis, and fights fungal infections such as athlete's foot.

BEAUTY BENEFITS

Cedarwood oil contributes to clear skin by healing skin rashes and clearing blemishes. It reduces excessive secretions of sebum, or oil, and normalizes both dry and oily skin and hair. Cedarwood oil controls dandruff and seborrhea, improves the condition of the hair, and stimulates the scalp and hair follicles. It helps reduce cellulite by increasing circulation and releasing wastes. It can minimize hair loss, and some men claim that it even promotes hair growth.

EMOTIONAL EFFECTS

Cedarwood calms the mind and eases anxiety, hyperactivity, nervous tension, and stress-related conditions. It helps defuse aggression, anger, and fear. It also helps stabilize energy imbalances. Cedarwood oil can comfort you during difficult times, provide clarity during crisis, and reinforce resolve and independence. It can help you see situations more objectively while remaining emotionally composed and confident. Even when external events, your own emotions, or other people cause you to doubt yourself and your capabilities, cedarwood can help you maintain proper perspective and faith. It restores esteem and confidence. In foreign environments or strange situations, it helps you adapt while diminishing culture shock and disorientation. Many people claim that cedarwood oil is an aphrodisiac.

HYDROSOL USES

Cedarwood hydrosol can be used to treat dandruff, dry hair, oily hair, acne, cold sores, dermatitis, eczema, and psoriasis, and as a scalp tonic to prevent hair loss. It is for topical use only—do not take it internally.

PRECAUTIONS

Cedarwood oil can stimulate menstrual flow; avoid using it during pregnancy.

CHAMOMILE

Two species of chamomile—German chamomile and Roman chamomile—yield essential oils. Both belong to the *Asteraceae* family and share similar properties.

The fine, feathery leaves of the Roman chamomile plant *(Chamaemelum nobile* or *Anthemis nobilis)* surround tiny daisylike flowers that are white with bright-yellow centers. This perennial plant attains a height of nine to twelve inches. Native to southern and western Europe, Roman chamomile is now cultivated in many countries, including Belgium, Bulgaria, England, France, Hungary, and Italy. Steam distillation of the flowers renders a yellow essential oil with a sweet, warm, herbaceous odor.

German chamomile *(Matricaria chamomilla* or *Matricaria recutita)* is similar in appearance to Roman chamomile, except that it is taller (it grows about two feet tall) and its flowers have smaller heads and fewer petals. German chamomile is an annual. Once native to Europe and parts of Asia, it now grows in eastern Europe, Egypt, North America, and in areas of the former Soviet Union. German chamomile oil has a characteristic deep blue or bluish-green color and for this reason is sometimes referred to as blue chamomile. This color comes from its high content of azulene, a chemical component that is produced during the distillation process and that also has a strong anti-inflammatory action. Stronger in smell than Roman chamomile oil, German chamomile oil has a sweet, slightly fruity, slightly spicy scent that is almost intoxicating.

Many people consider *Anthemis mixta* to be a third type of chamomile. Although called chamomile mixta, or Moroccan chamomile, it is not a true chamomile. It is a member of the same botanical family, *Asteraceae,* and is a distant relative to German and Roman chamomile. It bears no physical resemblance to them. *Anthemis mixta* has hairy leaves and tubular yellow flowers. This native of northwestern Africa and southern Spain also grows in Egypt, Israel, and Morocco. Its oil smells spicy and fresh, with a balsamic undertone.

FOLKLORE AND HERBAL HERITAGE

The ancient Egyptians offered chamomile to Ra, their sun god, to honor and appease him. They also massaged chamomile into their skin to cool fevers, to alleviate aches and pains, and to relieve muscle soreness and spasms.

The ancient Greeks gave chamomile its name. They called it *kamai melon,* which means "ground apple." Although the chamomile plant looks nothing like an apple tree, its sweet scent is reminiscent of fresh-cut apples. In Spanish, the herb and a chamomile-flavored sherry share the name *manzanilla,* meaning "little apple." Greek herbalists and physicians prescribed chamomile baths and poultices to relieve headaches and to dissipate disorders of the kidneys, liver, and bladder.

During the Middle Ages, Europeans scattered chamomile flowers on their floors. Stepping on the flowers released a sweet fragrance into the atmosphere. Chamomile purportedly possessed the power to replenish a person's energy when he or she was confronted with adversity. In Beatrix Potter's famous children's story *The Tale of Peter Rabbit,* Peter's mother gave him a dose of chamomile tea to calm and comfort him after a day of mischief in the garden. Chamomile tea has long enjoyed popularity as a nighttime beverage because it helps to induce restful sleep.

For centuries, herbalists have recommended chamomile for colic, gout, head-aches, heartburn, indigestion, and loss of appetite, as well as to promote urination and relieve diarrhea. They have also suggested using it to prevent nightmares or to calm a person who has suffered from a nightmare. Chamomile poultices were applied for abscesses, swelling, and pain. Chamomile has long been a favorite of English country gardeners. Besides adding color and fragrance to the garden, this hardy plant repels insects. In fact, chamomile was nicknamed the "plant's physician" because it supposedly cured any ailing plant placed near it.

MEDICINAL USES

Modern European doctors recommend chamomile to treat many of the same conditions for which traditional herbalists recommended it. Doctors regularly prescribe it as a sedative, stress-reducer, and digestive aid, as well as for healing skin problems. Chamomile oil reduces any kind of inflammation. In addition, chamomile fights infection and irritations and speeds up the healing process. Chamomile oil relieves injuries such as bruises, inflamed tendons, sprains, and swollen or overexerted muscles. It soothes muscle pain and inflamed joints and reduces the discomfort of arthritis, backache, bursitis, carpal tunnel syndrome, rheumatism, and sciatica.

Many Germans believe that chamomile oil is capable of healing almost any problem. Chamomile aids digestion, relieves gas, decreases constipation, eases heartburn, and soothes nausea. Medical practitioners in Germany recommend it for female disorders such as painful or irregular periods, scanty periods, vaginitis, menopausal problems, and premenstrual syndrome (PMS). Its diuretic properties reduce the fluid retention that often accompanies PMS, while its antidepressant action helps alleviate feelings of depression, irritability, and stress. Chamomile oil minimizes the pain of headaches, including migraines. It is often effective in treating symptoms of candidiasis and chronic fatigue syndrome.

Chamomile oil is mild enough to use on infants and children. For centuries, mothers have used chamomile to calm crying children, ease earaches, fight fevers, soothe stomachaches and colic, and relieve toothaches and teething pain. Chamomile oil safely and effectively can reduce irritability and minimize nervousness in children, especially hyperactive children.

BEAUTY BENEFITS

Azulene, the chemical component that gives German chamomile oil its characteristic blue color, is largely responsible for chamomile's anti-inflammatory action. By reducing swelling and calming irritated skin, chamomile oil relieves the discomfort of psoriasis, eczema, dermatitis, and sunburn. Scientific studies have shown that chamomile reduces dryness, itching, redness, and sensitivity in irritated and inflamed skin. Chamomile oil soothes dry or sensitive skin. With regular treatment, it can reduce the redness of fragile or broken capillaries. Chamomile oil conditions the hair and scalp and adds shine, silkiness, and luster to the hair.

EMOTIONAL EFFECTS

Chamomile oil's subtle sedative action is much milder than that of harsh and potentially habit-forming prescription tranquilizers. Because it is calming and relaxing, it can combat depression, insomnia, and stress. It eliminates much of the emotional charge of anxiety, aggression, irritability, and nervousness. Chamomile oil can dispel anger, stabilize the emotions, and help to release emotions linked to the past. Applied over the throat, it can help a person express his or her true feelings. Chamomile silences self-criticism and softens harsh criticism from others. Its nurturing nature allows you to accept compassion from others and especially from yourself. Chamomile helps regain composure during times of grief, hysteria, and shock while releasing nervous tension.

Chamomile oil helps resolve control issues. If you feel the need to control other people or situations, if you feel frustrated by other people's attempts at controlling you, or if you simply feel out of control, chamomile can help.

HYDROSOL USES

Chamomile hydrosol is beneficial for inflammation and itching. It is a digestive aid that can also be used in baby and child care and in breast care for nursing mothers. It promotes relaxation, making it useful for anxiety, depression, emotional upsets, and insomnia. In skin care, chamomile hydrosol is helpful for many skin disorders and as a skin spray, facial toner, and aftershave lotion. It is healing for burns and sunburn.

PRECAUTIONS

Because chamomile has the ability to induce menstruation, avoid it during pregnancy.

CLARY SAGE

From May to September, the clary sage plant displays hardy whorls of pale blue, purple, or pink blossoms atop long spikes. Heart-shaped green leaves with soft and fuzzy crinkled surfaces surround the flowers. This stout biennial or perennial is a member of the *Lamiaceae* family and attains a height of three to five feet.

Steam distillation of the flowering tops and leaves of *Salvia sclarea* yields a colorless or pale yellowish-green oil. The aroma of clary sage oil is sweet, fresh, and clean, with warm, herblike, nutty, and balsamic undertones.

Native to southern France, Italy, and Syria, clary sage is now cultivated worldwide, especially in Mediterranean climates, central Europe, England, Morocco, Russia, and the United States. Superior oils come from England, France, and Morocco.

FOLKLORE AND HERBAL HERITAGE

Herbalists throughout the ages have used clary sage to treat digestive disorders, kidney diseases, respiratory infections, and sore throats. It cooled and calmed inflammation and brought relief for abscesses, skin disorders, swelling, and wounds. The herb was a common remedy for female complaints.

Clary sage derives its name from the Latin *clarus,* meaning "clear," and was famous for its ability to clear eye problems such as tired or strained eyes or blurred vision. In fact, its nickname during the Middle Ages was *clear eyes.* Mucilage from clary sage seeds was inserted into the eye to expel any foreign matter. Other names were *Christ's eye* and *Ramona.* Germans called it *muscatel sage* due to its similarity in taste to muscatel wine. Some wine merchants adulterated cheap wines with clary sage to impart the taste of the more expensive muscatel wine. Clary sage also substituted for hops in brewing beer. When added to or taken with any alcoholic beverage, clary sage tends to exaggerate drunkenness and increases the discomfort of the hangover that follows.

MEDICINAL USES

Clary sage oil possesses many of the same attributes and healing properties of common sage oil, *Salvia officinalis,* which often has skin-irritating or toxic side effects. Clary sage makes a safer choice for aromatherapy. It is an all-around tonic and is especially useful for toning the liver and kidneys.

Clary sage oil contains hormonelike components that can balance female hormones. In Europe, physicians prescribe it to diminish menopausal discomfort, ease menstrual cramps, encourage delayed or scant periods, minimize the symptoms of premenstrual syndrome (PMS), and regulate menstrual cycles. It can cool hot flashes and ease migraines that are related to menopause or menstruation. Clary sage oil relaxes abdominal and lower-back muscles and reduces the pain of menstrual cramps. It also relaxes muscular aches and pains resulting from mental or emotional stress and nervous tension.

Clary sage oil strengthens the immune system and is helpful in treating chronic fatigue syndrome and candidiasis. It restores and invigorates the body during convalescence from illness. Clary sage helps regulate blood pressure; high blood pressure often decreases after clary sage baths and inhalations. As a muscle relaxant, clary sage oil helps soothe spasms and tightness in the muscles surrounding the bronchial tubes of asthma sufferers. In addition, it alleviates the anxiety and emotional tension that frequently accompany asthma attacks. Clary sage oil relieves respiratory ailments such as bronchitis, colds, coughs, sore throats, laryngitis, and tonsillitis. It encourages better digestion by soothing the muscles of the digestive tract, stimulating digestion, and calming such digestive disorders as colic, gas, and stomachache.

Psoriasis responds well to clary sage's ability to reduce inflammation, as do eczema and other types of dermatitis. Clary sage oil also helps cuts, wounds, and burns to heal. It minimizes the pain, itching, and irritation of herpes and candida outbreaks.

BEAUTY BENEFITS

Clary sage oil promotes the regeneration of skin cells, helping to ward off wrinkles and keep skin looking healthy and youthful. It helps oily skin and hair by controlling excessive oil secretions. It also improves acne and seborrhea. It is equally effective in treating dandruff, dry skin, and dry hair. Used as a scalp massage, clary sage oil reputedly encourages hair growth and minimizes hair loss.

EMOTIONAL EFFECTS

Clary sage oil balances the extremes of emotions and restores emotional equilibrium. It alleviates melancholy and lifts depression. As a nervous system tonic, it eases fear and nervousness. Clary sage oil helps both men and women become more aware of their feminine qualities. It can increase concentration, improve memory, and stimulate mental activity without being overstimulating. Clary sage oil inspires creativity and awakens intuitive powers. Many people report that they have very vivid dreams after using it. Clary sage oil makes an ideal companion in times of personal challenge or change, especially when there is external stress and extreme pressure. In situations of midlife crisis, clary sage oil can exert a balancing, inspiring, and revitalizing influence.

In stressful situations, clary sage oil reduces deep-seated tension, slows a racing mind, and calms nerves. By restoring inner tranquility, clary sage oil minimizes the debilitating effects of stress and stress-related disorders. It reduces irritability, anxiety, and feelings of panic or hysteria as it revives frazzled nerves. It revives cases of mental and emotional exhaustion. It restores a sense of direction and purpose to people suffering from indecision and indifference. Clary sage oil can even create a state of euphoria, and many people consider it an aphrodisiac. European physicians and psychotherapists have successfully treated cases of frigidity and impotence with clary sage oil.

Hydrosol Uses

Clary sage hydrosol balances female hormones, making it useful for bloating, cramps, hot flashes, and PMS. It is a whole-body tonic that helps to counteract moodiness. In skin care, it is beneficial for acne and oily skin, and can be used as a facial spray and facial toner. Clary sage hydrosol also has uses in cooking.

Precautions

Clary sage oil should be avoided during pregnancy because of its ability to stimulate menstrual flow. Also, you should avoid alcohol when using it. Clary sage oil can ex-aggerate the effects of alcohol and intensify drunkenness and hangovers. It can also cause drowsiness.

CORIANDER

The bright-green, feathery leaves of the coriander plant are delicately lobed. After its tiny, lacy white or pale-pink flowers bloom, they turn into green seeds that eventually become brown or brownish gray. At maturity, the plant reaches a height of two to three feet.

Steam-distilling the crushed ripe seeds produces a colorless or pale-yellow oil with a fresh, spicy fragrance that is sweet, woody, and slightly balsamic. It takes about 45 pounds of seeds to produce 1 pound of coriander oil.

Known also as Chinese parsley or cilantro, *Coriandrum sativum* is a member of the *Apiaceae* family. Coriander is indigenous to Morocco and the Middle East, and is now grown commercially in India, North Africa, Russia, South America, southern Europe, and western Asia. Romania, Russia, and the other former Soviet republics produce the majority of coriander oil. Coriander leaf oil is also available. It smells similar to the seed oil but is stronger, greener, and not as sweet.

Folklore and Herbal Heritage

Coriander is one of world's oldest flavorings and has been cultivated for more than 3,000 years. The ancient Egyptians called it the "spice of happiness" and used it as an aphrodisiac. They also presented coriander seeds as funeral offerings to deceased pharaohs.

The ancient Greeks and Romans flavored wines with coriander and also used it as a medicinal herb. The Chinese incorporated coriander into their medical practice as long ago as 207 B.C.E., and believed that coriander could bestow immortality. Coriander reportedly grew in the Hanging Gardens of Babylon; the Hebrews supposedly used it as one of the bitter herbs in Passover rites.

After coriander was mentioned as an aphrodisiac in *The Arabian Nights,* numerous love potions containing coriander appeared. In India, coriander was a remedy for constipation and insomnia, as well as for easing the pain of childbirth. In magical and religious ceremonies, Indians offered the seeds as gifts to their deities. Women consumed the seeds regularly to promote fertility. Coriander was a popular potted plant in England. During the Elizabethan era, candy-coated coriander seeds were served as a sweet after meals and to guard against gas. Besides being an integral part of many ethnic cuisines, coriander adds a distinctive flavor to Benedictine and Chartreuse liqueurs and a savory scent to some tobacco blends.

MEDICINAL USES

Like many other culinary herbs and spices, coriander improves digestion and alleviates such disorders as colic, diarrhea, gas, heartburn, indigestion, nausea, and stomach cramps. Coriander oil stimulates the appetite and can help people with anorexia to overcome their eating disorders. Chinese physicians prescribe it for dysentery and nausea. Chewing on the seeds after a meal prevents indigestion and freshens the breath. Coriander oil can also stop hiccups.

As a circulatory stimulant, coriander oil encourages the release of toxins from the body, thereby improving conditions such as arthritis, chronic fatigue syndrome, gout, rheumatism, and a sluggish lymph system. It also helps regulate breathing and may prevent fainting and dizziness. Coriander oil's antispasmodic and analgesic actions relieve muscular aches and pains and stiffness in the joints. It can diminish facial tension from stress and relax the facial muscles, and is therefore effective in relieving TMJ, facial neuralgia, and nervous facial cramps. In general, coriander is very cleansing and toning for the body and for increasing physical energy.

Chinese doctors recommend coriander for hemorrhoids, hernias, measles, and toothaches. European physicians use coriander oil to treat fatigue, flu, physical exhaustion, and migraines and other headaches. It is an overall tonic for the glands and can encourage estrogen production, helping to regulate the menstrual cycle and alleviate symptoms of premenstrual syndrome (PMS) and menopause. It also helps to reduce fluid retention.

BEAUTY BENEFITS

Coriander oil is a natural deodorant. It is also frequently used in perfumery, particularly in men's fragrances. It imparts a fresh, clean note to any blend. Because it stimulates circulation and fights fluid retention, it is helpful in reducing cellulite and fights the fungus that causes athlete's foot.

EMOTIONAL EFFECTS

Coriander oil stimulates the central nervous system and relieves lethargy, mental fatigue, and nervousness. Some people say that it decreases dizziness. It improves the memory and mental functions. Coriander oil can even inspire creativity. It promotes happiness and joy, reduces worries, and helps provide a sense of security and stability.

Coriander oil refreshes and energizes, yet it is also relaxing and calming for anxiety, hyperactivity, irritability, and stress. It is especially revitalizing during recovery from illness. Coriander oil offers comfort in times of emotional shock or fear. Due to its estrogenlike component, it balances female hormones and can stimulate erotic feelings. It also reputedly helps overcome impotence.

HYDROSOL USES

A digestive aid, coriander hydrosol is helpful for bloating, gas, and constipation. It also has detoxifying properties.

PRECAUTIONS

Because coriander oil can promote menstruation, it should not be used during pregnancy.

CYPRESS

Pointing upward toward the heavens, the cone-bearing cypress maintains an erect shape even at heights of over eighty feet. This evergreen, *Cupressus sempervirens,* has slender horizontal branches that bear small, round gray-brown cones, dark-green needles, and small flowers. Originally from southern Europe and western Asia Minor, this member of the *Cupressace* family now grows wild in France, Italy, North Africa, Portugal, Spain, and some of the Balkan countries. France, Italy, Morocco, and Spain are the primary producers of cypress oil.

Cypress oil is clear, light yellow, or greenish yellow in color. Its fragrance is sharp and smoky, warm and woody, resinous and spicy, with a lemony and balsamic undertone. Steam-distilling about 30 pounds of cypress needles, twigs, and cones yields 1 pound of oil.

FOLKLORE AND HERBAL HERITAGE

Ancient civilizations valued cypress for both medicinal and religious reasons. The Egyptians dedicated the cypress tree to the gods of death; the Greeks dedicated it to Pluto, the god of the underworld. In Greek mythology, when Cyparissus, a beloved of Apollo and Zephyrus, accidentally killed his favorite stag, his grief transformed him into a cypress tree. The evergreen branches of the cypress tree were symbolic of life after death. In fact, *sempervirens* means "ever-living." People of many cultures have planted cypress trees in cemeteries.

The ancient Egyptians treated urinary problems with cypress. They also used cypress to control problems involving excessive secretions of bodily fluids such as bloating, diarrhea, heavy menstrual flow, and perspiration. The Chinese found cypress beneficial for the liver and respiratory system, and ate cypress nuts for their nutritional value. In the early twentieth century, one brand of French cough lozenges contained cypress.

MEDICINAL USES

Cypress oil stimulates circulation and has a detoxifying effect on the entire body. It relieves congestion and eases coughing. It can also stop cuts and wounds from bleeding. Cypress oil soothes bleeding gums and periodontal disease. It provides relief from hemorrhoids. A cypress foot bath will ease tired, swollen feet and reduce foot odor and perspiration. Cypress oil can decrease any excessive flow of fluids, whether a runny nose, diarrhea, excessive menstrual flow, perspiration, or urine. It may even help control incontinence.

Cypress oil releases muscle spasms and can avert an attack of asthma or bronchitis when used in a diffuser or as an inhalant. Cypress oil also relieves muscular cramps and sore muscles. It balances female hormones, eases heavy menstrual flow, relieves cramping, and reduces hot flashes during menopause. Massaged over the area above the ovaries, it reportedly can inhibit the growth of cysts. Used in a sitz bath, it speeds recovery from cystitis or jock itch.

BEAUTY BENEFITS

Cypress oil regulates oil production, making it a useful treatment for oily skin, oily hair, acne, and dandruff. Its deodorizing action and its ability to control excessive bodily secretions make it beneficial as a deodorant. Cypress oil acts as a styptic and is ideal for stopping the bleeding of nicks and cuts from shaving. Broken capillaries and varicose veins respond well to cypress oil's stimulating properties and its ability to constrict blood vessels. It may prevent or diminish stretch marks. It makes an effective treatment for cellulite because it strengthens weak connective tissues, improves circulation, and helps release toxins. It also repels insects.

EMOTIONAL EFFECTS

Cypress oil helps revitalize a nervous system that is overloaded with stress and tension. It calms the mind, increases objectivity, and decreases indifference. It soothes upset emotions and helps stop crying fits. Cypress oil also improves concentration and helps focus thoughts. It helps to provide support and a sense of structure and stability during major transitions, such as a career change, changes in relationships, divorce, midlife crisis, loss of a loved one, or a change in residence. It helps you learn to flow with the ever-changing nature of life and to see crisis or change as lessons to learn and as opportunities for personal growth. Cypress diminishes the dread and fears associated with making changes, allowing new adventures and exciting experiences into your life. It encourages an optimistic outlook, healthy self-esteem, and freedom of self-expression by releasing repressed feelings, resentment, and self-doubt. It gives comfort, strength, and endurance in times of grief or mourning.

HYDROSOL USES

Cypress hydrosol is a diuretic that helps to relieve cystitis, bloating, and swelling. Because it decreases joint inflammation, it eases symptoms of arthritis and rheumatism. It releases mucus and phlegm and aids in detoxification. Other conditions for which it is useful include acne, broken capillaries, varicose veins, eczema, and psoriasis.

ELEMI

As it sprouts new leaves, the elemi tree exudes a white resin with a pungent aroma. When exposed to the air, the resin hardens and turns yellow. Steam distillation of this resin yields a clear or light-yellow oil with a fresh, slightly sweet aroma that is citrusy and spicy. Sometimes the oil is called Manila elemi or gum elemi. The elemi tree, *Canarium luzonicum,* is a member of the *Burseraceae* family and is a relative of the plants that produce frankincense and myrrh. The tree, which reaches heights of up to ninety feet, originated in the Philippines, and the Moluccas, a group of islands in Indonesia. Brazil and Central American countries also cultivate it commercially.

FOLKLORE AND HERBAL HERITAGE

In Arabic, *elemi* means "above and below," which has spiritual connotations. Ancient Turks and Arabs used elemi as an ingredient in incense, probably because it can heighten a meditative state. The ancient Egyptians included elemi in embalming because of its preservative properties.

Beginning in the fifteenth century, Europeans incorporated elemi into medicinal balms, liniments, and unguents. They also used it to treat respiratory problems. A topical plaster of elemi helped knit broken bones. Soldiers suffering from sword wounds supposedly found speedy relief by applying elemi to their wounds. Skin-care products and cosmetics also frequently contained elemi for its skin-healing qualities.

MEDICINAL USES

Elemi oil activates the immune system. In Europe, physicians and aromatherapists use it to treat and tone the thymus gland, a key organ of the immune system. A good general stimulant for the entire body, elemi oil reinforces the body's ability to resist disease and restores physical strength, especially after an illness. It energizes people suffering from physical fatigue.

Elemi oil possesses many of the same properties as its relatives, frankincense and myrrh. It helps fight respiratory ailments such as bronchitis, colds, coughs, and the flu. It eases congestion and helps the body to expel excess mucus. Elemi oil tones the urinary tract, helps to cure cystitis, and may control incontinence. Massaging elemi oil onto the area above a broken or fractured bone will hasten healing and minimize aches and pains, especially when applied before the bone is set in a cast. Continued treatment with elemi may prevent rheumatic arthritis from developing in the area of the break. Elemi oil also hastens the healing of cuts, sores, and wounds, and encourages the development of new skin cells. It cools inflamed skin and can help clear chronic skin conditions such as eczema, especially weeping eczema, and other types of dermatitis. Fungal infections such as athlete's foot, candida infections of the skin, and fungal infections of the fingernails also respond well to elemi oil.

BEAUTY BENEFITS

Elemi oil has cell-regenerating properties that benefit dry or mature skin. It makes a rejuvenating treatment for wrinkled or sagging skin. By balancing sebum secretions, elemi oil helps to normalize both oily and dry skin. It can also control heavy perspiration.

EMOTIONAL EFFECTS

Elemi oil balances the nerves. It calms nervousness and promotes harmony within oneself and with others. It energizes and revitalizes a mind overwhelmed by mental fatigue or stress. Its sedative effect helps in overcoming stress-related disorders. Elemi oil strengthens, centers, and focuses the mind and emotions. It brings peacefulness and clarity, and acts as an aid to meditation and spiritual development.

PRECAUTIONS

Elemi oil may irritate sensitive skin.

EUCALYPTUS

As eucalyptus trees mature, their young, round, silvery blue-green leaves turn into long, swordlike, deep-green leaves that emit the characteristic camphoraceous odor of eucalyptus. Woody seed pods dangling down from the creamy-colored branches almost completely cover the budding blossoms; hence the tree's name, which comes from the Greek word *eukalypto*, meaning "covered" or "wrapped."

Eucalyptus oil has a refreshing, penetrating, and stimulating aroma that enters into the respiratory tract, bringing a fresh vitality to mind, body, and spirit. Its scent is somewhat medicinal. About 50 pounds of eucalyptus leaves yields 1 pound of clear or pale-yellow eucalyptus oil.

Australia is the original homeland of eucalyptus, the tallest deciduous tree on earth. Some species of eucalyptus stretch skyward nearly 500 feet. More than 75 percent of all the trees in Australia are eucalyptus; in all, there are more than 500 varieties of eucalyptus worldwide. They thrive in the Mediterranean-like climates of Algeria, California, Egypt, Hawaii, India, Portugal, South Africa, and Spain. Eucalyptus trees also are cultivated in India, Latin America, South Africa, southern Europe, and Tahiti.

Eucalyptus globulus is the most common species employed in aromatherapy, although over a dozen others—including *Eucalyptus australian, Eucalyptus baker, Eucalyptus citriodora, Eucalyptus dives, Eucalyptus polybrachtea, Eucalyptus radiata,* and *Eucalyptus smithii*—also yield essential oils. The oil of *Eucalyptus citriodora* has a citruslike aroma; *Eucalyptus dives* yields an oil with a smell reminiscent of peppermint. All of these trees are members of the *Myrtaceae* family.

FOLKLORE AND HERBAL HERITAGE

Many mothers have massaged away their children's cold symptoms with rubs containing medicinal-smelling eucalyptus. Inhaling its fresh, camphorlike aroma opens up sinuses and clears congestion. Eucalyptus's action in fighting colds, coughs, and other respiratory conditions is well known. During the 1940s and 1950s, cold and cough medicines commonly contained eucalyptus for its strong antibacterial, expectorant, and cough-suppressant properties.

Australian aborigines bound eucalyptus leaves around serious wounds to prevent infection and expedite healing. Water stored in the roots of eucalyptus trees provided liquid for native peoples and early European settlers in Australia. The settlers cultivated the trees for their hardwood and for their ability to fight malaria. The trees' massive root systems absorb large amounts of water, so they were able to drain the mosquito-infested marshes that fostered malaria. In addition, insects dislike the strong camphorlike odor that the leaves emit; this may explain the trees' success as insect repellents. Veterinarians have administered eucalyptus to horses with influenza, dogs with distemper, and a variety of animals with parasitic skin afflictions. Koala bears thrive off the eucalyptus tree.

MEDICINAL USES

Eucalyptus oil fights bacterial and viral infections that can cause colds, coughs, the flu, laryngitis, sinusitis, sore throats, and tonsillitis. It loosens and expels mucus and reduces inflammation. Eucalyptus oil eases nasal congestion and hay fever, and can prevent asthma attacks and bronchitis. It increases the blood's oxygen supply so that more oxygen and nutrients can be delivered to cells throughout the body. Eucalyptus oil also stimulates the regeneration of lung tissue. Dispersed through the air in a spray, diffuser, or vaporizer, it can inhibit the spread of infection.

Many popular topical medications rely on eucalyptus oil to relieve the joint pains, muscular aches, and swelling that accompany arthritis, backaches, rheumatism, sprains, strains, and other injuries. Eucalyptus oil can reduce the pain of headaches, including migraines. It kills germs and disinfects skin abscesses and wounds. It fights fevers by cooling down the body.

Used in sitz baths, eucalyptus oil can treat urinary tract infections such as cystitis. It encourages urination and fights bacteria that contribute to infection. It also helps improve immunity. Reports from Europe state that eucalyptus oil, especially when used together with geranium oil and juniper oil, can help to lower or regulate blood sugar levels. Used alone or with bergamot, eucalyptus oil minimizes the pain and hastens the healing of cold sores, herpes outbreaks, chickenpox, and shingles. It speeds the process of recovery from burns and wounds, particularly slow-healing ones, and fights fungal infections such as athlete's foot, facial candida, and fungal infection of the fingernails. Eucalyptus oil repels insects and helps to reduce the sting of insect bites. Many commercial air fresheners and insecticides contain eucalyptus oil.

Beauty Benefits

Eucalyptus oil clears acne and skin blemishes by reducing excessive oiliness. It promotes the regeneration of skin tissue and can also soothe the pain of sunburn.

Emotional Effects

Eucalyptus oil's stimulating and refreshing nature helps overcome sluggishness. If you feel stifled or smothered by a confining situation or overbearing person, use eucalyptus to give you "room to breathe." It overcomes melancholy and increases optimism. During times of emotional overload, it can restore balance, improve concentration, and increase intellectual capacity. Eucalyptus oil can cool the heat of anger. After a fight or conflict, diffusing eucalyptus oil through the room will cleanse the environment. Eucalyptus encourages spirituality and purity of thought and purpose.

Hydrosol Uses

Eucalyptus hydrosol is beneficial for respiratory ailments, including colds, flu, allergies, hay fever, and sinusitis. It also boosts immune function. Dilute it for internal or topical use by a child or a sensitive individual.

Precautions

Eucalyptus oil can irritate sensitive skin.

FENNEL

Umbrellas of delicate yellow flowers rise above the gray-green feathery fronds stemming from the celerylike stalks of the fennel plant. After blooming, the flowers turn into grayish-brown seeds with a licoricelike flavor. At maturity, fennel stands about four feet tall. Fennel oil, steam-distilled from the crushed seeds, smells similar to anise. It has a sweet and zesty, sharp and spicy, fresh and warm aroma.

Indigenous to the Mediterranean area, fennel flourishes in environments near the sea. Sweet fennel, or *Foeniculum vulgare dulce,* is a member of the *Apiaceae* family and is now cultivated in China, France, Germany, India, Iran, and Russia.

FOLKLORE AND HERBAL HERITAGE

The ancient Chinese cured snake bites with fennel. The ancient Egyptians and Romans ate it after meals to tone their digestive tracts and release toxins from their bodies. Garlands of fennel were customarily awarded as praise to victorious warriors because fennel was believed to bestow strength, courage, and longevity.

The word *fennel* derives from the Latin *fenuculum,* which means "hay." The plant probably got its name from fennel's frequent use as fodder. The ancient Greeks called it *marathon,* meaning "to grow thin." Wealthier Greeks supposedly ate fennel as a slimming aid because of the feeling of fullness it gave. For the same reason, poor people chewed fennel seeds to hush growling stomachs; Roman soldiers chewed the seeds to stave off hunger during long marches when meals were sporadic. Devout Christians often ate fennel seeds when fasting.

Women have taken fennel for thousands of years because of its toning effect on the female reproductive system. Physicians and herbalists have treated earaches, eye problems, insect bites, kidney complaints, and lung infections with fennel. It has also been used to expel worms. Medieval Europeans often hung bunches of fennel over doorways or stuffed it into keyholes to ward off evil spirits and block spells cast by witches.

MEDICINAL USES

Fennel oil helps rid the body of accumulated toxins, particularly after overindulgence in foods, spirits, or drugs. Its detoxifying properties are helpful for controlling cellulite and for dieting. Fennel also suppresses the appetite. European doctors have successfully treated gout with fennel oil. They also use it to prevent and cure arthritis and rheumatism because it prevents the buildup of toxins in the body, especially in the joints.

Fennel oil fights infection in the urinary tract. Its diuretic action prevents the retention of urine and aids in eliminating bladder infections by flushing toxins from the body. Eating fennel seeds reputedly prevents the development of kidney stones. Fennel oil also soothes a variety of digestive difficulties. It tones the stomach, improves digestion, prevents heartburn, and eases stress-related indigestion. It relieves colic, gas, hiccups, nausea, and vomiting. By toning the smooth muscles of the intestines, fennel oil strengthens peristalsis and counteracts constipation.

Fennel contains a substance that is similar to estrogen and helps to regulate menstrual cycles, minimize symptoms of premenstrual syndrome (PMS), and reduce fluid retention. Fennel can increase scant menstrual flow and heighten low libido. It is also helpful for menopausal distress. Estrogen helps maintain good muscle tone, skin elasticity, good circulation, and strong bones, all of which deteriorate with degenerative aging. Perhaps the ancients claimed that fennel promoted longevity because of its similarity in action to estrogen. Athletes use fennel oil in baths or massage oils to tone their muscles. It also restores muscle tone and vitality to people convalescing after illness.

Bronchitis, colds, and coughs all respond well to fennel oil. It also helps fight gum infections. Fennel oil can pull poisons from insect and snake bites. In Europe, it is frequently used for its detoxifying action in the treatment and rehabilitation of alcoholics and drug abusers, and it can counteract alcohol poisoning. Fennel oil has a toning influence on the liver, kidneys, and spleen.

BEAUTY BENEFITS

Fennel oil's muscle-toning effect helps maintain youthful facial muscles. It reputedly wards off wrinkles and minimizes puffiness around the eyes. In addition, it restores moisture to dry and dehydrated skin. Some aromatherapists say that regularly massaging fennel oil into the breasts helps to keep them firm and attractive.

EMOTIONAL EFFECTS

Fennel oil has an overall calming effect on the emotions. It reduces hyperactivity, nervousness, and stress while revitalizing the mind and improving memory. Fennel oil provides a sense of protection, strength, and courage during vulnerable or emotionally low times. It encourages verbal self-expression and reduces fear. By releasing repressed emotions, fennel inspires artistic and intellectual creativity. It frees the mind from overanalysis and allows you to put into practice your ideas and inspirations. It can also increase sexual desire.

HYDROSOL USES

Fennel hydrosol is a digestive aid that is useful for bloating, gas, and constipation. It is also beneficial for cystitis, respiratory ailments, allergies, and congestion.

PRECAUTIONS

Persons with seizure disorders should use fennel oil with caution, because it may trigger epileptic seizures in susceptible individuals. If you have a history of seizures, consult with a health-care professional before using fennel. Pregnant women should avoid using fennel oil because of its capability to induce menstruation.

FRANKINCENSE

The small, shrubby frankincense tree bears abundant foliage and white or pale-pink blossoms. Gatherers gash and peel back the bark, which exudes a milky white juice. When it comes into contact with air, this sap solidifies into tear-shaped lumps that are amber or burnt orange and range from about ¼ inch to 1½ inches in size. Steam distillation of the gum resin of *Boswellia carteri* or *Boswellia thurifera* renders a clear, pale-yellow, or yellowish-green oil. It has a warm and woody, sweet and spicy, rich and resinous aroma, with a light, lemony undertone. Some frankincense oil is extracted with alcohol or a chemical solvent such as hexane. Only steam-distilled or alcohol-extracted frankincense resin should be used for aromatherapy purposes.

A member of the *Burseraceae* family, frankincense is native to areas in the Middle East around the Red Sea, as well as to China, Iran, Lebanon, and Oman. It grows wild throughout northeast Africa, primarily in Ethiopia and Somalia. Most of the distillation takes place in Europe. There is some distillation of frankincense oil in India as well.

FOLKLORE AND HERBAL HERITAGE

Since the beginning of recorded history, frankincense has been associated with spirituality. The sensuous, spicy fragrance of burning frankincense wafted through temples in ancient Egypt. During religious rituals, Egyptians offered it to their gods in hopes of expelling evil spirits.

Since antiquity, frankincense has been incorporated into incense in China, Egypt, and India. Worshippers in these cultures inhaled it to achieve deeper levels of meditation. Today, the tradition of burning frankincense continues in some churches.

Frankincense was a prized possession in ancient times, as valuable as many precious gems and metals. As a result, it exerted an influence on the political activities of many countries, and crises developed when various governments attempted to monopolize the frankincense market. It was the major economic resource of some Arabic countries. The Queen of Sheba, whose country was a main supplier of frankincense in ancient times, reportedly undertook a perilous journey to visit King Solomon in Israel to ensure his business.

Camel caravans voyaged through treacherous terrain and extremes of weather to deliver this beloved botanical from Arabia to other parts of the known world. Both the Egyptians and the Hebrews spent fortunes importing it from the Phoenicians. The Egyptians mixed it with cinnamon to soothe aching muscles and limbs. The Babylonians and the Syrians dedicated abundant amounts of frankincense to their gods. Besides burning frankincense for religious purposes, the Romans relied on it for government ceremonies, as well as for its many medicinal properties. According to the Bible story, it was given as a gift to the baby Jesus, probably because it was so cherished and valuable, and also because of its association with spirituality.

The ancient Chinese used frankincense to treat leprosy and tuberculosis. Both Eastern and Western medical practitioners treated such conditions as digestive disorders, nervous complaints, respiratory problems, rheumatism, skin diseases, syphilis, and urinary tract infections with frankincense. Frankincense was one of the first cosmetic miracle ingredients; it proved so successful when Egyptian embalmers used it to preserve the bodies of dead royalty and rulers that people decided to take advantage of its rejuvenating and restorative properties while alive. They began formulating cosmetics with frankincense to maintain soft and supple skin. One of its most popular applications was in a rejuvenating facial mask. Facial oils, ointments, and perfumes also contained frankincense.

MEDICINAL USES

Medical professionals in Europe and England today prescribe frankincense oil to treat many of the same disorders as the ancients did. It has a soothing and healing effect on mucous membranes, wounds, and inflammations. As an expectorant, it can clear congestion in the lungs. Frankincense oil reduces swollen lymph glands in the neck. It soothes respiratory problem such as colds, coughs, bronchitis, the flu, and laryngitis; it eases shortness of breath and helps avert asthma attacks.

Frankincense oil soothes stomach distress and eases digestive difficulties. It is frequently used in Europe to treat reproductive and urinary tract maladies. Medical practitioners say that it alleviates the discomforts of cystitis, genital infections, and kidney complaints. It may help control incontinence. Inflammation of the breast responds well to applications of frankincense oil. Some doctors use it to tone the uterus and relieve uterine hemorrhaging and heavy menstrual flow. Frankincense oil can also ease labor pains and decrease postnatal depression.

BEAUTY BENEFITS

Although well known to ancient peoples, frankincense oil's beautifying properties were practically forgotten for centuries. Its restorative, regenerating, and rejuvenating actions are especially useful for dry, mature, and/or sensitive skin. It smoothes lines and wrinkles, and soothes and softens raw, chapped skin. Frankincense oil's astringent properties help to balance oily skin. It accelerates the healing of blemishes, inflammations, sores, scars, skin ulcers, and wounds. Frankincense was one of the first botanical essences to be used in fragrances. It has a powerful fixative quality and is still used to add "staying power" to perfumes.

EMOTIONAL EFFECTS

Frankincense oil helps to fortify a mind burdened with mental anxiety, nervous tension, panic, or stress. In cases of mental or physical exhaustion, it revitalizes both body and mind. It soothes the emotions, comforts during transition and change, and heals emotional wounds. Frankincense oil can help sever ties with the past that contribute to depression and hamper personal growth. By slowing respiration, frankincense oil produces a sense of serenity. It eases hyperactivity, impatience, irritability, and restlessness. It helps to focus energy, minimize distractions, and improve concentration. Frankincense allows freedom from attachments to material objects and to outcomes. Self-discipline in spirituality can then translate into purposeful endeavors in the outer world.

HYDROSOL USES

Frankincense hydrosol improves breathing and eliminates mucus and phlegm, making it helpful for respiratory infections. It is also used for urinary tract infections, in oral hygiene, and as a skin toner and spray.

GERANIUM

Of the more than 700 varieties of geranium, only a few—*Pelargonium roseum, Pelargonium graveolens, Pelargonium odorantissimum,* and *Pelargonium radula*—produce essential oils. The entire plant, including leaves, stalks, and flowers, is steam-distilled to produce a pale greenish-yellow oil with a sweet scent that is sometimes rosy, sometimes minty.

Originally native to southern Africa, these members of the *Geraniaceae* family now flourish in many countries. China, Egypt, Morocco, Russia, and the island of Réunion in the southwestern Indian Ocean, specialize in the commercial cultivation of geraniums. Many authorities believe that the world's finest geranium oil comes from Réunion.

FOLKLORE AND HERBAL HERITAGE

For centuries, geraniums have adorned window boxes, walkways, gardens, and homes around the world with splashes of brilliant red, lavender, pink, and white blossoms. Both the showy flowers and serrated-edged leaves of these tender perennial plants can emit delightful fragrances. Dutch sailors transported geraniums to Europe from Africa during the 1600s. Europeans appreciated them for their delightful fragrance and their adaptability to the European climate. Many gardeners planted geraniums to ensure that no evil spirits would enter their homes. Colonial American housewives lined baking pans with rose geranium leaves to impart a delicate rose flavor to their cakes.

Herbalists and doctors treated such maladies as dysentery, hemorrhoids, inflammations, and heavy menstrual flow with geranium. Some folkloric sources claimed geranium as a cure for cancer; others stated that it was a remedy for bone fractures, tumors, and wounds. Nineteenth-century perfumers discovered to their delight that inexpensive rose geranium oil smelled similar to costly rose oil. Few of their customers could detect the difference in the final fragrances.

MEDICINAL USES

European physicians today prescribe geranium oil to treat such ailments as diarrhea, gallstones, kidney stones, and urinary tract infections. It relieves respiratory problems, particularly sore throats and tonsillitis. Geranium oil can balance hormones; it stimulates the adrenal cortex, which regulates the balance of hormones secreted by other organs. Some European physicians recommend it for treating diabetes. Geranium oil improves immune function and is helpful for relieving some of the symptoms of chronic fatigue syndrome and candidiasis.

Geranium oil provides many European women with relief from female problems such as painful periods, premenstrual syndrome (PMS), and menopausal difficulties. It normalizes fluctuating hormones during menopause. In addition, geranium oil is a diuretic and diminishes fluid retention, a common source of discomfort associated with PMS. It can ease inflammation of the breast and reduce breast engorgement. Geranium oil stimulates both the lymphatic and circulatory systems, making it useful for boosting circulation and for reducing or eliminating edema. It helps to ease skin disorders such as eczema and other forms of dermatitis, herpes infections, and seborrhea, and accelerates the healing of bruises, burns, cuts, skin ulcers, and other wounds.

BEAUTY BENEFITS

Geranium oil helps almost any skin type or skin condition. Its stimulating action promotes the regeneration of skin cells and speeds the healing of acne and blemishes. It also soothes dry, sensitive skin. Geranium oil imparts a healthy glow to the complexion, making the skin appear radiant and more youthful. It improves the appearance of broken capillaries and varicose veins. Because it stimulates both the lymphatic and circulatory systems, geranium oil helps to combat the kind of sluggish circulation and waste accumulation present with cellulite, and it clears skin that is blemished or dull and dry as a result of the accumulation of toxins. Geranium oil also helps control excessive oiliness of the skin.

EMOTIONAL EFFECTS

Inhaling geranium oil eases the anxiety, tension, and irritability resulting from mentally and physically demanding days. As an antidepressant, geranium has an uplifting effect that frees the mind from negative or depressing thoughts. Almost any stress-related condition responds to a few whiffs of it. As an added bonus, geranium oil can stimulate feelings of sensuality.

Geranium oil encourages self-expression, increases confidence, and helps overcome the fear of speaking, particularly in public. It promotes harmony in male-female relationships by balancing aggressive and passive tendencies and by improving intimate communication. Geranium heightens sensitivity to pleasurable sensations and enjoyable activities. It liberates creativity, revitalizes imagination, and invites spontaneity. Some people respond to geranium oil's sedative, somewhat analgesic effect; others say it stimulates them. For most people, it simultaneously calms and energizes through its balancing actions.

HYDROSOL USES

Geranium hydrosol equalizes the emotions and is beneficial for hot flashes, PMS, skin irritation and inflammation, sunburn, and insect bites. It can be used in skin care for all skin types as a skin mist, facial toner, and/or aftershave lotion.

PRECAUTIONS

Geranium oil can lower your blood sugar level. Use it with caution (or avoid it) if you have hypoglycemia, or low blood sugar.

GINGER

The glossy grasslike spears of this tropical perennial protrude upward two to four feet from thick, spreading tuberous roots called rhizomes. Erect reedlike spikes with compact white, yellow, or yellow-green conical flowers stem directly from the rhizomes, which look like white or beige hands with multiple fingers.

Sharp and spicy, peppery and pungent, warm and wonderful, the aroma of golden-yellow or amber ginger oil has slightly woody and lemony undertones. Ginger oil is steam-distilled from the unpeeled dried ground roots of the plant.

Native to southern Asia, China, India, and Java, *Zingiber officinale* is a member of the *Zingiberaceae* family. Ginger is now cultivated in the tropical regions of Central America, China, India, Jamaica, Japan, Nigeria, and the West Indies. Many experts claim that the finest ginger grows in Jamaica. Most ginger oil comes from China, England, and India.

FOLKLORE AND HERBAL HERITAGE

For thousands of years, ginger has been treasured as a spice and medicinal remedy. More than 4,000 years ago, the enticing aroma of warm gingerbread emanated from Greek ovens. The Greeks treated stomach disorders with ginger and administered it as an antidote to poison. The ancient Egyptians incorporated ginger into their cuisine to ward off epidemics, and it was a staple in Arabian pharmacies. Romans took advantage of its aphrodisiac powers and added it to wine. Indians drank ginger tea to soothe upset stomachs.

Chinese doctors prescribed ginger as a tonic to strengthen the heart, relieve head congestion, and fortify the constitution. They treated any illness associated with cold, damp conditions—such as colds and flu—as well as rheumatism, headaches, and muscle tension with ginger.

Hawaiians scented their clothing with ginger root. They also cooked with ginger and used the fresh root to cure indigestion. They made shampoos and massage oils from the secretions of ginger flowers.

During the Middle Ages, ginger found its way to Europe via the spice route. From there, it crossed the Atlantic Ocean with Spanish explorers headed for South America and the Caribbean.

MEDICINAL USES

Today, European physicians prescribe ginger oil for conditions ranging from digestive disorders to respiratory ailments, jet lag to motion sickness, sore throats to menstrual cramps. Ginger oil increases immunity and often can ward off colds and the flu. It warms chills caused by dampness, and it reduces fevers and cools down the body by inducing sweating. Ginger oil soothes the pain of sore throats and tonsillitis. It also reduces the drainage of a runny nose and eases respiratory infections.

Ginger helps to calm an upset stomach and alleviate nausea, and may reduce dizziness. It can avert the discomfort and queasiness of a hangover, motion sickness, or morning sickness. Ginger promotes better digestion by stimulating the secretion of digestive juices. It also increases appetite, relieves gas and heartburn, diminishes diarrhea, and soothes cramps, whether intestinal or menstrual. The *British Herbal Pharmacopoeia* indicates ginger for gas and colic.

As an analgesic, ginger relieves the pain of arthritis and soothes sprains and muscle spasms, especially in the lower back. It stimulates circulation and is useful for treating varicose veins. Chinese doctors use fresh ginger to treat a wide variety of conditions, including chills, colds, coughs, congestion, diarrhea, dysentery, the flu, malaria, rheumatism, sinusitis, and toothaches. Ginger oil can also speed the healing of bruises, sores, and blemishes.

BEAUTY BENEFITS

Ginger oil is widely used in perfumery to impart a sharp green, spicy note to fragrances, particularly men's colognes. It is rarely used in skin care because of its tendency to irritate sensitive skin, but because it increases circulation, ginger oil is sometimes used to treat varicose veins and cellulite.

EMOTIONAL EFFECTS

Ginger oil's warming tendency can heat up a cold, dull, or fearful emotional nature. It warms the heart and opens up feelings of love, helping to improve communication and increase self-confidence and self-esteem. Ginger oil sharpens the senses, improves memory, and aids in recall. It stimulates vitality and energy, assisting recovery from emotional or mental fatigue or nervous exhaustion. By helping you to overcome self-doubt and procrastination, ginger can increase courage and personal achievement. Ginger improves concentration and focus. Its aphrodisiac qualities may help in cases of impotence, especially when ginger is combined with coriander and rosemary.

PRECAUTIONS

Ginger oil can be irritating to sensitive skin.

HELICHRYSUM

Shiny golden daisylike flowers sit atop the ball-shaped flower heads of the helichrysum plant, which is also known as *immortelle* and *Italian strawflower.* These papery flowers emit an enticing, almost intoxicating fragrance with the essence of honey. The pale-yellow or yellowish-green essential oil they yield has a sweet, warm, and woody scent, with spicy and rosy undertones.

Due to its dry nature, helichrysum produces a limited quantity of oil. Several species of the flowering tops of helichrysum may be codistilled to increase yields of this essential oil.

Indigenous to Africa and Australia, helichrysum will grow almost anywhere, even in poor soil conditions, although it prefers a hot, dry climate with abundant sunlight. *Helichrysum angustifolium, Helichrysum gymnocephalum, Helichrysum orientale, Helichrysum italicum,* and *Helichrysum kilimandjarum* all are members of the *Asteraceae* family, and they prosper in Italy, Spain, the south of France, and other Mediterranean countries, both in the wild and as cultivated crops.

FOLKLORE AND HERBAL HERITAGE

Early herbalists recommended helichrysum for many respiratory conditions, such as asthma, bronchitis, and whooping cough; as a relief for headaches; and as a cure for liver ailments and skin disorders. Helichrysum is more popular, and probably more familiar, to many people today, as an ornamental dried flower. Commonly called *everlasting,* it lives up to its name by retaining its fragrance, color, and shape almost forever.

MEDICINAL USES

European physicians prize helichrysum oil as a treatment for any skin disorder or irritation because of its ability to reduce inflammation, fight bacterial infection, balance energy, and regulate blood flow. Helichrysum is also recommended for abdominal or stomach cramps, irritable bowel syndrome, bronchitis, colds, coughs, gallbladder infections, menstrual cramps, and sinus infections. Helichrysum oil stimulates digestion and improves the function of the liver and the pancreas. It can ease digestive, facial, or pulmonary spasms, as well as other muscle spasms. It also reduces the swelling and inflammation of arthritis, backache, carpal tunnel syndrome, rheumatism, and sciatica. Some people claim that helichrysum can improve hearing and reverse some loss of hearing.

BEAUTY BENEFITS

Helichrysum helps to decrease the inflammation of acne. In addition, helichrysum oil encourages regeneration of the skin and helps it adapt to stress. Mature skin responds especially well to helichrysum oil's restorative properties. It may help reduce scars and skin discolorations.

Helichrysum oil has virtually unlimited value in treating dermatitis and other skin disorders. Its ability to reduce inflammation exceeds that of any other essential oil. It improves the itching, redness, scaliness, and puffiness of psoriasis, as well as that of eczema and other forms of dermatitis. It relieves the discomfort of athlete's foot. Helichrysum also relieves the pain and redness of sunburn. Recent research suggests that helichrysum oil may serve as an effective sunscreen or sunblock when used in a dilution of 3 to 6 percent, or 3 to 6 drops of helichrysum in 100 drops of sesame oil.

EMOTIONAL EFFECTS

Helichrysum oil helps clarify thought processes and opens the mind to new concepts and ideas. During times of transition, it helps to instill self-confidence and provide the illumination necessary to accept change. It restores the emotions and nerves in mental and emotional exhaustion. Helichrysum oil activates the right side of the brain, elevating awareness, awakening intuitive and creative processes, and inspiring personal growth. It also helps improve meditation and visualization. Some people report that helichrysum oil increases their dream activity and helps them to remember their dreams, which sometimes deliver important messages to them.

Turn to helichrysum when the tension from doing too much, trying to control everything, and taking too little time out for yourself cause resentment, frustration, irritability, and moodiness. Anger, bitterness, and a negative attitude brought on by the vulnerability of emotional trauma—in childhood or adulthood—respond to the fresh scent of helichrysum. It allows you to release repressed emotions, even if you

deny them or are unaware of their hold on you. It can gently guide you to a place of understanding and compassion for yourself and other people.

HYDROSOL USES

Helichrysum hydrosol is helpful for inflammation, swelling, bruises, aches and pains, postsurgical recuperation, oral hygiene, gingivitis, receding gums, scars, and ingrown hairs. Appropriate even for sensitive skin, it can be used as a skin spray or toner.

JASMINE

Delicate white star-shaped jasmine flowers fragrance the air with their exotic, erotic, and nearly narcotic aroma. Shiny green leaves cover the large evergreen shrub *Jasminium officinalis* or *Jasminium grandiflorum,* which can reach 20 to 30 feet in height. Jasmine can also grow along the ground or cascade downward in vines. Native to China, India, and Iran, this member of the *Oleaceae* family is chiefly cultivated in China, India, the Mediterranean countries, and northern Africa.

Working at night, gatherers pick these flowers by hand, making the production of jasmine essence very labor-intensive. About 1,000 pounds of flowers—or more than 3.5 million blossoms—yields just 1 pound of precious jasmine essence. While jasmine is commonly considered together with the essential oils, it is more accurate to refer to it as jasmine enfleurage or jasmine absolute because of the way in which it is extracted. For simplicity's sake, however, jasmine enfleurage and jasmine absolute are referred to as jasmine essence in this section.

Jasmine essence is a thick, mahogany-colored oil that has a rich, warm, floral scent with tealike undertones. This intensely sweet "king of essential oils" smells of mystery and magic. Its long-lasting fragrance has a pheromonelike quality, perhaps due to its chemical similarity to human perspiration, which some scientists speculate may contain pheromones.

FOLKLORE AND HERBAL HERITAGE

In India, jasmine was called *queen of the night* and *moonlight of the grove*, and was used both as an aphrodisiac and as an aid to spiritual growth. For millennia, women have adorned their bodies with perfumes and cosmetics made with jasmine. In many religious traditions, the jasmine flower symbolizes hope, happiness, and love. The Chinese treated hepatitis, cirrhosis of the liver, and dysentery with jasmine. They also used it to help overcome nervous system disorders, including depression and nervousness, and to ease coughs and improve breathing. For centuries, the Chinese have enjoyed drinking jasmine tea. Jasmine was a favorite fragrance of the Japanese for both perfumes and incense. The Japanese used jasmine as a remedy for reproductive problems and to stimulate uterine contractions in pregnant women as childbirth approached.

MEDICINAL USES

In Europe, many physicians use jasmine essence to ease labor pains and encourage contractions. It helps to speed the expulsion of the afterbirth and the overall recovery from giving birth. It also helps to relieve postnatal depression. Jasmine essence stimulates the production of milk, tones the uterus, and can induce menstrual flow. It can also soothe and comfort women going through menopause.

Jasmine is helpful for men as well as for women. It strengthens the male reproductive system and can relieve the discomfort of an enlarged prostate gland. As an aphrodisiac, jasmine stimulates desire and helps overcome impotence and frigidity.

Jasmine essence also helps to soothe muscle spasms and sprains. It can calm coughs, ease hoarseness and laryngitis, and act as an expectorant to help the body clear excess mucus. Jasmine essence calms skin inflamed as a result of a skin disorder such as dermatitis or eczema, or as a consequence of stress or an emotional upset.

BEAUTY BENEFITS

The hormone-balancing action of jasmine essence affects the condition of the skin. Jasmine benefits any skin type—whether dry, oily, irritated, or sensitive. It inhibits bacteria and regulates oil production, thereby helping acne and oily skin. Jasmine essence also helps to moisturize dry, dehydrated, or mature skin. Jasmine imparts a soft and seductive floral note to many fine fragrances.

EMOTIONAL EFFECTS

Jasmine essence benefits almost any nervous condition. It decreases anxiety, depression, emotional fatigue, nervous exhaustion, and stress. It elevates spirits and balances moods. Jasmine encourages love, pleasure, optimism, and self-confidence while diminishing fear, shyness, jealousy, and anger. It is both emotionally and physically relaxing. Jasmine essence warms the emotions and helps counteract apathy and indifference. In times of grief, it eases sadness. It spurs creativity, inspires artistic expression, and awakens intuition. By opening the heart, it arouses an appreciation of the beauty in the world and helps dissolve emotional blocks such as disappointment and frustration that hinder personal growth. The sensual and inspirational aroma of jasmine essence creates a sense of euphoria that engenders trust, passion beyond the physical realm, and true love. As a sensual stimulant, jasmine promotes feelings of attractiveness and allure.

PRECAUTIONS

Jasmine can stimulate menstruation; avoid it during pregnancy.

JUNIPER

Of the more than fifty species of juniper, only one—*Juniperus communis*—yields the berries that render juniper oil. This evergreen member of the *Cupressaceae* family bears green needles, yellow flowers, and round bluish-green berries that turn black upon maturity. Juniper may sprawl near the ground as a prickly shrub two to four feet high or stand erect as a bush of six to twelve feet tall. Some wild junipers grow as high as thirty feet.

Fresh ripe, black berries, when steam-distilled, produce a clear or yellowish-green oil that has a pinelike aroma with spicy, peppery, and earthy undertones. Juniper trees, which are native to Europe, have become naturalized throughout the Northern Hemisphere. They flourish in the forests of Canada, Korea, and Sweden, and atop mountains in Hungary and Scotland. Austria, Canada, France, Germany, Italy, Slovakia, and Spain produce the most juniper oil.

FOLKLORE AND HERBAL HERITAGE

Ancient Egyptians anointed their bodies with juniper and used it to embalm the bodies of the dead. They burned juniper incense for physical and spiritual purification. During biblical times, juniper was often used to banish evil spirits. According to one traditional story, Mary hid the baby Jesus under a juniper tree to protect him from King Herod, earning the juniper the reputation of affording protection against harm.

Because black pepper was expensive and difficult to obtain, ancient Romans used juniper berries in place of pepper to flavor their food. They added the crushed berries to wine and drank it to treat liver ailments and for its diuretic action. The ancient Greeks burned juniper berries to discourage epidemics.

Juniper has been used in many parts of the world to fight the spread of plagues, epidemics, and contagious diseases. As late as 1870, French hospitals burned juniper wood for this purpose during a smallpox epidemic. During the Middle Ages, people found multiple uses for juniper: as a cure for headaches as well as kidney and bladder problems; as a treatment for pulmonary infections; and as a fever reducer. Bundles of juniper berries were hung over doors to ward off witches, while burning juniper wood supposedly deterred demons. Many medieval Europeans considered juniper a panacea. The Dutch were probably the first to flavor gin with juniper berries. Native Americans ate juniper berries alone or added them to their food. They drank tea made from the stems and leaves of the plant to relieve arthritis and urinary tract infections. They also applied juniper topically to cleanse infections and heal wounds, and they burned the needles and branches for purification.

MEDICINAL USES

For centuries, juniper's primary medicinal application has been for urinary tract problems, particularly cystitis and prostate problems. Juniper oil encourages urination, fights infection, and helps the body to eliminate wastes, especially after indulgence in rich foods and/or alcohol. It is useful for menstrual difficulties; it eases painful menstrual cramps, promotes menstruation for women with scant or late periods, helps to regulate the menstrual cycle, and reduces fluid retention. Juniper oil is also useful in treating leukorrhea, or yeast infection, and vaginitis. In sitz baths, it can ease the pain of hemorrhoids.

Juniper can minimize the pain of muscle spasms and the aches of arthritis, backaches, and rheumatism. It speeds the healing of bruises, skin ulcers, and wounds. Respiratory problems such as bronchitis, colds, and coughs respond to inhalations of juniper oil. Juniper oil tones the digestive tract, stimulates or regulates appetite, and combats sluggish elimination, especially when one is recovering from illness. By encouraging the elimination of wastes and stimulating circulation, juniper oil helps to improve such conditions as arthritis, bloating and fluid retention, and sluggish lymph glands. It accelerates healing, particularly of slow-healing wounds, and is helpful for psoriasis and dermatitis.

BEAUTY BENEFITS

Juniper oil is good for any kind of skin inflammation. Because juniper oil promotes the elimination of cellular wastes and stimulates circulation, varicose veins and cellulite conditions often respond to it. Juniper oil enlivens dull skin and helps to clear acne. It can regulate oiliness, making it useful in treating acne, oily skin, oily hair, and seborrhea. Juniper is frequently added to fragrances, cosmetics, aftershaves, and men's colognes.

EMOTIONAL EFFECTS

Juniper oil helps to fight anxiety, mental fatigue, nervous tension, and stress. It can clear mental clutter and confusion, revive exhausted emotions, and strengthen nerves. Juniper oil helps to neutralize negative emotions, particularly anger, aggression, or confusion, and imparts a feeling of emotional cleanliness and spiritual purity. It strengthens resolve while freeing the mind from thoughts and worries of the past and present that prevent success and purposeful action. Juniper provides stamina and support to overcome obstacles.

HYDROSOL USES

As a diuretic, juniper hydrosol helps to relieve bloating and aids in weight loss. It is also good for circulatory problems, arthritis, and rheumatism. It promotes detoxification. In skin care, juniper hydrosol reduces cellulite, puffiness, acne, and oily skin, and it can be used as a hair tonic for seborrhea that affects the scalp. It also provides emotional protection.

PRECAUTIONS

Juniper should be avoided during pregnancy because it can stimulate menstrual flow. Also, juniper activates the kidneys, so people with kidney problems should consult with a health-care professional before using it.

LAUREL

Creamy yellow flower clusters grow on both male and female laurel trees. This hardy evergreen tree produces large, glossy, dark oval leaves—bay leaves—the same popular spice that flavors foods all around the world. Female trees produce small oval berries that turn blue-black when ripe.

Native to Asia and introduced to the Mediterranean in antiquity, *Laurus nobilis,* a member of the *Lauraceae* family, grows wild in Italy, Greece, and southern France. In warm subtropical climates, it attains a height of sixty feet, but it flourishes as a shrub in gardens and potted plant in homes around the world. Commercial crops come from countries such as Algeria, Belgium, the Canary Islands, France, Greece, Guatemala, Portugal, Spain, Turkey, and the United States, where it is grown in southern California.

In the early hours of morning during late summer or autumn, workers hand-harvest the leaves that are dried for the spice and steam-distilled for this essential oil. The shiny leaves yield a clear oil with a fresh and spicy scent similar to a blend of cinnamon, clove, allspice, and pepper. Its penetrating aroma has a subtle hint of menthol mixed with a floral sweetness. Many names identify laurel, including bay, bay tree, bay laurel, sweet bay, true laurel, Roman laurel, noble laurel, and daphne. Common laurel, however, is a different plant.

FOLKLORE AND HERBAL HERITAGE

Laurus derives from the Latin, meaning "to praise" while *nobilis* means "renowned" or "famous." Ancient Greeks and Romans venerated laurel in mythology and their daily lives. They believed that it possessed powers to protect against evil, to safeguard social status, and to bestow the gifts of culture, music, and poetry. To Romans, laurel was a symbol of wisdom and glory; to Greeks, it signified military victory. The Greeks thought that laurel had powers to divine or prophesy the future.

In Greek mythology, Apollo—the god of light, poetry, prophecy, and healing—claimed the laurel tree for himself. After he encountered Daphne, goddess of the mountains, in the forest, she transformed herself into a laurel tree rather than surrender to his seduction. Later, Apollo dedicated the plant to his son, Aesculapius, the Greek god of medicine. Before revealing the oracles of Apollo, priestesses at Delphi ate bay leaves. So revered was laurel that the entire roof at the Delphi temple was fashioned from its leaves to provide protection against evil and disease.

Both Greeks and Romans adorned the heads and homes of praiseworthy people with garlands and wreaths woven from laurel leaves to symbolize victory, glory, and heroism. They honored philosophers, poets, and orators with laurel crowns encircling their foreheads, a sign of consecration to the gods. Caesar wore a garland of laurel to celebrate triumph in battles and conquests.

In biblical times, people believed that laurel would bring health and happiness. Architects incorporated the design of laurel garlands into moldings of buildings. Arabs rendered an oil from both leaves and berries to incorporate into fragrances and soaps. Bay fat, made from the berries, is still a component of some soaps. The medicinal virtues of laurel were many. It protected against contagious diseases. In his *Natural History*, the ancient Roman scientist and scholar Pliny the Elder recommended it as an insect repellent and in massages to ease the pains of rheumatism. Dioscorides, a Greek physician, attributed to laurel the ability to stop vomiting and to soothe the stomach. He said that the roots could dissolve kidney stones. For centuries, people have used bay to prevent plague and fight diseases. The Greek doctor and anatomist Galen, who was known as "the Great Physician," suggested it for stimulating vital functions and correcting liver disorders.

During the Middle Ages, homeowners customarily planted laurel trees near their front doors for protection against evil, witchcraft, disease, and lightning. Dying or dead laurel trees foretold death and disaster. Writing in the early twelfth century, St. Hildegard of Bingen praised laurel as a universal remedy for many ailments: angina, asthma, fever, gout, heart palpitations, migraines, and spleen and liver conditions. In Tudor times, bay laurel trees provided pleasure and profit for both ornamental and practical uses by the sick and the well, the living and the dead. Elizabethan housekeepers strewed bay laurel leaves upon floors both for their fragrance and for their antiseptic properties. People averted attacks of weevils and other insects by placing leaves among dried fruits, flour, and beans. From *laurel* derives the title *laureate,* which means "crowned with laurels." During the French Renaissance, gifted scholars were crowned with wreaths of laurel. To this day, *baccalaureate* is the term for the bachelor's degree, earned upon completion of college.

European restaurants and hotels often adorn entryways with laurel trees shaped into globes, cones, and topiary shapes. Chefs and cooks around the world add bay leaves to flavor many dishes—sauces, soups, stews, marinades, meats, poultry, pâté— and as a pickling spice. Homemakers add the dried leaves to potpourri and sachets to impart a spicy scent.

MEDICINAL USES

Like other culinary herbs, laurel aids digestion. It stimulates appetite and improves sluggish or poor digestion. It relieves bloating, gas, and colic. The essential oil enjoys a reputation as an antibacterial and antifungal agent that can help control athlete's foot and candida. It depresses heart rate, lowers blood pressure, stimulates the liver, and works as a diuretic. Laurel helps to regulate energy while promoting proper circulation. Its anti-inflammatory action reduces swelling, making it a remedy for arthritis, bursitis, carpal tunnel syndrome, rheumatism, and sciatica, as well as for sprains, sore muscles, and edema. Massage oil that contains laurel oil can relieve the muscular dis-

comfort of chronic neck, shoulder, and lower back pain. Laurel stimulates a sluggish lymphatic system. It can produce sweating that assists the body in releasing wastes from illness or a general toxic state.

Laurel has preventive and restorative properties useful for maintaining and regaining health. For respiratory ailments, its antiseptic and antiviral actions reduce phlegm, relieve congestion, and ease symptoms of asthma, bronchitis, colds, the flu, and sore throat. It may also help with symptoms of chronic fatigue syndrome. It is useful as an ingredient in insect repellents, as well as for relieving the itching and stinging of insect bites. Some people report that it helps heal scabies.

BEAUTY BENEFITS

Laurel stimulates circulation and therefore may help reduce hair loss with regular use. Some dandruff treatments contain laurel. Fragrances include laurel oil to impart a spicy masculine note.

EMOTIONAL EFFECTS

Laurel has stimulating qualities that help to release repressed emotions or blocked energy, while helping to warm the spirit and enliven the personality. It can help overcome sadness and emotional exhaustion. It invigorates the mind, improves memory, and heightens concentration. It replaces self-imposed limitations with greater self-confidence and can diminish nervousness. Laurel inspires lost confidence by restoring your belief in your capabilities and enhancing self-esteem. It awakens your creative spirit, inspires originality, and sparks an inner vision that gently guides you toward higher spirituality.

HYDROSOL USES

Laurel hydrosol is a lymphant stimulant. An antiseptic, antibacterial, and antiviral, it is useful against infections and in oral hygiene. It is an intestinal tonic that helps relieve digestive disorders and constipation, and it can be used in cooking. Laurel hydrosol is unstable—it is susceptible to going rancid more quickly than other hydrosols. Never use a hydrosol if it does not look or smell fresh.

PRECAUTIONS

Use laurel oil in low concentrations to avoid skin irritation. Avoid it during pregnancy.

LAVENDER

Beautiful blue-violet or deep-purple blossoms resembling tiny purple pine cones grow in whorls around a single lavender stalk. The abundant branches have long, narrow pale silvery-green leaves. This woody evergreen shrub grows three or four feet tall.

Lavender smells clean and fresh and permeates the air with a delightful aroma that simultaneously stimulates and relaxes. Steam-distilling the flower tops and stalks produces a colorless, pale-yellow, or yellow-green oil. It has a sweet, floral, and herbaceous scent with a balsamic, woody undertone. An acre of lavender plants will yield about 15 to 20 pounds of essential oil. Distilling only the blossoms produces a superior oil. Of the more than thirty different species of lavender, *Lavandula officinalis, Lavandula angustifolia,* and *Lavandula vera* are the most popular varieties for producing essential oils. French lavender *(Lavandula stoechas)* is also used in aromatherapy.

A member of the *Lamiaceae* family, lavender thrives high atop the dry, rocky, sun-drenched mountain slopes in its native France, Persia (now Iran), Mediterranean countries, and Tasmania. It is now also cultivated commercially in Bulgaria, England, Greece, Italy, Russia, Spain, and Turkey. France is the primary producer of lavender oil.

FOLKLORE AND HERBAL HERITAGE

The ancient Greeks and Romans prized lavender for its perfume and for its cleansing properties. They lavished it upon their bodies in scented soaps and baths. The Romans are credited with naming it, although there are two different theories of the name's derivation. One theory holds that lavender comes from the Latin word *lavare,* meaning "to wash," while according to the other, it derives from the Latin word *lividula,* which means "bluish in color." Ancient Romans added lavender to their baths to relieve fatigue and stiff joints. Despite their enjoyment of lavender, however, the plant symbolized mistrust to them, probably because they believed the deadly asp inhabited lavender bushes.

Medieval Europeans considered lavender an herb of love. Many claimed that it had aphrodisiac properties; others touted its ability to keep the wearer chaste. England's Queen Elizabeth I supposedly ate lavender conserves most mornings. Lavender flowers freshened sickrooms and were added to potpourris for their fragrance. They were commonly strewn on floors so that, when stepped upon, the flowers would release their essence into the air. This tradition continues today in Portugal and Spain.

For centuries, lavender was a remedy for ailments as diverse as insect bites, lice, muscular aches and pains, nervous disorders, scabies, sprains, and toothaches. Herbalists frequently prescribed it to fight fatigue, relieve respiratory ailments, and soothe stomachaches. Women relied on lavender to keep their skin clean, clear, soft, and supple.

Early twentieth-century medications for colic, coughs, headaches, hoarseness, nervous palpitations, sore joints, and toothaches contained lavender oil. Chinese white flower oil included lavender oil. It was also an ingredient in smelling salts. In homes throughout Europe, delicate lavender sachets lined linen closets, scented lingerie drawers, and protected clothing from moths and insects. During World Wars I and II, soldiers and medics carried lavender oil with them onto the battlefields for disinfecting wounds.

MEDICINAL USES

European health professionals prescribe lavender oil for an array of ailments—digestive disorders, earaches, respiratory illnesses, skin disorders, and sore throats. Lavender oil clears the congestion and stuffiness of sinusitis and other respiratory ailments; it soothes sore throats, laryngitis, and tonsillitis. Lavender oil eases the pain and discomfort of muscular aches, spasms, and injuries, and helps to heal bruises, cuts, and insect bites. It relieves the pain of migraines and tension headaches. It is also useful in reducing some of the symptoms of chronic fatigue syndrome, and helps to boost immunity.

Lavender oil soothes the inflammation of skin disorders, including psoriasis, eczema, and other types of dermatitis. It cools burns and provides relief for facial candida, cold sores, and herpes. It may diminish the pain of hemorrhoids, and can relieve the itching and inflammation of jock itch. Lavender oil can treat many common childhood maladies. Its mildness makes it safe for infants and children.

BEAUTY BENEFITS

Lavender oil calms and soothes the skin. It balances oil production, helps heal blemishes, and stimulates circulation to the skin. Lavender oil reduces the inflammation of acne and soothes the pain of sunburn. It regulates the oil secretions of the scalp and helps repair damaged or overprocessed hair.

EMOTIONAL EFFECTS

Throughout Europe, physicians and psychologists recommend lavender oil for emotional difficulties such as depression, fear, hysteria, insomnia, irritability, melancholy, mood swings, nervousness, and stress. They say that it strengthens the nervous system. Lavender oil clears thinking, dissipates fears, releases repressed emotions, minimizes anger, and reduces worry. By balancing extremes of emotion, it contributes to emotional equilibrium. Lavender can avert anxiety or panic attacks. When being overwhelmed or frustrated leads to irritability, breathe in the soothing scent of lavender. It relaxes the mind and promotes physical and mental well-being. It nurtures creativity and self-expression. Lavender oil can neutralize sensory overload and balance either a racing or sluggish mind. It helps reduce hyperactivity, especially in children. Used at bedtime, it helps overcome insomnia.

HYDROSOL USES

Lavender hydrosol can be used as a gargle for sore throat and in treatments for insect bites, ingrown hairs, menstrual cramps, premenstrual syndrome (PMS), and sunburn. It acts as a mood stabilizer and can be used in skin care as a facial spray and toner. It is gentle enough for use in baby and child care.

LEMON

The small, evergreen lemon tree has serrated-edged oval leaves, stiff thorny branches, and fragrant white or pale-pink flowers. The round or oval green fruits of *Citrus limon* or *Citrus limonum* turn sunshine-yellow when ripe. A native of India and Asia, this member of the *Rutaceae* family grows to about 18 feet tall. Lemon trees grow wild in Mediterranean climates and are cultivated in Guinea, Israel, Italy, and North and South America. Cold expression of the fresh peels of the fruit renders a pale greenish-yellow oil. Its scent is fresh and light, slightly sharp but sweet, with the tart and tangy smell of fresh lemons. About 1,000 lemons will yield one pound of oil.

FOLKLORE AND HERBAL HERITAGE

The ancient Egyptians used lemons to fight food poisoning and typhoid epidemics. Romans revered the goddess of youth, Juventas, and symbolized her with the lemon, which enjoyed a reputation as a cure-all and a health tonic and preserver. Inhabitants of Spain and some other European countries regarded lemon as a panacea for infectious illnesses. Europeans used it to resist malaria and typhoid fever. Lemons and limes were carried on English ships to control scurvy on long voyages. Credit goes to Christopher Columbus for carrying lemon seeds to the New World.

Historically, herbalists have used lemons to lower blood pressure and suggested fresh lemon juice for internal cleansing, for clearing excess toxins from the liver, and for providing relief from arthritis and muscular aches and pains.

MEDICINAL USES

French physicians treat disorders such as diabetes, gonorrhea, high blood pressure, malaria, syphilis, tuberculosis, and typhoid with lemon oil. It fights the infection of bronchitis, coughs, and sore throats and relieves the discomfort of colds, fevers, and the flu. It can also avert asthma attacks. Because lemon oil can kill bacteria and other germs in minutes, many European hospitals use it to sanitize hospital rooms and kill airborne germs.

Lemon oil enhances immunity by stimulating white blood cell production and improving the body's ability to combat infection. It helps in treating disorders that may be related to a weakened immune system, such as chronic fatigue syndrome and sluggish lymph system. As a digestive aid, lemon oil counteracts acidity in the body, calms an upset stomach, and helps heartburn. It encourages the elimination of wastes, reduces constipation, and eases arthritis. It tones the heart, kidneys, liver, and pancreas. Lemon oil helps lower blood pressure and stimulates circulation.

Lemon oil can stop the bleeding of cuts and wounds. It helps with shaving nicks, nosebleeds, and bleeding gums from gingivitis or tooth extractions. Lemon oil also diminishes the pain of cold sores, herpes, and mouth ulcers. It relieves some of the symptoms of eczema and other types of dermatitis and can help relieve headaches.

BEAUTY BENEFITS

Lemon oil balances overactive sebaceous glands that lead to oily or blemished skin, helps clear acne, and controls oily hair and dandruff. It revitalizes sluggish or mature skin and helps reduce cellulite by improving circulation and encouraging the elimination of wastes. Lemon oil encourages the exfoliation of dead skin and enlivens the complexion. Long-term treatment with lemon oil reduces broken capillaries and varicose veins, softens scar tissue, and minimizes warts and corns. Lemon oil can also strengthen brittle nails.

EMOTIONAL EFFECTS

Lemon oil is cooling, refreshing, and uplifting. It encourages clarity, concentration, and recall. It can calm anxiety, hysteria, or shock and prevent emotional outbursts. It subdues aggressive behavior. It fights depression, eases fear, strengthens resolve, and assists in communication and decision making. Lemon inspires trust and a sense of security; it relieves confusion and worry. It can help you overcome obstacles and provide a clearer perspective. Lemon helps to open up the heart, especially if there is a fear of intimacy, a fear of commitment, or a fear of being consumed by the relationship. It purifies and promotes spirituality.

PRECAUTIONS

Lemon oil may be irritating to sensitive skin. It may also promote photosensitivity, leading to sunburn or uneven darkening of the skin.

MARJORAM

Marjoram is a bushy tender perennial that grows up to 1 foot in height. Its many branches have square stems and tiny oval gray-green leaves that may be fuzzy. Knot-like buds borne on spikes open to form clusters of white or pink flowers. When in full bloom, marjoram branches are steam-distilled to produce an oil with a warm, woody, spicy, slightly peppery, camphor-like, and nutty aroma that is calming and comforting.

Thymus mastichina is commonly called Spanish marjoram or Spanish wood marjoram. As the name implies, it grows primarily in Spain. Its oil is pale orange to amber in color and has a distinctive eucalyptuslike aroma. Sweet marjoram *(Origanum majorana* or *Majorana hortensis)* is native to the Mediterranean, North Africa, and southwest Asia. It produces a bright-yellow oil that often darkens with age.

Marjoram, a member of the *Lamiaceae* family, grows in gardens around the world and is a favorite in English country gardens. Most of the marjoram oil used for aromatherapy is produced in Bulgaria, Egypt, France, Germany, Hungary, Morocco, and Tunisia.

FOLKLORE AND HERBAL HERITAGE
Aphrodite, the Greek goddess of love, allegedly endowed marjoram with a spicy and sweet scent to symbolize happiness. The ancient Romans called marjoram the "herb of happiness." Greek and Roman newlyweds wore garlands of marjoram upon their heads to bless them with marital bliss. Wreaths and garlands of marjoram served as decorations at weddings and at funerals, where they were used to bestow peace upon the deceased. Marjoram warmed both the body and the emotions. Greek physicians treated rheumatism, muscle spasms, and fluid retention with marjoram. They also used it to regulate breathing and as an antidote for poisoning.

Many cultures believed that marjoram could increase longevity. Growing it on a gravesite was meant to comfort the departed one buried there. People used water scented with marjoram for washing and personal hygiene. In the Elizabethan era, the English would brew a blend of marjoram, rosemary, and sage with wine to treat blackened teeth. Women fashioned marjoram into nosegays to mask unsavory smells. Those curious about their futures anointed themselves with marjoram at bedtime so that they might dream of their future mates.

MEDICINAL USES
Physicians in Europe today use marjoram oil to treat high blood pressure and heart conditions. Marjoram oil dilates blood vessels, reducing the strain on the heart and creating warmth beneath the skin. It eases the pain of arthritis, muscular aches and

tension, and muscle spasms. Its warming action increases flexibility and range of motion, and it can prevent or reduce the pain of sports injuries. By improving circulation, marjoram oil encourages the removal of wastes from the muscles following physical exertion. It also relaxes overworked muscles and soothes sprains and strains. Marjoram can provide relief for backaches, carpal tunnel syndrome, sciatica, and temporomandibular joint (TMJ) syndrome.

Marjoram oil can counteract the symptoms of premenstrual syndrome (PMS), ease menstrual cramps, and stimulate menstrual flow. It stimulates appetite, improves digestion, reduces intestinal cramps from colic, and soothes an upset stomach or heartburn. By strengthening peristalsis, it reduces gas and relieves constipation. Marjoram oil eases asthma, bronchitis, colds, and sinusitis. It calms coughs and soothes sore throats. Its calming and sedative actions help to alleviate migraines, tension headaches, and insomnia. Marjoram oil also reduces some of the symptoms of chronic fatigue syndrome and candidiasis.

BEAUTY BENEFITS

Marjoram facilitates the drainage of blood from bruised areas, helping to minimize bruising and speed healing time. It also helps release tension from facial muscles, especially those associated with TMJ syndrome.

EMOTIONAL EFFECTS

Marjoram oil relaxes the body and mind and helps relieve insomnia. It calms emotions and minimizes emotional upsets, making it useful for relieving anxiety, aggression, anger, emotional exhaustion, hyperactivity, nervousness, and stress. Because of its balancing and regulating actions, it can ease obsessive behavior and negative thoughts. Marjoram oil provides comfort during times of grief, loneliness, and sadness. By helping to nurture and comfort yourself and others and to encourage affection, it eases loneliness and diminishes feelings of neediness. It strengthens willpower and confidence. Marjoram oil gives you greater control over sexual desire, but regular use can permanently numb erotic sensations, diminish sex drive, and decrease sexual function.

PRECAUTIONS

Marjoram oil can cause drowsiness, so you should avoid driving or operating machinery when using it. It should also be avoided during pregnancy because it stimulates menstruation. Long-term use may permanently inhibit sex drive.

MELISSA

From melissa wafts the delicate and delightful scent of fresh lemons. Clusters of white, pink, or yellow blossoms burst forth from bright-green foliage. Its crinkled leaves are oval- or heart-shaped with scalloped edges.

Among the many common names for

Melissa officinalis, a member of the *Lamiaceae* family, are balm, lemon balm, balm mint, and honey balm. This tender perennial grows upright to a height of three feet. Native to Europe, Mediterranean countries, and the Near East, melissa now grows easily in gardens, in fields, and along roadsides worldwide.

Steam distillation produces a golden-yellow essential oil that smells distinctly of lemons. Because the plants yield small amounts of essential oil, melissa oil is costly. Much of the essential oil sold as melissa oil is either entirely synthetic or adulterated with lemongrass, a less expensive oil that smells similar to melissa but lacks many of its therapeutic properties.

FOLKLORE AND HERBAL HERITAGE

Early beekeepers smeared melissa leaves on beehives because their fresh lemon fragrance lured bees back to the hives. Attracting bees was its main attribute until Arabs discovered its power to relieve anxiety and depression. They used it as a sedative and nerve tonic. Since then melissa has alleviated such ailments as asthma, bronchitis, colic, cramps, digestive disorders, dizziness, hyperactivity, insomnia, migraines, mumps, and nausea.

Avicenna, the eleventh-century Persian physician, praised melissa for relieving melancholy and making the heart and mind merry. In fourteenth-century France, King Charles V drank daily doses of melissa tea to preserve his health. Paracelsus, the noted sixteenth-century German scientist, recommended it for revitalizing the entire body. Carmelite water, a seventeenth-century tonic used to treat nervous headaches, contained primarily melissa. This formula continues to be popular in Germany today. Colonists in America lifted their spirits with melissa. Thomas Jefferson grew melissa at Monticello, his home in Charlottesville, Virginia. In 1988, Europeans honored melissa as the medicinal plant of year.

MEDICINAL USES

Melissa oil is calming and relaxing. As a tonic for the entire nervous system, it soothes such conditions as nervousness, nervous tension, nervous indigestion, and nervous asthma. Melissa makes a mild tranquilizer without dangerous and addictive side effects. As a sedative, it can help overcome insomnia without the harsh, hangover effect of synthetic sleeping pills. It is potent, yet mild enough for children, especially those with hyperactive tendencies.

Melissa soothes symptoms of colds, flu, and fevers, and can induce sweating necessary to release toxins. It relieves congestion, calms coughing, and eases attacks of asthma and bronchitis. Its ability to fight viral infections helps reduce the impact of mumps, herpes simplex, and other viruses. It also fights bacteria.

Melissa eases many symptoms associated with premenstrual syndrome (PMS), menstrual difficulties, and menopause; its cooling action can dissipate hot flashes. Its analgesic and antispasmodic actions alleviate the pain of menstrual cramps. It relieves headaches, including migraines. It soothes stress and releases tension. Melissa reduces vomiting and nausea and may relieve morning sickness.

Melissa can stimulate the appetite, soothe the digestive tract, and provide relief for colic, indigestion, gas, and stomachaches. It lowers blood pressure. Melissa can help restore equilibrium in cases of dizziness, shock, and vertigo. Studies indicate that melissa may help hyperthyroid conditions by inhibiting the production of a thyroid-stimulating hormone.

BEAUTY BENEFITS

Melissa soothes and calms the skin, while reducing the stress associated with many skin problems. In treatment of skin allergies or disorders such as eczema, psoriasis, and dermatitis, melissa can calm inflammation that contributes to redness, swelling, and itchiness. Melissa has antiviral action that offers relief of cold sores and other manifestations of herpes simplex virus infection. It shortens the duration of outbreaks, increases the length of intervals between outbreaks, and may discourage recurrences. It speeds healing of wounds. Its antihistaminic activity helps in relieving the sting and itch of insect bites. Melissa makes a lovely and therapeutic addition to perfumes and cosmetics.

EMOTIONAL EFFECTS

Melissa is a tonic for the entire nervous system. It provides a safe alternative to harmful or habit-forming drugs used to treat such problems as anxiety, depression, mood swings, nervousness, and panic. Melissa gently calms emotional upset while revitalizing your capacity to cope under pressure or during confrontations. It replaces confusion and disorientation with understanding and clarity. It engenders trust and courage. Melissa oil's soothing and sedative activity helps overcome agitation, hyperactivity, insomnia, and restlessness. It eases grief and soothes sadness. In cases of emotional oversensitivity or overexcitation, melissa brings back a sense of balance.

HYDROSOL USES

Melissa hydrosol is useful for calming emotional upsets, stress, and hyperactivity. It helps to ease morning sickness and can be used in baby care. In skin care, it can be used as a facial mist. It relieves the irritation caused by eczema, psoriasis, and poison ivy or poison oak. It fights viral infections such as cold sores and herpes. Melissa hydrosol also can be used in beverages and foods.

PRECAUTIONS

Because melissa can irritate skin, use in weak dilutions of 1 percent or less. In large doses, it can contribute to headache. Because melissa oil is very expensive, be aware that it is often adulterated with lemongrass or synthetic fragrances.

MINT

See PEPPERMINT.

MYRRH

Myrrh has a sweet, smoky, slightly musky, slightly spicy aroma with a warm, rich, timeless quality. To some people, the incenselike odor smells medicinal; others consider it soulful. Its taste may explain the origin of its name, which comes from an Arabic word meaning "bitter."

Myrrh oil comes from a thorny, sparse, and scraggly shrub or tree, known as either *Commiphora myrrha* or *Balsamodendron myrrha*. There are several different varieties, growing to heights of about nine to fifteen feet in dry climates. The trees' sturdy branches are knotted with aromatic leaves and small white flowers.

Also called true myrrh or herrabol myrrh, this member of the *Burseraceae* family is native to Arabia, northern Africa, southwestern Asia, and the region around the Red Sea, especially Ethiopia, Somalia, and Yemen. Historians believe that myrrh grew in the Tigris and Euphrates valleys, now thought to be the site of the biblical Garden of Eden. Today, most myrrh is obtained from the Middle East, particularly Iran. Making incisions into the gray bark of the trunks allows the sap to flow forth from the myrrh trees. This pale yellowish-white fluid hardens into reddish-brown tears.

Steam-distilling the resin renders a pale-yellow or amber oil. Myrrh oil may also be extracted from the tears of resin by means of alcohol or a chemical solvent such as hexane. Only steam-distilled or alcohol-extracted myrrh oil is suitable for aromatherapy.

FOLKLORE AND HERBAL HERITAGE

From antiquity, ancient cultures made myrrh an integral part of religious rituals, medical practice, beauty treatments, and perfumery. Writings from more than 2,700 years ago mention myrrh and its uses in embalming, perfumery, and incense. Originally, myrrh was collected from the beards of goats that grazed on the tasty leaves of myrrh bushes. Ancients used myrrh to cure cancer, leprosy, and syphilis. More than 2,000 years before the Biblical story told of the Magi presenting myrrh, frankincense, and gold to the baby Jesus, myrrh was already a precious commodity along the spice route. Demand far exceeded supply, making myrrh one of the most expensive items in the world.

References in the Bible, the Vedas, ancient Egyptian papyri, and the Koran link myrrh to religious rituals. The Egyptians burned myrrh incense in their temples. They burned Kyphi, an incenselike substance that contained myrrh, every day at noon in sun-worshipping rituals; during evening ceremonies, they offered myrrh as a consecration to the moon. The Egyptians believed that, in addition to appeasing the gods, Kyphi incense quelled fear and anxiety, improved meditation, and induced restful sleep with pleasant dreams.

The Egyptians employed myrrh in mummification because it kept skin and body tissues intact. Embalmers would smear a thin coat of myrrh resin over the skin to preserve it before wrapping the body in cloth. Such expensive treatments were usually reserved for pharaohs and high officials. Eventually, when clever cosmetic chemists realized that myrrh would work similar wonders on living skin, they incorporated it into balms, facial masks, pomades, and unguents.

Young Persian girls, preparing for court, used myrrh as part of a ritual purification. The ancient Hebrews created a holy anointing oil from myrrh, cinnamon, calamus, cassia, and olive oil; Moses consecrated his priests with it. Israelite women wore myrrh sachets next to their bodies, probably to have their body heat release myrrh's fragrant aroma and mask body odor. An unguent of myrrh, coriander, and honey was used to treat herpes. Prior to his crucifixion, Jesus drank wine mixed with myrrh, probably as a form of sedative.

In Greek mythology, Aphrodite forced the goddess Myrrha into an incestuous relationship with her father, Cinyras, who avenged the act by turning his daughter into a myrrh tree. When the tree sprouted its blooms, their child Adonis was born. The resinous drops that exude from cuts in the tree's bark were said to be Myrrha's tears.

Myrrh held a prominent place as one of the most important aromatic materials in ancient perfumery. Alexander the Great became enamored of myrrh and burned myrrh incense incessantly in his court. Greek and Roman perfumers created myrrh resins that were the longest-lasting perfumes of the day. Regarded highly for its fixative properties, myrrh could last for up to ten years, often improving with age. Myrrh continues to lend its fixative powers and its smoky, balsamic undertones to about 7 percent of the perfumes produced today, particularly ones with exotic or heavy floral fragrances.

MEDICINAL USES

In Europe, physicians prescribe myrrh oil for arthritis, inflammation, gum disorders, menstrual difficulties, prostate problems, and urinary tract infections. Myrrh oil boosts immunity by stimulating the production of white blood cells. It fights infection and speeds recovery from illness. It tones the digestive tract, stimulates appetite, reduces stomach gas and acidity, and alleviates diarrhea. European gynecologists use myrrh oil to treat scanty menstrual periods, leukorrhea, and thrush, and to cleanse obstructions in the womb. Chinese doctors treat arthritis, hemorrhoids, menstrual problems, and wounds with myrrh. Myrrh may help lower blood cholesterol levels and may help people wanting to lose weight.

Doctors prescribe myrrh oil for such respiratory ailments as asthma, bronchitis, colds, coughs, flu, and sore throat. It clears excess mucus, eliminates congestion, and soothes inflamed membranes. Myrrh oil relieves the itching and irritation of psoriasis and weeping eczema and fights the fungal infection of athlete's foot, candida, jock itch, and ringworm. The *British Herbal Pharmacopoeia* lists myrrh as a treatment for gingivitis and mouth ulcers. Many health-care practitioners claim that myrrh oil is the best treatment for oral ulcers, gingivitis, periodontal disease, and other gum disorders. It can relieve toothache and prevent bad breath.

BEAUTY BENEFITS

Myrrh oil maintains healthy skin and reputedly prevents premature aging of the skin. Many people claim that it wards off wrinkles. Myrrh oil soothes and softens rough, cracked, or chapped skin. It stimulates the regeneration of skin cells, reduces inflammation, fights infection, and helps to heal wounds. It improves circulation, imparting a healthy glow to the complexion and helping the skin look smoother and more youthful. Myrrh oil also helps heal blemishes, skin ulcers, and wounds.

EMOTIONAL EFFECTS

Myrrh oil fortifies the nerves and emotions. It replaces feelings of apathy, weakness, and lack of initiative with motivation, power, and strength. Myrrh oil provides the clarity, focus, and strength to pull through troubled times. It eases grief and sorrow in loss or separation from a loved one. As it restores tranquility and peace of mind, you can discover how to find solace in solitude and enjoy time alone. Its cooling and calm-ing effect subdues angry or inflamed emotional states and helps calm hyperactivity.

PRECAUTIONS

Because of its ability to stimulate menstrual flow, myrrh oil should be avoided during pregnancy.

NEROLI

Pale-yellow neroli oil emits a sweet, full-bodied citrus aroma with a slightly spicy, slightly bitter undertone. Delicate white blossoms of the bitter orange or Seville orange tree produce neroli oil. This evergreen tree bears glossy, dark-green oval leaves. In May and October, an abundance of small white flowers appears. One ton of hand-picked blossoms from *Citrus aurantium, Citrus bigaradia,* or *Citrus vulgaris* yields only one quart of neroli oil, or orange blossom oil. This makes neroli oil comparatively expensive. Unfortunately, distillers and suppliers often adulterate neroli due to its high cost.

The bitter orange tree, which grows to heights of twenty to thirty feet, belongs to the *Rutaceae* family. Once native to central Asia and China, these trees now grow in subtropical regions of California, Mexico, and South America, as well as in areas surrounding the Indian Ocean and the Mediterranean. Farmers in Egypt, Italy, Morocco, Sicily, southern France, Spain, Tunisia, and the Comoro Islands, located off the southeast coast of Africa, cultivate commercial crops of bitter orange trees.

Many experts claim that the best neroli oil comes from Tunisia.

FOLKLORE AND HERBAL HERITAGE

So enamored of the smell of orange blossoms was Anna Maria de la Trémoille, a seventeenth-century princess of Nerola (in what is now Italy), that she adorned herself and almost everything in her environment with its fragrant oil. Elite members of the court followed her lead, making orange blossom oil the most sought-after scent of the time. In praise of the princess, orange blossom oil was reputedly given the name *neroli*. Another account suggests that the name derives from Nero, the Roman emperor.

Throughout history, brides have crowned their heads with garlands of orange blossoms and woven the blossoms into bridal bouquets. Orange flowers symbolized chastity; brides wore them to signify that their purity equaled their loveliness. Their ability to calm nerves probably helped compose many brides on their wedding nights.

On the other hand, neroli oil purportedly possessed aphrodisiac and euphoria-inducing properties. Prostitutes supposedly wore it to distinguish themselves; prospective customers could easily detect them by the unique smell of neroli emanating from their bodies.

Herbalists often recommended orange flower water, a byproduct of the steam distillation of neroli, to aid digestion. For centuries, people in North Africa and the Middle East have added orange flower water to various foods, both to impart a delightfully sweet flavor and to increase their digestibility. Mothers would give babies a spoonful of orange flower water to induce sleep or overcome insomnia. People drank orange flower tea for its enjoyable flavor, to fight off fevers, and to protect against plagues.

Neroli was a component of Hungary water, reputedly created by Queen Elizabeth of Hungary. The queen claimed that the formula healed her of crippling, disfiguring arthritis; afterward, she won the love of a man many years her junior. The original *eau de cologne,* formulated in the eighteenth century, contained neroli, along with bergamot, lavender, lemon, and rosemary.

MEDICINAL USES

Pharmacies still sell orange flower water as a digestive aid and sedative. European physicians and aromatherapists use neroli oil to settle heart palpitations and gently calm a person suffering from shock. Some health-care practitioners use it to lower blood pressure. Neroli oil is helpful in alleviating diarrhea, especially if related to nerves or stress. It soothes tense muscles and muscle spasms. It can bring relief of menstrual cramps and premenstrual syndrome (PMS). Neroli also soothes the irritation and itching of psoriasis, eczema, and dermatitis.

BEAUTY BENEFITS

Neroli oil increases circulation and stimulates new cell growth. It can prevent scarring and stretch marks. It is useful in treating skin conditions linked to emotions or stress, as it calms the emotions as well as the skin. Any type of skin can benefit from neroli oil, although it is particularly good for dry, irritated, or sensitive skin. It regulates oiliness and minimizes enlarged pores. Neroli oil helps to clear acne and blemished skin, especially if the skin lacks moisture. With regular application, it can reduce the appearance of fragile or broken capillaries and varicose veins.

EMOTIONAL EFFECTS

Neroli oil soothes emotional upsets and eases anger, depression, grief, hysteria, mood swings, nervousness, and shock. Health-care practitioners and aromatherapists in Europe use it to bring quick relief for anxiety and panic attacks and to treat chronic anxiety. Neroli oil subdues stress and tension. Its hypnotic effect helps to induce sleep. It encourages confidence, courage, creativity, esteem, joy, love, peace, and sensuality. Neroli oil can provide the strength and support to get through difficult or trying times.

HYDROSOL USES

Neroli hydrosol calms the nerves and is useful for hyperactivity, hysteria, and shock. As a digestive aid, it eases bloating and gas. It can be used as a douche for vaginitis and in skin care as a toner or skin spray.

NIAOULI

White, yellow, or purplish flowers form long spikes atop long lancelike leaves. The spongy bark of the *Melaleuca quinquenervia viridiflora* peels back from the trunk of the tree, which can reach twenty-three feet in height.

Niaouli is indigenous to Australia and New Caledonia and is a cousin to cajeput, eucalyptus, and tea tree. All belong to the *Myrtaceae* family. Madagascar cultivates and distills niaouli oil. This durable tree can survive severe droughts or extreme rainy seasons. Even forest fires cannot destroy it. Some tropical places, such as Florida, report that once these trees take root, they stay. Despite attempts to cut them down, felled trees simply sprout new shoots.

Steam distillation of the tree's twigs and needlelike leaves produces an oil that smells antiseptic, medicinal, and camphoraceous. Its balsamic note hints of an evergreen forest and leaves a cooling sensation in the nostrils and respiratory tract. Oils may range from clear to a pale or golden-yellow, which may reflect the copper content of the soil. Niaouli often is called *MQV,* an abbreviation for its Latin name. Another name, *gomenol,* is derived from the early site of distillation in Gomen, New Caledonia.

FOLKLORE AND HERBAL HERITAGE

Local residents of New Caledonia applied niaouli on wounds to accelerate the healing process. They also reduced fevers with it. By massaging niaouli into sore muscles and stiff joints, they relieved the pain of arthritis and rheumatism. It eased the symptoms of diarrhea. During epidemics, they breathed into niaouli-soaked handkerchiefs to prevent the spread of germs and disease. Local folks credited their absence of malaria to their use of niaouli. Niaouli purified their drinking water. Middle Easterners drank niaouli tea to stimulate peristalsis for maintaining healthy bowels. French obstetricians relied upon it for its antiseptic qualities.

MEDICINAL USES

Niaouli offers relief for a variety of respiratory conditions. Its antibacterial and antiviral actions help to reduce the duration of colds and flu, while offering relief from scratchy or sore throats, stuffy or runny noses, and coughs. As an expectorant, it releases the congestion and accumulation of phlegm common in many respiratory ailments, such as asthma, bronchitis, and sinusitis. Inhaling niaouli oil directly from the bottle or in a steam bath can quickly open sinus passages and improve breathing. A gargle of niaouli in water can soothe sore throat.

Niaouli oil helps to relieve ear infections and earaches. Niaouli boosts immunity and can help ward off sickness. As a tonic for the lymphatic system, it reduces infection and stimulates the removal of wastes that interfere with the flow of lymphatic fluids. Niaouli gives gentle but effective relief for allergies.

As an endocrine tonic, niaouli shows an affinity for the pituitary gland and ovaries, probably due to its estrogenlike constituents. Niaouli relieves genitourinary tract infections. As a vaginal douche, niaouli fights yeast infections and vaginal candida while reducing offensive odors. Its antiseptic properties help overcome cystitis and other urinary tract conditions, especially when used in sitz baths. It can diminish hemorrhoids. Applied topically in low dilutions, niaouli oil offers relief from the pain and irritation of genital herpes. Its antifungal action helps to reduce the spread of athlete's foot and jock itch.

French aromatherapists and doctors use niaouli oil for hepatitis and some intestinal problems. Cancer patients shield their skin against burns from radiation treatment with a preparation of niaouli. Niaouli helps counteract symptoms of chronic fatigue syndrome and candidiasis.

Diffusing niaouli throughout your house can cleanse and purify the air, especially after exposure to cigarette smoke. It counteracts air pollution while discouraging the spread of infection.

BEAUTY BENEFITS

Niaouli hastens the healing of wounds and skin ulcers by relieving inflammation, reducing infection, and stimulating new cell growth. As an astringent, niaouli helps to tighten and tone the skin. It promotes the regeneration of damaged tissue as it encourages formation of new cells. It soothes burns and relieves the pain of sunburn, especially when used with lavender. Cold sores and fever blisters respond well to niaouli; it speeds healing, minimizes the spread, and diminishes the pain. Niaouli is mild on the skin and on mucous membranes.

Through its regulating action on the skin's secretion of oil, or sebum, it helps to reduce oiliness and outbreaks of blemishes. It provides relief for sufferers of seborrhea. Niaouli is an ideal treatment for oral hygiene. Massaged into the gums, it can relieve inflammation and swelling.

EMOTIONAL EFFECTS

Niaouli is invigorating to the mind without being too stimulating. Its fresh, sharp scent increases alertness. It exerts a pleasant balancing effect on emotions.

ORANGE

Smooth and shiny oblong leaves, fragrant white flowers, and sweet-tasting, nutritious fruit adorn the bounteous orange tree. The bitter orange tree, *Citrus aurantium,* yields orange oil from its fruit, neroli oil from its flowers, and petitgrain oil from its foliage. The sweet orange tree, *Citrus sinensis,* yields orange oil from its fruit and, occasionally, an oil called neroli Portugal from its blossoms.

Cold-expressing either whole oranges or orange peels, by hand or machine, yields a yellow or orange oil with a zesty, refreshing, slightly green-smelling, and very citrusy aroma. Some orange oil is steam-distilled from fresh orange peels. Approximately fifty oranges render one ounce of orange oil.

Native to China and India, the orange tree belongs to the *Rutaceae* family. Oranges grow abundantly in the Americas, Israel, and Mediterranean countries. Brazil, Cyprus, Israel, Mexico, and the United States are the primary producers of orange oil.

FOLKLORE AND HERBAL HERITAGE

From early times, oranges have been associated with generosity and gratitude. Ancient practitioners of Chinese medicine prescribed oranges for digestion. To the Chinese, oranges represented prosperity and good luck. Once called "golden apples," oranges symbolized innocence and fertility. According to tradition, Mary fed the baby Jesus, Joseph, and herself with three oranges from a tree inhabited by a sleeping eagle. The original pomanders were oranges pierced with clove buds. The word *orange* comes from the Persian *narang* by way of the Arabic word *narandj.* In the sixteenth century, Portugese ships returned carrying orange trees from China. Later, missionaries transported oranges to California, which now has a thriving orange industry. Orange peels provide a tangy taste to orange marmalade, and they flavor curaçao, a West Indian liqueur.

MEDICINAL USES

Orange oil relieves the discomfort of bronchitis and the flu. It aids in the absorption of vitamin C, boosts immunity, helps prevent colds and flu, and relieves some of the symptoms associated with chronic fatigue syndrome. Orange oil heals mouth ulcers and gingivitis. It also soothes painful muscles and joints. The Chinese treat anorexia nervosa, colds, coughs, and malignant breast sores with dried orange peels.

Orange oil calms an upset stomach, especially if nerve or stress related, and can aid in digestion and restore appetite. It regulates the bowels and relieves diarrhea and constipation. Orange oil encourages the elimination of wastes and promotes urination, making it helpful in treating obesity, fluid retention, and premenstrual syndrome (PMS). It regulates body temperature and either cools a fever or warms a chill. Orange oil soothes inflammation from psoriasis as well as eczema and other types of dermatitis.

Beauty Benefits

Orange oil restores balance to dry or oily skin. It maintains healthy, youthful skin by promoting the production of collagen. It reduces puffiness and discourages dry or wrinkled skin. Orange oil stimulates circulation to the skin surface and softens rough skin. It also clears blemishes and improves acne-prone skin. It tends to increase perspiration, thus assisting the release of toxins from dull or blemished skin. Orange stimulates the circulation of lymphatic fluids and helps relieve tissue swelling and fluid retention. It improves cellulite, which is sometimes called orange-peel skin.

Emotional Effects

Orange oil balances the emotions, either relaxing or stimulating as needed. It revitalizes and energizes when boredom and lethargy set in. Seek help from orange oil before perfectionism, overwork, or mental overexertion takes a toll on your psyche. Orange oil has a warm, happy, and light influence that prevents extreme seriousness. It calms the nerves and can combat anxiety, hysteria, and insomnia. Orange oil brightens gloomy feelings, dissipates depressing thoughts, and subdues tension and stress, particularly in wintertime with seasonal affective disorder or if the stress is related to premenstrual syndrome or menopause. It eases fear of the unknown and encourages a more adventuresome approach to life. It brings a more positive outlook, replacing sadness and negativity with warmth, optimism, and happiness. Orange oil awakens creativity, inspires harmony, and promotes self-awareness.

Precautions

Orange oil may irritate skin and promote photosensitivity, leading to sunburn and uneven darkening of the skin. Avoid using it if your skin will be exposed to sunlight.

OREGANO

Oregano emits a pungent and penetrating herbal scent, as does the essential oil. Whorls of petite white flowers cluster close together along spikes that spring from overlapping little leaflike bracts at the base of the stems. Glandular dots speckle the round green leaves and fine white hairs surround the stems. Oregano's appearance is similar to that of marjoram. It can creep low to the ground or reach eighteen inches in height. It can be classified as an annual, a biennial, or a perennial herb.

The essential oil is golden to dark yellow with a pungent phenol odor that is spicy, tangy, and hot. The smell is sharp and strongly medicinal. Within the *Lamiaceae* family, the *Origanum* genus has about thirty-six species native to Eurasia. Another thirteen species originated in Europe, primarily in the Mediterranean area. Confusion permeates this genus; oregano perplexes botanists and herbalists who wish to identify the plants. Botanical names become essential to distinguish which plants produced the essential oil you are using. Some varieties that are steam-distilled for use in aromatherapy include *Origanum elongatum, Origanum vulgare, Origanum heracleoticum,* and *Origanum compactum.* However, Spanish oregano, *Corydothymus capitatum,* is sometimes mistaken for oregano. *Origanum marjorana* is sweet marjoram.

Oregano grows wild throughout Europe, especially in Spain and Greece, and in North Africa. Most cultivated oregano and oregano oil come from Mediterranean countries. Sometimes oregano is called *shepherd's thyme.*

FOLKLORE AND HERBAL HERITAGE

Oregano derives from the Greek words *oros,* meaning "mountain," and *ganos,* signifying "joy"—it was once known as "joy of the mountain." Indeed, joyous describes the feeling of standing high atop a mountainside carpeted in oregano as its scent suffuses through the air and wafts deep into the lungs. Egyptians valued oregano for its ability to disinfect wounds and speed the healing process. They used in it preservation, perhaps in mummification.

After Aristotle observed that tortoises ate snakes and then ate oregano to avoid dying, he recommended it as an antidote for poisoning. Oregano also soothed coughs, calmed digestive disorders, and assisted digestion. Doctors respected oregano as an antiseptic for the respiratory system. They used it to heal wounds, burns, and skin ulcers. Oregano relaxed tension and could overcome insomnia. It also relieved nervous headaches, irritability, and general exhaustion. Women found relief for menstrual cramps and discomfort with oregano.

The famous Roman gourmet Apicius prized oregano in his culinary creations. Oregano plays a vital part in Mediterranean cuisine. Post–World War II GIs returned from overseas relishing the taste of oregano they had enjoyed in Italian cuisine. Their demand for the herb helped make it a popular seasoning in the United States. Before they began using hops, brewers flavored beer and ale with oregano. An old tradition continues in Mediterranean countries such as Turkey, Lebanon, and Greece in which restaurants serve oregano as a health-promoting beverage.

MEDICINAL USES

Oregano oil is one of the strongest antiseptic and antiviral essential oils. It boosts immunity and is especially effective against allergies, candidiasis, chronic fatigue syndrome, and fungal infections. It stimulates sluggish lymphatic circulation. During convalescence or in states of general weakness, the body can be strengthened and energized by oregano. Its antibacterial action makes oregano ideal for spraying in a sickroom to cleanse or sterilize it and to prevent the spread of infection.

Respiratory ailments as asthma, bronchitis, colds, flu, sore throat, and even whooping cough respond well to oregano oil's ability to fight bacterial and viral infections, relieve congestion, loosen and release phlegm, and soothe coughs, while it eases aches and pains and reduces muscle spasms. Oregano alleviates the pain and inflammation of joint and spinal problems such as arthritis, backache, bursitis, carpal tunnel syndrome, rheumatism, and sciatica. It is often used in a pack or poultice to treat sprains, swelling, and stiffness.

Oregano is helpful for all digestive disorders, particularly those resulting from nervousness. It eases indigestion that results from eating too rapidly. It calms the stomach, can stimulate appetite, relieves diarrhea, and can even cure hiccups. Oregano can soothe headaches, migraines, and nervous tension. Its antiseptic abilities help to fight the infection of earaches. Some people report success in preventing or minimizing motion sickness by drinking oregano herb tea. Others recommend chewing fresh oregano leaves to provide temporary relief from a painful toothache.

The anti-inflammatory action of oregano oil helps to heal wounds and skin infections, as well as to relieve skin disorders such as dermatitis, eczema, psoriasis, and seborrhea. Because it has strong antifungal and antiseptic properties, it can fight fungal infections of the skin such as athlete's foot and jock itch. Massage diluted oregano oil into the fingernails to fight fungal infection there. Applied topically, it helps reduce chronic skin afflictions. Oregano is a powerful insect repellent; it may help to alleviate skin parasites, such as lice, because of its antiparasitic activity.

Oregano can often stimulate the flow of menstruation when used in a sitz bath or when massaged on the abdomen. It also relieves the pain of menstrual cramps and helps to overcome insomnia.

BEAUTY BENEFITS

Oregano is a powerful oil that can burn or irritate skin if applied directly to it. Highly diluted in a carrier oil, oregano oil can stimulate skin cells and promote healthy circulation, making it useful for eliminating cellulite.

EMOTIONAL EFFECTS

As a nervine, or nerve tonic, oregano calms and quiets almost any nervous upset. It is relaxing and can help overcome insomnia. It can ease irritability and tension. It reduces stress and anxiety while restoring emotional balance. It helps to clarify thinking and promote a positive attitude.

HYDROSOL USES

Oregano hydrosol is a digestive aid, intestinal cleanser, and immune tonic. It can be used as a douche for vaginitis and for urinary tract infections. It is also useful in oral hygiene and as a gargle for sore throat. Oregano hydrosol can be added to beverages and used in cooking.

PRECAUTIONS

Avoid using oregano during pregnancy due to its ability to stimulate menstruation. It can irritate skin and mucous membranes. Use very dilute solutions on the skin. One drop in an ounce of carrier oil is often sufficient.

PALMAROSA

Palmarosa is a sweet-smelling grass that grows wild in tropical climates. Clusters of bluish-white flowers rise out of its long, slender leaves. As they mature, the flowers turn dark red.

Harvesting, drying, and steam-distilling palmarosa grass before the flowers mature assures a higher yield of superior palmarosa oil. This pale yellowish-green oil has floral notes reminiscent of roses or geraniums. Originally from central and northern India, *Cymbopogon martini* is a member of the *Poaceae* family. It now grows in Africa, Java, Madagascar, and the Seychelles.

FOLKLORE AND HERBAL HERITAGE

Since the eighteenth century, the Turks have distilled palmarosa oil to adulterate costly Turkish rose oil. Palmarosa was once known as Turkish or Indian geranium oil because of its geraniumlike odor. Indian doctors prescribed palmarosa to prevent infections and fight fever. Palmarosa was also added to Indian curry dishes and some West African meat dishes to kill bacteria and aid digestion.

MEDICINAL USES

Indian doctors use palmarosa oil to fight bacteria and infection. It can help fight the pain, discomfort, and infection of cystitis, urethritis, and vaginitis. Palmarosa oil cools fevers and eases the discomforts of colds and the flu. It can hasten recovery from illness and relieve malaise. It accelerates the healing of cuts and wounds. Palmarosa oil can also help the body restore healthy intestinal flora. It stimulates the appetite and helps in cases of anorexia nervosa.

BEAUTY BENEFITS

Palmarosa oil enhances any skin type. It regulates the production of sebum, or oil, helping to normalize oily skin; in dry or mature skin, it stimulates sebum production and helps replenish moisture. It helps clear acne and blemishes; with regular application, it can fade old acne scars. It stimulates the regeneration of cells, discourages wrinkles, heals wounds and sores, and soothes inflamed or irritated skin. Palmarosa oil also minimizes the appearance of broken capillaries with long-term use.

EMOTIONAL EFFECTS
Palmarosa oil promotes recovery from mental fatigue, nervous exhaustion, or stress. It calms and uplifts the emotions while refreshing the mind and clarifying thoughts. It reduces stress and tension and encourages feelings of freedom and flexibility. It expands feelings of love and romance by discouraging the oppressive nature of insecurity, jealousy, and possessiveness.

PATCHOULI
Patchouli oil is pungent and powerful, mossy and musty, earthy and exotic, sweet and spicy. It is steam-distilled from the dried and fermented fuzzy young leaves of *Pogostemon patchouli* or *Pogostemon cablin,* a three-foot-tall perennial bush with white flowers that have a purplish or mauve hue. Age enriches the heavy herbal odor of its viscous amber, orange, or dark-brown oil.

A member of the *Lamiaceae* family, patchouli is native to tropical Asia and is cultivated in India, Indonesia, Malaysia, the Philippines, and Singapore. Patchouli oil is produced in Burma, India, Malaysia, and some South and Central American countries.

FOLKLORE AND HERBAL HERITAGE
For centuries, the people of China, India, Japan, and Malaysia have relied on patchouli for various medicinal purposes. They used it to fight infection and cool fevers and to tone the skin and, indeed, the entire body. It was also used as an antidote for insect and snake bites. It is the combination of patchouli and camphor that gives India ink its characteristic smell.

During the Victorian era, British manufacturers imported patchouli oil to fragrance machine-made cashmere shawls, in the hope that buyers could not distinguish the difference between their wares and authentic handmade cashmere shawls from India, which had a lingering odor of patchouli. In India, patchouli sachets scented clothes and protected them against insects. Patchouli perfume also provided the persistent and unforgettable fragrance associated with the "flower power" movement of the 1960s and 1970s.

MEDICINAL USES
Patchouli oil helps with weight loss: It curbs the appetite and it tones and tightens skin to prevent sagging after weight is lost. It can improve the appearance of cellulite and varicose veins. By increasing urination, it discourages bloating and water retention associated with premenstrual syndrome

(PMS). It may also reduce hot flashes during menopause. Patchouli diminishes the distress of diarrhea. It fights fungi and is useful in treating athlete's foot, jock itch, vaginitis, and fungal infections of the skin, such as candida. Patchouli oil reduces the inflammation of skin disorders such as acne, psoriasis, sunburn, skin allergies, and eczema and other forms of dermatitis. It can relieve the swelling and inflammation of hemorrhoids.

BEAUTY BENEFITS

Patchouli oil regenerates skin cells and may ward off wrinkles. It also tightens and tones sagging skin. Patchouli oil speeds the healing of sores and wounds and helps to fade scars. It cools and calms inflamed skin and sunburn; it soothes and smoothes rough, dry, and cracked skin. At the same time, it regulates the oiliness of skin and hair and helps control acne and scalp disorders such as dandruff and seborrhea. It also repels insects. By reducing fluid retention and tightening saggy skin, patchouli oil helps combat cellulite. It acts as a deodorant and helps control perspiration.

EMOTIONAL EFFECTS

Patchouli oil diminishes depression and eases anxiety by heightening a sense of joy in life. It helps recovery from nervous exhaustion, stress, and stress-related conditions. It reduces mental fatigue and banishes lethargy. In low doses, it acts as a sedative, while in larger quantities, it is stimulating. It can sharpen intelligence, improve concentration, and provide insight. It cools and calms during physically or emotionally hot situations. It is a stabilizing and balancing oil with aphrodisiac attributes that can heighten libido, combat impotence and frigidity, and decrease sexual anxiety about performance. It replaces fear with confidence, indecision with motivation, and indifference with compassion. Patchouli expands sensuality, inspires creativity, and encourages freedom of expression of the imagination.

PEPPER

See BLACK PEPPER.

PEPPERMINT

Compact, serrated-edged leaves on short, square stems contrast with the long, spear-like spikes bearing the tiny purple, pink, or white flowers of the peppermint plant. Originally, some twenty-five species of peppermint were native to Asia and Europe, but hybridization has reduced this number. Now this member of the *Lamiaceae* family grows commercially in humid regions of Australia, Brazil, China, England, France, Japan, Morocco, Spain, and the United States, which is the primary producer of peppermint oil. Steam-distilling 1,000 pounds of mature *Mentha piperita* plants in full bloom will produce about 1 pound of peppermint oil. This clear or pale-yellow oil emits a strong, sharp menthol aroma that is pungent and powerful, even overwhelming.

FOLKLORE AND HERBAL HERITAGE

In Roman mythology, when Pluto professed his love for the nymph Mentha, his wife Persephone, afire with jealousy, crushed Mentha into dust on the ground. Pluto, unable to change her back, transformed her into a peppermint plant and gave her a fresh fragrance so that she would smell sweet whenever stepped upon.

The ancient Hebrews added peppermint to perfumes, possibly for its aphrodisiac attributes. Peppermint played a prominent part in Greek and Roman religious rites. For thousands of years, Asians, Egyptians, and Native Americans have soothed digestive difficulties with peppermint and used it to freshen their breath.

During the eighteenth century, peppermint became a well-known medicine throughout Europe and North America. It relieved such common complaints as colic, gas, headaches, heartburn, and indigestion. Today some pharmacists still suggest peppermint oil for upset stomach and indigestion. Overindulgent diners sip peppermint tea to soothe bloated bellies, stimulate sluggish digestion, and reduce heartburn and gas. For decades, peppermint has added a refreshing punch to numerous commercial products, including breath mints, chewing gums, toothpastes, toothpicks, after-dinner mints, and mouthwashes. In addition, the food industry utilizes its invigorating taste and strong aroma to enliven foods, teas, candies, and pastries.

MEDICINAL USES

Peppermint oil stimulates the central nervous system and counteracts drowsiness and fatigue by increasing alertness and promoting clear thinking. It calms and soothes muscles, particularly those of the digestive tract when they are affected by stress and poor diet. It stimulates the appetite and increases stomach acidity necessary for digestion. It balances intestinal flora and relieves colon spasms and irritable bowel syndrome. Peppermint reduces the inflammation and irritation of gout and stomach ulcers.

It eases motion sickness and nausea and can revitalize some symptoms of jet lag. Chronic fatigue syndrome also responds to its stimulating action.

Peppermint oil relaxes tense muscles and muscle spasms. It eases painful menstrual cramps, cools hot flashes and fevers, and reduces the inflammation and swelling of muscular aches, pains, sprains, and strains. Peppermint oil relieves the itching and swelling of dermatitis and sunburn. It also relieves headaches, whether from tension or migraine. It clears sinuses and can improve breathing, particularly in asthma and bronchitis. It also serves as an insect repellent and soothes the itching and swelling of insect bites.

BEAUTY BENEFITS

Peppermint oil fights bacterial infection and reduces the oiliness present with acne and blemishes. It stimulates circulation and helps enliven dull, dry skin. Peppermint oil leaves skin feeling soft and silky. It also regulates and normalizes oily skin and hair. It constricts capillaries and minimizes the redness of broken capillaries and varicose veins.

EMOTIONAL EFFECTS

Peppermint oil cools emotions and dissipates anger, hysteria, and nervousness. It energizes and relieves mental fatigue. It diminishes depression while increasing joy. It inspires confidence and esteem. It provides focus while diminishing indecision. Peppermint oil increases alertness and improves concentration. It awakens the central nervous system, stimulates the brain, improves memory, and clarifies thought processes. It increases insight and inspires new thoughts and ideas.

HYDROSOL USES

Peppermint hydrosol is a digestive aid and intestinal cleanser that is effective for heartburn and irritable bowel syndrome. It relieves muscular aches, pains, and strains. It calms nerves and is a mental and physical stimulant. In skin care, peppermint hydrosol is helpful for insect bites, inflammation, irritation, and acne. It also has uses in beverages and foods. Peppermint hydrosol is susceptible to going rancid more quickly than other hydrosols. Never use a hydrosol if it does not look and smell fresh.

PRECAUTIONS

Peppermint oil may elevate blood pressure, so you should avoid using it if you have high blood pressure. It may irritate sensitive skin. It can stimulate menstrual flow and stop the flow of milk, so women who are pregnant or nursing should avoid it. Peppermint oil can counteract homeopathic remedies. If you are using both peppermint oil and a homeopathic remedy, allow at least one hour between the two.

PINE

Majestic, aromatic Scotch pine trees tower above the forest, reaching heights of 65 to 115 feet. Deep fissures mark the reddish-brown bark of this large evergreen, *Pinus sylvestri,* also known as the Norway pine. Yellow-orange flowers and pointed amber, green, or brown cones cluster around gray-green or blue-green needles. Native to Europe and Asia, this member of the *Pinaceae* family is now found in northern Europe, northeastern Russia, Scandinavia, and the eastern United States. Pine needles, twigs, and cones are steam-distilled to produce pine oil. This colorless or light-yellow oil emits an earthy, resinous, and medicinal odor that is strong, fresh, and balsamic. Trees grown in more northerly climates produce superior oils.

FOLKLORE AND HERBAL HERITAGE

The ancient Greeks dedicated pine trees to the sea god, Neptune, because they built the first Greek ships with pine wood. They also honored the gods Bacchus and Pan with it. In Greek mythology, Pitys, one of Pan's many nymphs, escaped the embraces of Boreas by becoming a pine tree. According to folklore, the sayings "pining for" and "pitying" someone may have come from that incident.

One Christian tradition holds that Jesus was crucified on a cross made from a pine tree. In some cultures, mourners placed pine branches on the coffins of loved ones to signify immortality. To the Japanese, pine trees symbolized constancy and fidelity because they are always green.

Native Americans stuffed pine needles into their mattresses to repel lice and fleas. Arabs treated pneumonia and other lung infections with pine. Pine branches have been bruised and floated in baths to revitalize people suffering from mental or emotional fatigue and nervous exhaustion. Pine helped to improve circulation and relieve aching muscles; in the nineteenth century, pine was a popular diuretic. It could induce perspiration and helped to break fevers. Pine-tar ointments relieved skin disorders such as psoriasis and eczema and healed sores. Pine was also a remedy for constipation.

MEDICINAL USES

Pine oil fights any type of respiratory infection, especially asthma, bronchitis, colds, the flu, laryngitis, and sore throats. It encourages the release of mucus; it relieves congestion and clears the sinuses; it eases coughing and improves breathing. Pine oil can either warm a chill or cool a fever, depending on what the body needs. It soothes muscle aches and pains and stiffness in joints, providing relief for arthritis, backaches, carpal tunnel syndrome, gout, rheumatism, and sciatica. Pine also stimulates circulation, raises blood pressure, and activates the adrenal glands. It acts as a kidney and liver cleanser and can help treat cystitis and prostate problems. It soothes the itching and inflammation of eczema and psoriasis, and helps to heal cuts and sores. Pine oil has a revitalizing effect on the entire body and helps fight fatigue. It tones and regulates the endocrine system. As an insect repellent, it protects against bug bites.

BEAUTY BENEFITS

Pine oil encourages the elimination of toxins from the skin, making it useful for clearing dull, dry skin as well as acne. It improves oily scalp conditions, dandruff, and seborrhea. It also reduces excessive perspiration.

EMOTIONAL EFFECTS

Pine oil is refreshing and revitalizes a body and mind suffering from general malaise or mental fatigue. It restores strength after physical weakness or during convalescence. Because it has a balancing effect on the endocrine glands, it can help combat emotional upsets due to hormonal imbalances. It helps purify thoughts and promote positive attitudes.

Hydrosol Uses

Pine hydrosol is an immune stimulant, body tonic, and physical and mental energizer. It is useful for respiratory ailments, muscular and joint aches and pain, and skin care. It is also used in oral hygiene and hair care, especially for dandruff.

Precautions

Because pine oil can increase blood pressure, you should avoid using it if you have high blood pressure. Pine oil may be irritating to sensitive skin.

ROSE

Of the estimated 5,000 or more species of roses that grace our environment, the damask rose *(Rosa damascena)* and the cabbage rose *(Rosa centifolia)* are the most fragrant, and they are the two primary roses that produce essential oils for aromatherapy. At one time, the red rose *(Rosa gallica)* supposedly yielded rose oil as well, but it is rarely available today.

Native to the Orient, Persia (now Iran), and Syria, these members of the *Rosaceae* family are now cultivated in the temperate regions of Bulgaria, China, France, India, Italy, Morocco, Russia, Tunisia, and Turkey. These bushy deciduous shrubs grow three to six feet tall or taller. Their sweet-scented blossoms range in color from white to pink to red.

Steam-distilling more than 60,000 fresh-picked roses will yield only one ounce of rose oil. Pale-yellow or deeper yellow rose oil, or rose otto, has a rich, sweet, and spicy floral fragrance. Rose absolute, a reddish-orange oil with a heavier, sweeter scent, is extracted with solvents. Because residues of solvent may remain in rose absolute, rose oil or rose otto is more desirable for aromatherapy purposes.

Folklore and Herbal Heritage

Fossils reveal that roses have existed for 32 million years. More than 3,000 years ago, the rose was christened the "queen of flowers."

Throughout history, roses have been the subject of art, literature, poetry, medicine, and love. There are many myths and legends surrounding the rose. In Roman mythology, the goddess Venus was presented with a rose as she arose from the sea; according to Greek mythology, the blood of Aphrodite, who pricked her finger on a thorn of the rosebush while helping Adonis, colored roses red. The rose was sacred to both Aphrodite and Eros.

One tradition holds that thorns appeared on rosebushes only after the Fall, when God expelled Adam and Eve from the Garden of Eden. Another myth attributes the thorns to Cupid's arrow, which accidentally punctured the rosebush, permanently endowing it with thorns.

In ancient times, roses meant confidence. The practice of hanging a rose over a meeting table signified that everything said would be held in strictest confidence; hence the term *sub rosa*. Other meanings attributed to roses included beauty, enjoyment, fertility, joy, love, and pleasure. In addition, each color of rose was supposed to have its own special meaning: red for passion and desire; pink for simplicity, happiness, and love; white for innocence and purity; yellow for jealousy or achievement. Egyptian art and architecture contained depictions of roses; Cleopatra's cosmetics contained actual roses. She supposedly employed the seductive powers of the rose when entertaining Mark Antony by carpeting her floors knee deep with red rose petals.

Roses became an integral part of Roman culture. Lavish displays of roses decorated banquet tables, and rose petals covered floors at feasts. Romans crowned newlyweds with garlands of roses. In conquered lands, they planted gardens of roses for use in bathing, confectionery, cosmetics, medicine, and perfume, and as a cure for hangovers. Rose petals floated atop rose water in canals in the Shalimar Gardens for the wedding of Shah Jahan and his bride, in whose honor the shah later built the Taj Mahal. Legend has it that when his wife noticed the rose oil particles surfacing on the water, she ordered them collected for her perfume.

For centuries, roses have soothed the pain of fever blisters and cold sores. Until the Middle Ages, roses were a chief cure for digestive disorders, eye infections, headaches, menstrual difficulties, nervous tension, and skin disorders, and as a treatment for respiratory ailments and asthma. In Elizabethan England, cooks flavored many foods with roses. Middle Eastern cuisine still employs rose water in some dishes and beverages.

MEDICINAL USES

Physicians in Europe prescribe rose oil for mouth sores and to heal wounds. It clears congestion, eases coughs, and soothes sore throats. Rose water relieves conjunctivitis, helps heal herpes outbreaks, and soothes gingivitis. Rose oil strengthens the digestive system and helps overcome constipation, nausea, and vomiting. It can also relieve the pain of migraine and other headaches.

Rose oil helps balance female hormones. It regulates the menstrual cycle, reduces menstrual cramps, and eases the discomforts of premenstrual syndrome (PMS) and menopause. It is also helpful in treating genitourinary conditions. Sexual difficulties such as frigidity and impotence respond to rose oil, particularly if they are stress related. It stimulates circulation and tones the capillaries. It soothes and comforts psoriasis, eczema, dermatitis, and other skin disorders by reducing inflammation. Rose oil is gentle enough to use on babies and children.

BEAUTY BENEFITS

Rose oil benefits all skin types, especially mature, sensitive, dry, or damaged skin. It helps restore the moisture balance and smoothes wrinkles. It constricts tiny blood vessels, thus helping to diminish the redness of broken capillaries. Rose water is a soothing and nourishing treatment to use as a skin toner or facial mist.

EMOTIONAL EFFECTS

Rose oil nurtures the heart and encourages feelings of love and trust. It supports and soothes the emotions. It lifts depression, eases anxiety and panic, elevates spirits, and reduces stress and tension. It stabilizes mood swings, particularly if they are related to postnatal depression. It calms the nerves and helps to overcome hyperactivity and insomnia. Rose oil can ease grief and subdue sadness. It helps to eliminate feelings of disappointment, jealousy, resentment, and anger, and can help dissolve emotional blocks standing in the way of happiness. It inspires creativity and activates intuition. Rose oil symbolizes love, purity, and innocence, yet it is a sensual and stimulating aphrodisiac. It may help overcome impotence or frigidity.

HYDROSOL USES

Rose hydrosol balances the emotions and female hormones. It promotes relaxation and is helpful for PMS and stress. It is very useful in skin care as a facial mist and skin toner, and is appropriate for all skin types as well as for many skin disorders. Rose hydrosol can be used in eyewashes. It induces feelings of compassion and love, and can be used in cooking.

ROSEMARY

Cascades of rosemary emit a pungent, pinelike aroma with a woody, camphoraceous note. This aromatic shrub, *Rosmarinus officinalis,* has scaly bark and dense leathery, needlelike leaves. Tiny pale-blue blossoms abound from December through spring. Rosemary can grow to heights of five to six feet.

Steam distillation of 100 pounds of rosemary in bloom will yield 1 pound of strong, clean, and potent rosemary oil. Rosemary oil from varieties grown in Spain and North Africa smell similar to eucalyptus oil, while the scent of oil from plants grown in France is reminiscent of frankincense. Rosemary has several chemotypes; the plants are alike in physical appearance, but they produce essential oils with different chemical compositions. Moroccan rosemary, Spanish rosemary, rosemary Provence, and rosemary verbenone are four chemotypes of rosemary used in aromatherapy.

A member of the *Lamiaceae* family, rosemary is native to the Mediterranean regions of Europe. The Dalmatian islands, France, Spain, and Tunisia produce the majority of rosemary oil.

FOLKLORE AND HERBAL HERITAGE

Rosemary, whose name comes from the Latin *ros marinus,* meaning "dew of the sea," was one of the first plants used for medicine, food, and religious rituals. In ancient times, it was a part of almost all feasts and festivals. Rosemary reminded people of the cycle of life and death.

In flower lore, rosemary means "remembrance," possibly because of its ability to improve memory. In fact, to reinforce recall, students in ancient Greece wore garlands of rosemary on their heads while studying. Both the Greeks and the Romans associated rosemary with love and marriage. On her wedding day, a bride would wear a wreath woven with sprigs of rosemary and scented with rosemary oil. Brides carried rosemary in their bouquets. At a Greek or Roman funeral, friends and family members would toss rosemary into the grave to express the hope that the departed would be remembered.

During the sixteenth century, refreshing rosemary incense was a luxury of the wealthy, who paid perfumers to scent their homes with it. Hospitals burned rosemary to purify the air and prevent the spread of infection. People placed sprigs of rosemary under their pillows to ward off demons and to prevent bad dreams during the night. Priests used rosemary extensively in exorcisms to expel evil spirits. One of rosemary's most famous uses was in a therapeutic formula called Hungary water, named for Queen Elizabeth of Hungary. After bathing in this formula, drinking it, and having it massaged it into the joints of her paralyzed limbs, the queen—then in her seventies—supposedly recovered from her many ailments, and soon thereafter, she won the heart of a man many decades her junior.

Herbalists have long recommended rosemary to stimulate the activity of the stomach, the liver, and the gallbladder, as well as to improve circulation. Elizabethan physicians used rosemary to treat headaches, brain disorders, and toothaches. Paracelsus, the sixteenth-century German physician who first introduced the disease theory of illness, regarded rosemary as a most essential component in his medicines. He and other healers of his time treated disorders affecting the brain, heart, eyes, and liver with rosemary. Arab herbalists used it to restore memory, speech, and strength. Rosemary also improved the condition of the hair and scalp.

MEDICINAL USES

European doctors use rosemary oil in medical treatments for arthritis, colds, coughs, depression, diabetes, headaches, the flu, memory loss, migraines, and muscle spasms. British physicians prescribe rosemary oil to lower blood cholesterol levels and strengthen people with cardiovascular weaknesses. They also use rosemary oil to treat colic, cirrhosis of the liver, gallbladder infections, gallstones, and hepatitis. Digestive disorders such as colitis, gas, and indigestion often improve with rosemary, as do liver problems and jaundice. It stimulates the appetite and can improve food absorption by stimulating digestion. It tones the intestinal tract. Rosemary oil also relieves respiratory ailments such as asthma, bronchitis, colds, sinusitis, and whooping cough. It can inhibit the formation of stones in the bladder and kidneys. It fights infection and helps the body to expel excess mucus.

Rosemary oil stimulates circulation and helps raise low blood pressure. It relieves the pain and swelling of arthritis, muscle aches and spasms, injuries, and sprains and strains. It encourages cellular metabolism and assists in the drainage of lymphatic fluid. Rosemary oil tones the entire body and is helpful in treating candidiasis, chronic fatigue syndrome, and weakened immunity. It soothes the itching and inflammation of psoriasis, eczema, and other types of dermatitis. Recent studies indicate that it may discourage the spread of cancer cells.

BEAUTY BENEFITS

Rosemary oil stimulates cell renewal. It improves dry or mature skin, eases lines and wrinkles, and heals burns and wounds. It can also clear acne, blemishes, or dull, dry skin by fighting bacteria and regulating oil secretions. It improves circulation and can reduce the appearance of broken capillaries and varicose veins by strengthening fragile vessels. Rosemary oil nourishes the scalp and keeps hair looking healthy and shiny. Many users claim that it promotes hair growth. It normalizes excessive oil secretions and improves most scalp problems, particularly dandruff and seborrhea. Rosemary oil is also helpful in treating cellulite.

EMOTIONAL EFFECTS

Rosemary oil helps to overcome mental fatigue and sluggishness by stimulating and strengthening the central nervous system. It enhances mental clarity while aiding alertness and concentration. Rosemary oil can help you cope with stressful conditions and see things from a clearer perspective. It relaxes nerves and restores nerve health, especially after long-term nervous or physical ailments.

Rosemary oil balances intense emotions, such as aggression and anger, and controls mood swings. It lifts spirits and counters depression. It assists in managing stress and overcoming stress-related disorders and nervous exhaustion while restoring vitality. Rosemary oil can open the heart and bring the wisdom and discrimination necessary to establish healthy boundaries in relationships while retaining individuality. Rosemary oil arouses ambition and drive, inspires enthusiasm and the desire to achieve, and strengthens willpower and confidence. It also reputedly helps in overcoming impotence.

HYDROSOL USES

Rosemary hydrosol is a mental stimulant and digestive aid. It is good for respiratory ailments because it reduces mucus and congestion, and it is beneficial for earache and ear infections. Used in skin care and for skin disorders, it is helpful for treating acne, oily skin, or congested skin, and in skin toners.

PRECAUTIONS

Rosemary oil elevates blood pressure; avoid using it if you have high blood pressure. It may be irritating to sensitive skin. Rosemary oil may trigger epileptic seizures in susceptible individuals.

ROSEWOOD

Rosewood oil's subtle smell is soft, sweet, and spicy, with fresh floral notes. It is reminiscent of rose, citrus, and wood. This colorless or pale-yellow oil is distilled from the heartwood of the evergreen rosewood tree, *Aniba roseaodora*. Reaching heights of 125 feet, this member of the *Lauraceae* family has reddish bark and yellow flowers. It is native to the tropical areas around the Amazon river.

Rosewood trees grow and are harvested in the rain forests of South America. During the yearly flood season, huge rosewood tree trunks float downstream headed for the distilleries. Peru and Brazil supply most of the world's rosewood oil. So that the harvesting of rosewood trees does not lead to their extinction or to deforestation of ecologically sensitive areas, Brazilian legislation now requires that one new tree be planted for each one cut down.

FOLKLORE AND HERBAL HERITAGE

The original site of production of *bois de rose,* as the French called rosewood, was French Guiana, on the northern coast of South America. So great was the demand among the French for rosewood oil, which was used to create lily of the valley and lilac-type fragrances, that the French depleted the colony's rosewood forests. Carvings and chopsticks were commonly made from rosewood; the rose-scented heartwood was frequently used in cabinetmaking and to make handles for cutlery and hairbrushes. As an aphrodisiac, rosewood oil reputedly could restore a lost or diminished sex drive and overcome frigidity and impotence.

MEDICINAL USES

Rosewood oil is an overall tonic for balancing the body; it is neither too stimulating nor too sedating. By boosting the immune system, it deters colds and the flu, subdues coughs, and fights fever. It clears the head and eases headaches, especially those caused or accompanied by nausea. Rosewood oil promotes alertness and can diminish jet lag. It helps to heal cuts and wounds, and reduces the itching and inflammation of psoriasis, eczema, and other forms of dermatitis.

BEAUTY BENEFITS

Until relatively recently, rosewood oil was used primarily in perfumery. When used in skin care, it stimulates new cell growth, regenerates tissue, and minimizes lines and wrinkles. Rosewood oil can balance either dry or oily skin. It soothes sensitive and inflamed skin; it also clears blemishes and improves acne. With regular application, it helps to diminish scars.

EMOTIONAL EFFECTS

Rosewood oil calms and steadies the nerves and helps relieve anxiety, hyperactivity, and stress. It strengthens the nervous system and balances the emotions. Rosewood oil arouses alertness, especially under stressful circumstances. It encourages self-acceptance and the appreciation of others. As a subtle aphrodisiac, it stirs positive sensual feelings, especially in people whose past sexual experiences were traumatic.

SAGE

See CLARY SAGE.

ST. JOHN'S WORT

During the summer months, the bright-yellow star-shaped flowers of St. John's wort send out the subtle fresh aroma of lemon. If crushed, these flowers ooze a blood-colored liquid that stains the finger a shade of blue-purple. Oil glands are visible as tiny perforations on the pale-green oval leaves. This fragrant multibranched perennial grows as a hardy shrub to three feet in height. It is weedy-looking yet ornamental.

Steam distillation of the plant renders a pale-yellow essential oil that emits an oily herbal odor that smells fresh and pungent, medicinal, and balsamic. Once native to Europe, *Hypericum perforatum,* a member of the *Hypericaceae* family, now grows in meadows and along roadsides in Asia, Africa, Australia, and North America. Canada distills much St. John's wort oil.

Ancients nicknamed this plant *sol terrestris,* meaning "terrestrial sun," for its brilliant yellow blossoms with glistening golden stamens. Other names include sweet amber, common tutsam, goatweed, klamath weed, and tipton weed.

FOLKLORE AND HERBAL HERITAGE

The word *Hypericum* derives from Greek and means "over an apparition." This plant's popularity began with the ancient Greeks and continues to the present. Ancient Greeks believed that its fragrance forced evil spirits or ghosts to fly away.

During the summer solstice, the hypericum plant bloomed a golden hue; sun-worshippers revered the herb and used it as a totem to the gods. Romans burned it in bonfires as part of the celebration of Mid-summer Day. St. John's wort has been used as a health-enhancer since the time of the ancient Greeks. Galen, a great Greek healer, suggested it for the same purposes it is still used for today. Dioscorides claimed it would heal wounds. Turks took it to protect the liver against toxicity.

In England, before the arrival of Christianity, St. John's wort figured in ceremonies to celebrate the earth and the changes brought on by the summer season. On mid-summer's eve, or summer solstice, people decorated their homes with St. John's wort to protect against the evil eye. After the English converted to Christianity, they continued to celebrate the summer solstice, but now the holiday commemorated the birthday of John the Baptist, for whom the plant was given its common name. (*Wort* is an Anglo-Saxon word that means "herb.") The English continued to protect themselves by draping branches of St. John's wort in doorways and over windows, or even on their bodies, using the herb as a charm to protect them against witchcraft, evil, and enchantment, as well as storms and thunder. They believed that sleeping with a sprig of the plant under their pillows on St. John's Eve would ensure a vision of the saint and his blessing. People once believed that the red oil glands that dotted the leaves were actually drops of blood, to remind them of the beheading of St. John. Priests exorcised demons with St. John's wort. On the Isle of Man, there was a superstition that whoever trod on St. John's wort after sunset would be whisked away on a fairy horse and ride throughout the night until sunrise.

Most likely, Europeans introduced St. John's wort to America. Native Americans sipped the tea as a respiratory remedy, particularly for fighting tuberculosis. Herbalists and doctors suggested the herb as a treatment for anxiety, tension, neuralgia, and other nerve-related conditions. Homeopaths recommended the remedy following surgery to reduce inflammation and speed the healing of incisions. People brewed the flowers in teas to cure stomach ailments. One folk remedy suggested that children could overcome bedwetting by drinking the tea before bedtime.

MEDICINAL USES

Exciting evidence reveals the potential antiretroviral activity of hypericin, one component of St. John's wort, including its ability to inhibit spread of viruses. Scientists are investigating the herb's effect on human immunodeficiency virus (HIV), the flu, herpes simplex, and cancer. They suspect that it works by hampering the reproduction of viruses. It also stimulates immune function. Laboratory experiments show that the antibacterial action of St. John's wort may suppress tuberculosis bacteria. It can benefit any respiratory condition.

Hypericum is a valuable homeopathic remedy used in both pill and cream form for its anti-inflammatory action. Externally, it serves as a remedy for the joint and muscle pain of arthritis, rheumatism, and sciatica. Homeopathic physicians frequently recommend taking hypericum tablets before and after surgery to prevent hemorrhaging, to reduce swelling, and to promote rapid healing.

St. John's wort can relieve headaches and minimize migraines. It eases menstrual cramps and reduces bloating. It may provide some relief for incontinence and urinary tract problems such as cystitis. St. John's wort has helped many children triumph over bedwetting. It can relieve diarrhea and dysentery, and can reduce the inflammation of hemorrhoids.

St. John's wort is a tonic for the nervous system. It supports nerve tissues and nervous system functions throughout the body.

It acts as a mild sedative and helps overcome insomnia. The anti-inflammatory activity of St. John's wort oil reduces the swelling and pain of skin irritations, dermatitis, and disorders such as eczema, psoriasis, and seborrhea. It relieves the itching and inflammation of insect bites.

BEAUTY BENEFITS

St. John's wort oil tones the skin and improves the complexion. It heals wounds and skin ulcers, diminishes bruises, and soothes burns. It helps to minimize the appearance of varicose veins.

EMOTIONAL EFFECTS

Researchers speculate that depression occurs when natural body chemicals known as neurotransmitters in the brain are deficient, inefficient, or ineffective. St. John's wort may contain chemical components that, through a chain of chemical reactions, can increase the efficiency of these neurotransmitters. St. John's wort can relieve depression and is proving especially effective in treating seasonal affective disorder (SAD). SAD occurs during wintertime, when days are shorter with less sunlight.

Studies show that herbal extracts of St. John's wort relieved anxiety in women after four to six weeks of use. St. John's wort can benefit some of the emotional disturbances, such as anxiety, depression, irritability, and nervousness, that frequently accompany menopause.

St. John's wort provides general support to the nervous system and can repair damaged nerves. It restores balance after emotional, mental, or nervous exhaustion. It helps reestablish normal sleep patterns. Though the herbal form of St. John's wort may take several weeks or longer to show results, the essential oil usually produces effects more rapidly, even immediately after inhaling.

HYDROSOL USES

St. John's wort hydrosol gives emotional support and elevates mood. It is helpful for depression and seasonal affective disorder. It is also good for back problems, helps minimize scarring, and can be used in skin care as a skin spray and toner.

PRECAUTIONS

St. John's wort may cause photodermatitis or sun sensitivity in some individuals.

SANDALWOOD

An abundant array of small blossoms, ranging in color from red to yellow to pinkish-purple, sprout forth from the leathery leaves and the yellowish limbs of the sandalwood tree. This slow-growing evergreen, *Santalum album,* grows to a height of twenty-four to thirty feet over the course of thirty to sixty-four years. These heavy, somewhat parasitic members of the *Santalaceae* family obtain much of their nourishment by sending out suckers that tap into roots of other nearby trees.

Pale or golden-yellow sandalwood oil

emits a sweet, woody, velvety fragrance that is warm, rich, and exotic. Steam-distilling 25 pounds of crushed heartwood yields about 1 to 1½ pounds of thick, viscous oil.

Sandalwood is native to tropical Asia; India is the main producer of sandalwood oil. The finest sandalwood comes from the area of Mysore, in southern India. The Indian government now permits the harvesting only of mature trees that are approaching the end of their long lives. Once the trees are felled, ants eat away the outer bark and expose the heartwood, which contains the essential oil.

FOLKLORE AND HERBAL HERITAGE

Sweet, sacred-smelling sandalwood oil has played an integral part in Indian religion and culture for millennia. Indians made furniture and even built entire temples from the heartwood of sandalwood trees because it could resist attack by insects.

Sandalwood incense permeated Indian temples, helping worshippers to relax and achieve higher states of meditation. Sandalwood was closely associated with yogic, tantric, and other spiritual practices. It purportedly awakened *kundalini,* or the latent life-force energy, of anyone who breathed it during meditation. At funerals, mourners burned sandalwood incense to free the soul of the deceased.

Indians anointed their bodies with the seductive scent of sandalwood. Sandalwood oil's sultry smell has an erotic quality that has earned it a reputation as an aphrodisiac.

Many people claim that its aroma is similar to the masculine hormone androsterone. Indeed, for centuries, men have worn sandalwood-based scents to elicit desired responses from women.

In ancient times, caravans carried sandalwood from India to Egypt, Greece, and Rome. The Egyptians used sandalwood in the embalming process. Sandalwood's popularity in religious ceremonies, especially in India and China, continues today, and many Eastern cultures still consider sandalwood sacred.

The Polynesians added powdered sandalwood to massage oils to treat earaches, headaches, and skin ailments. Unfortunately, during the 1800s, greedy traders traveled to such places as India, Indonesia, and Hawaii, where flourishing forests of sandalwood trees embellished the local landscapes. These traders ravaged entire forests, leading to the extinction of some species of sandalwood and the endangered status of others.

MEDICINAL USES

Ayurvedic doctors in India still use sandalwood oil to fight infection and to treat urinary problems such as cystitis and urethritis, as well as prostate problems. They rely on sandalwood to relieve diarrhea, earaches, and respiratory infections. Chinese doctors prescribe sandalwood to cure cholera, gonorrhea, stomachaches, and vomiting. Other health-care practitioners also treat gastritis and nausea with it.

Sandalwood oil stimulates the immune

system, benefiting the entire body. Respiratory ailments such as bronchitis, coughs, laryngitis, sinusitis, and sore throats respond to sandalwood oil treatments. It also eases a variety of skin complaints. It helps to heal cuts and wounds, soothes skin, and relieves the itching and inflammation of psoriasis, eczema, and other types of dermatitis.

It alleviates insomnia and promotes restful sleep.

BEAUTY BENEFITS

Sandalwood oil nourishes dry, dehydrated, and mature skin. It smoothes and softens lines and wrinkles. It can balance either oily or dry skin and benefits any skin type or condition. Sandalwood oil helps to clear acne and blemishes by regulating oil production and fighting bacteria. It also makes an effective deodorant. It calms barber's rash, relieves itching and irritation after shaving, and inhibits the growth of bacteria that can cause infection of ingrown hairs. Sandalwood oil is mild enough even for sensitive skin.

EMOTIONAL EFFECTS

Sandalwood oil soothes emotions that are exhausted from a hectic lifestyle. It relaxes the body and mind, relieves stress and tension, and can lift depression. Sandalwood oil also subdues aggression and irritability. It helps to release confusion, fear, and nervousness. Sandalwood oil promotes compassion, openness, and understanding. It helps

reduce unrealistic expectations of self and others. It can help an introverted person to become more sociable and outgoing. Sandalwood elevates spiritual awareness by calming the mind, encouraging peace and tranquility, and allowing detachment from the dependence upon material goods. It stimulates the senses and clears thought processes. Sandalwood oil strengthens your resolve during times of emotional turmoil, and allows you to accept reality while enjoying your many blessings. As an aphrodisiac, sandalwood oil helps overcome frigidity and impotence while raising lovemaking to a spiritual realm.

HYDROSOL USES

Sandalwood hydrosol is an emotional equalizer that is also useful for urinary tract infections. Used in skin care, it benefits mature or aged skin, acne, broken capillaries, and skin disorders such as eczema and psoriasis. It can be applied as a skin spray, facial toner, or aftershave lotion. Unfortunately, sandalwood hydrosol is rarely available.

SPRUCE

Like a tall, thin pyramid, spruce rises from the forest floor reaching upward for sunlight. Beneath bristly, needlelike blue-green leaves, wispy branches terminate in coppery cones. Its reddish-brown trunk grows from twelve to eighteen inches annually until it attains a height of about thirty-five feet. At maturity, *Picea mariana* or *Picea negra* has a spread of only ten feet.

This hardy evergreen in the *Pinaceae* family tolerates the cold, wet climate of northern North America. It appears in Canada from the Atlantic coast to the Pacific coast, in some of the northern states of the continental United States, and in Alaska, Labrador, and Newfoundland.

Harvesting of the leaves occur between January and April, when essential oil levels are highest. Branches that bask in the sun yield more oil than ones confined to the dense forest. The twenty-five-year-old trees produce twice as much oil as those forty-five years or older.

Botanists believe that this narrow, sparse specimen is not as beautiful nor as ornamental as many of its conifer cousins—cedars, firs, pines, and other spruces. Whatever spruce lacks in looks, it compensates for in the healing qualities of its essential oil. Spruce oil smells sweet and soft, warm and inviting, like an evergreen forest that wants to envelop, protect, and bring you back into balance. Spruce oil is similar in scent to fir or pine, yet much smoother and milder. It is crystal clear in color.

FOLKLORE AND HERBAL HERITAGE

Native Americans chewed the balsam of spruce as a chewing gum and spread spruce gum as caulking or glue. They ate the inner bark and young shoots for food. From strips of spruce they wove watertight baskets for storage, big baskets for cooking, and mats to sleep and eat on. They concocted ointment, salves, and lotions from spruce, honey, and alum to treat skin problems such as boils, burns, skin inflammation, sores, and wounds. Sprucewood powder reportedly kept their hair dark. They fashioned canoes from the bark and stitched them together with needles made from splinters of spruce.

Throughout history, spruce has contributed to folk remedies for a wide array of ailments. People used spruce to relieve the pain and inflammation of arthritis and rheumatism, and to ease headache. Respiratory problems such as congestion, cough, sore throat, and tuberculosis responded to treatment with spruce. It soothed digestive distresses such as diarrhea, dyspepsia, and stomachaches. Spruce resin, seeds, and shoots served as treatments for cancers, tumors, and ulcers.

Spruce saved many a sailor and pioneer from scurvy. They brewed spruce tea or beer and sipped it to ward off the dreaded disease brought on by a lack of vitamin C in the diet. One recipe for the beer combines extracts of spruce shoots and leaves with a sugary substance. In the seventeenth century, folks boiled the tops of spruce boughs in beer and drank the refreshing beverage. Captain James Cook carried spruce on his sailing voyages to prevent scurvy. Miners in the California gold rush of 1849 also took spruce tea to prevent scurvy.

Leather tanners used spruce bark in preparing hides. Spruce resin was once used to hold together false teeth. The lumber industry valued spruce as a soft lumber that took a fine finish. Stringed instruments are sometimes shaped from spruce. It is a favorite miniature tree in bonsai gardening.

MEDICINAL USES

As a tonic, spruce improves many functions of the body. It stimulates and fortifies the immune system. It regulates hormones and tones the endocrine system, which controls all the glands. Its hormone-mimicking action helps reestablish balance, especially in the pituitary, thyroid, adrenal, and reproductive glands. It may help control some cases of hyperthyroidism. Spruce helps to stimulate or regulate the production of adrenaline to help the body deal with stress and "fight-or-flight" situations. External application over the kidneys helps to revive depleted or exhausted adrenal glands.

The antiseptic action of spruce oil relieves respiratory tract infections such as bronchitis and asthma. As an expectorant, it gently expels excess mucus. It soothes coughs. Spruce is stimulating and can improve circulation. It relieves inflammation and eases the pain of joint and muscle problems such as arthritis, backache, bursitis, carpal tunnel syndrome, rheumatism, and sciatica. It fights fatigue, including nervous exhaustion and chronic fatigue. It also has antifungal attributes that fight candidiasis.

BEAUTY BENEFITS

Acne can benefit from the skin-stimulating, antibacterial, and hormone-balancing actions of spruce. Spruce can also soothe other skin conditions, such as dermatitis, eczema, psoriasis, and seborrhea. It calms outbreaks triggered by hormonal imbalances, nerves, or stress. Because it fights fungi, spruce may help clear up fungal skin infections such as athlete's foot, facial candida, jock itch, and fingernail fungi. It improves skin tone and accelerates cell renewal. It reduces cellulite by encouraging waste removal and improving circulation. The refreshing scent of spruce makes a welcome and uplifting addition to perfume.

EMOTIONAL EFFECTS

Spruce promotes happiness and diminishes sadness. It revives weary emotions and gives a fresher outlook. It can regulate energy and restore equilibrium, even in cases of mood swings. It enhances memory functions. Spruce can help to release emotional blocks and to restore a sense of emotional balance. It is uplifting, liberating, and stimulating to the psyche. Spruce aids meditation and deepens spirituality.

HYDROSOL USES

Spruce hydrosol is an adrenal tonic, mental stimulant, and immune stimulant. It is helpful for relieving inflammation and pain of the joints and muscles, carpal tunnel syndrome, back pain, and insect bites. It can be used as a skin spray or aftershave.

TEA TREE

The swampy, flood-prone marshlands in the subtropical coastal areas of northeastern

New South Wales and southeastern Queensland, Australia, provide the perfect climate and growing conditions for tea trees, also called paper bark trees. Feathery bright-green leaves cover the branches of these small trees, which at maturity rarely reach more than twenty feet in height. Clusters of yellow flowers sometimes embellish these trees.

Of the 300 varieties of tea trees, one variety, *Melaleuca alternifolia,* produces the tea tree oil that is most commonly used for aromatherapy. Australian scientists are currently researching the therapeutic properties of essential oils from other tea trees. All tea trees are members of the *Myrtaceae* family.

Distilling the needlelike tea tree leaves yields a colorless or pale-yellow oil with a characteristic camphorlike odor. The aroma is spicy, strong, and pungent. It smells similar to its aromatic relative, eucalyptus.

FOLKLORE AND HERBAL HERITAGE

For centuries, Australia's Bundjalung aborigines have applied poultices of tea tree leaves to cuts, wounds, and skin infections, and have inhaled crushed tea tree leaves to treat respiratory problems. The tree supposedly received its common name in the eighteenth century, when Captain James Cook, after drinking a refreshing herbal tea brewed from the leaves of these hardy, disease-resistant trees, christened it "tea tree."

Modern science first acknowledged tea tree oil's medicinal properties in 1925. Laboratory experiments showed that it was twelve times stronger than phenol (carbolic acid), then the standard for antiseptic compounds. In the 1920s, dentists and surgeons began using tea tree oil to disinfect wounds and incisions. It became a customary dental treatment for bleeding gums, gingivitis, and periodontal disease. Physicians prescribed it for cystitis, fungal infections, skin disorders, throat infections, and yeast infections. During World War II, Australian soldiers were issued first-aid kits containing tea tree oil. Medics poured the oil directly into wounds to disinfect them and speed healing without damaging the surrounding tissues. The Australian government regarded tea tree oil as such an important contribution to the war effort that it exempted from military duty any workers employed in producing it.

Prior to tea tree oil's current popularity, farmers tried unsuccessfully to destroy the trees, which they considered a nuisance. Tea trees exhibit extraordinary persistence; some authorities liken the tea tree's own powers of recovery to its strong immune-stimulating abilities. Today, people visit coves of coppery-colored water formed by the flooded wetlands surrounding tea trees, seeking therapeutic benefits from soaking in the oily secretions floating atop the water.

MEDICINAL USES

Australians call tea tree oil a "first-aid kit in a bottle." Their claims may sound far-fetched, but they are not. Tea tree oil exhibits a broad spectrum of uses. It is effective for the treatment of abscesses, acne, bites, blisters, burns, cuts, dandruff, skin disorders, and scalp problems. It cleanses and disinfects wounds and soothes and heals burns. Like its cousin, eucalyptus oil, tea tree oil aids respiratory ailments. It relieves the symptoms of asthma, bronchitis, colds, congestion, coughs, earaches, fevers, laryngitis, sinusitis, sore throats, tonsillitis, and whooping cough. It boosts immunity and reduces the incidence of colds, fevers, the flu, and other infectious illnesses.

Reproductive and urinary tract infections, such as vaginitis and cystitis, respond to tea tree oil. It fights fungal infections such as athlete's foot, candida infections, and jock itch, and helps heal cold sores, herpes outbreaks, and hemorrhoids. It relieves the itching, redness, and scaling of psoriasis, seborrhea, and eczema and other types of dermatitis. Tea tree oil improves oral hygiene and relieves gingivitis, mouth ulcers, periodontal disease, and toothaches. Because it is nontoxic and nonirritating and exhibits powerful action against bacteria, fungi, and viruses, it has attracted the attention of medical researchers. Tea tree oil can also help relieve some of the symptoms of chronic fatigue syndrome.

BEAUTY BENEFITS

Tea tree oil works well on a wide range of skin problems, including blemishes, rashes, and warts. Clinical studies in Australia have shown that tea tree oil rivals benzoyl peroxide for effectiveness in fighting acne, but without causing dryness, itching, stinging, burning, redness, or other side effects. Men can prevent skin irritation from shaving and the infection of ingrown hairs by applying tea tree oil after shaving. Tea tree oil also provides an effective treatment for fungal infection of the fingernails, an increasing problem that may be linked to the growing use of artificial fingernails.

EMOTIONAL EFFECTS

Tea tree oil can restore energy depleted by everyday stress. By reviving mental energy it can reduce or alleviate mental fatigue and exhaustion. It is calming and centering during times of emotional shock. By easing the depleting effects of emotional disorders such as anxiety, depression, panic, and stress, tea tree can raise immune function and increase response. Its multifaceted healing abilities promote positive attitude and increase confidence while releasing the feelings of victimization or doom that can accompany and aggravate chronic illness.

HYDROSOL USES

Tea tree hydrosol is antibacterial, antifungal, antiseptic, and antiviral. It can be used to fight all kinds of infection, including respiratory ailments, sinusitis, and fingernail fungus. It is also useful in first aid and oral hygiene, and as a gargle for sore throat. Tea tree hydrosol is beneficial for skin disorders such as acne.

PRECAUTIONS

Tea tree oil may be irritating to sensitive skin.

THYME

Thyme grows as a small, woody evergreen shrub with many branches that are covered with fragrant foliage. Common thyme, *Thymus vulgaris,* has tiny gray-green oval leaves and pink, lilac, or white flowers. *Thymus citriodoria,* or lemon thyme, has lemon-scented leaves and lavender-colored flowers. These perennial members of the *Lamiaceae* family grow about one foot tall. Native to Spain and other Mediterranean countries, thyme is now cultivated in Algeria, central Europe, China, Israel, Russia, Turkey, Tunisia, and the United States.

The fresh or partially dried leaves and flowering tops of the plant are steam-distilled to produce thyme oil. The first distillation yields red thyme oil, which is red, brown, or orange in color and has an intense warm and spicy smell. Further distilling renders white thyme oil, a clear or pale-yellow oil with a sweet, fresh, and mild green aroma. White thyme oil contains fewer irritants than red thyme oil. There are several different *chemotypes* of the thyme plant. Chemotypes are plants that, although similar in appearance, produce essential oils with different chemical compositions. These chemotypes produce oils with different therapeutic properties. Some of these, such as *thymus vulgaris citral, thymus vulgaris geraniol,* and *thymus vulgaris linalool,* are less irritating than common thyme. France, Morocco, and Spain are primary producers of thyme oil, but Algeria, Germany, Greece, Israel, and the United States also produce it.

FOLKLORE AND HERBAL HERITAGE

Early inhabitants of Mediterranean countries used thyme for health and culinary purposes. Hippocrates, the ancient Greek physician known as the "Father of Medicine," spoke highly of thyme's healing properties. Thyme probably derives its name from one of two Greek words, either *thymos,* meaning "to fumigate" or "perfume," or *thymus,* meaning "courage."

According to Greek mythology, thyme developed from the teardrops of Helen of Troy. The Greeks created perfumes with thyme; they fumigated their houses with thyme to protect against infectious diseases. They also treated nervous disorders with it. They burned thyme incense at their altars to honor their gods. For millennia, thyme has enhanced foods with both its flavor and its digestive effects. Before refrigeration existed, thyme was added to meat to preserve it and prevent it from spoiling. The ancient Egyptians took advantage of thyme's preservative property in embalming.

In medieval Europe, sprigs of thyme were presented to chivalrous knights to reward them for courageous acts; judges carried thyme into their courtrooms for purification purposes. Sleeping on pillows stuffed with thyme reputedly relieved depression and epilepsy. Thyme was also supposed to cure leprosy, muscular atrophy, and paralysis. For centuries, herbalists treated colds, coughs, and sore throats with thyme. It combated the infection of many European plagues and served as a battlefield antiseptic during World War I.

MEDICINAL USES

The *British Herbal Pharmacopoeia* lists thyme as a remedy for asthma, bronchitis, diarrhea, dyspepsia, gastritis, laryngitis, and tonsillitis. European physicians use thyme oil to expel intestinal parasites. It combats infection and improves immunity by increasing the production of white blood cells. European physicians prescribe thyme oil for bronchitis, colds, coughs, the flu, laryngitis, sinusitis, sore throats, tonsillitis, and whooping cough. Lemon thyme oil is especially good for asthma and other respiratory conditions. Used in a mouthwash or gargle, thyme oil fights gum, mouth, and throat infections. It reduces the inflammation and irritation of skin disorders such as acne and psoriasis, as well as eczema and other types of dermatitis. It can accelerate the healing of bruises, burns, cuts, sores, and wounds. It makes an effective insect repellent and soothes the sting of insect bites.

Thyme oil helps to reduce some of the symptoms of chronic fatigue syndrome. It counteracts general sluggishness, making it particularly valuable in convalescence. It restores energy depleted by physical fatigue or exhaustion. It also stimulates the appetite and expels gas. Thyme oil reduces fluid retention and helps with obesity, premenstrual syndrome (PMS), and edema. A thyme sitz bath relieves the discomforts of cystitis or urethritis.

Thyme oil stimulates menstrual flow. It increases circulation and can elevate low blood pressure. It relieves the pain of arthritis, sore muscles, sprains, and injuries, and it can ease the pain of headaches, including migraines. Thyme oil also helps fight athlete's foot and jock itch.

BEAUTY BENEFITS

Thyme oil increases circulation to the skin and helps to improve sluggishness and to regulate oily skin. Thyme also encourages the elimination of wastes that contribute to cellulite.

EMOTIONAL EFFECTS

Thyme oil can strengthen your nerves when you are experiencing emotional fatigue. It eases nervousness, stress, and some stress-related complaints. It can reduce the severity or frequency of anxiety attacks. It enhances memory and increases concentration. Thyme oil is stimulating, although when used in a bath, it helps overcome insomnia. It can balance you, either keeping you alert or helping you to sleep. By promoting confidence, courage, and ambition, thyme can counteract fear, despondency, pessimism, and self-doubt.

HYDROSOL USES

Thyme hydrosol is an antiseptic, antiviral, digestive aid, intestinal cleaner, and immune stimulant. It is useful for fungal infections such as candidiasis, respiratory ailments, and skin problems such as acne. It is also used in first aid and oral hygiene and as a gargle for sore throat.

PRECAUTIONS

Thyme oil can irritate or sensitize skin and mucous membranes. Because it can stimulate menstrual flow, it should be avoided during pregnancy. People with hyperthyroidism or high blood pressure should avoid using this essential oil.

VALERIAN

Tiny pink or lilac flowers cluster atop feathery groups of narrow, dark, toothed leaves. The sharp scent of the earth infuses every part of the valerian plant, particularly the roots. Steam distillation of dried valerian roots renders a golden essential oil with a fresh and penetrating odor of damp earth.

Native to Europe and northern and western Asia, *Valeriana officinalis* belongs to the *Valerianaceae* family. This herb reaches a height of about three feet. Sites of commercial cultivation include Belgium, China, France, Hungary, Japan, Poland, and Russia. In the northern United States and parts of Canada, valerian grows in damp woods, meadows, and other habitats with partial shade.

FOLKLORE AND HERBAL HERITAGE

Throughout the ages, valerian has known numerous names: all-heal, amantilla, an accommodating disposition, bouncing Betty, blessed herb, capon's tail, charity, finger grass, kiss-me-quick, good neighbor, great wild valerian, poor man's remedy, setawale, and setwall. The word derives from the Latin *valere*, meaning "to be in health," and *valor*, meaning "courage." Some speculate that the Greek physicians Galen and Dioscorides named the herb *phu* to describe their opinion of its odor.

Hippocrates wrote about and recommended valerian. The plant served as a strong sedative that induced sleep, calmed nervous afflictions, and overcame hysteria. It relieved headaches and even migraines with its ability to relax muscles and sedate nerves. Often, herbalists recommended it to soothe stomachaches and aid digestion.

In pagan times, people added valerian to various kinds of potions as a mystic herb. Poor rural workers relied upon it for a variety of conditions, which earned it the names *poor man's remedy* and *all-heal*. In the Middle Ages, cooks simmered the leaves and roots in stews, soups, and other dishes to impart flavor and add nutrients. Housewives placed dried roots in drawers and closets to scent clothing.

Historically, valerian has been praised for its powerful action as a tranquilizer. Chinese, Nordic, and Persian herbalists have prescribed the root for centuries. In the fourteenth century, would-be fighters drank valerian juice to restore peace and dissipate animosity; it probably prevented many broken bones and bloody brawls. Reputedly, valerian could restore affection between man and woman, earning it the nickname of *accommodating disposition*. Valerian was dedicated to St. Benedict.

Legend suggests that the Pied Piper of Hamelin enticed rodents out of the town by toting valerian root while he played his flute as a decoy. In the seventeenth and eighteenth centuries, people suffering from insomnia and muscle spasms regularly sought relief from valerian. One nineteenth-century English physician noticed that cats liked it, often preferring it to catnip. He began rating the quality of his valerian roots according to which ones the cats most favored.

In World War I and World War II, weary soldiers received valerian to treat shell shock and nervous exhaustion. The U.S. Pharmacopoeia named valerian as an official remedy from 1820 to 1936. From 1888 to 1946, the U.S. National Formulary recognized it as a tranquilizer. Pharmacies sold tincture of valerian until the late 1970s. The U.S. government accepts the essential oils as a GRAS (generally recognized as safe) food ingredient for flavoring processed foods. Valerian flavors certain tobacco blends and is sometimes used as an ingredient in perfumery.

MEDICINAL USES

Nervous conditions such as nervous tension, nervous indigestion, nervous headaches, and restlessness respond to valerian's soothing and settling influence. European studies show that valerian can sedate the central nervous system. It fortifies the entire nervous system, reviving frazzled nerves and releasing tension. Valerian can relax the parasympathetic nervous system, thereby counteracting the stressful effects of the fight-or-fight response.

German pharmacists offer more than 100 remedies containing valerian and its derivatives. They sell teas and extracts as safe nighttime sleep aids to induce restful sleep without disturbing dreams or interfering with rising refreshed the following morning. Other over-the-counter valerian remedies ease agitation, excitation, and nervousness. Valerian diminishes the pain of headaches and even migraines. European doctors treat nervous heart conditions, high blood pressure, anorexia nervosa, trembling, and stomach complaints with valerian. For three decades, Germans have treated hyperactive children with valerian. Some people with learning disabilities experience improved muscle coordination after taking valerian.

Valerian possesses powerful antispasmodic properties that soothe cramping of the intestines and stomach, menstrual cramps, and strained muscles. Applied topically, it eases pain and relaxes muscle spasms and decreases the distress of joint pains associated with arthritis and rheumatism. As an antidiuretic, valerian may help people who suffer from incontinence. It also relieves irritable bowel syndrome and may expel worms and intestinal parasites.

BEAUTY BENEFITS

When added to facial massage oils, valerian can release tension and tightness in facial muscles that detract from the appearance and that contribute to muscle spasms, frowning, and temporomandibular joint (TMJ) syndrome. Some people claim that it can rid the scalp of dandruff. Frequently used for perfumes in India and the Far East, and in some Western blends, valerian imparts an enduring, earthy quality to fragrances.

EMOTIONAL EFFECTS

Valerian is a strong sedative that can soothe and restore balance in cases of anxiety, hysteria, panic, shock, and trauma. As a tonic to the entire nervous system, it eases nervousness. It can reestablish emotional equilibrium following any upset or distress. Valerian accelerates recuperation from nervous exhaustion and emotional fatigue.

Valerian can calm and bring focus. It minimizes feelings of aggression, anger, and fear. When you feel restless, fearful, or anxious, valerian can help you to detach, assess the situation, and gain new perspective so you can better cope with the circumstances. Valerian imparts a sense of peace to your personality, relieves agitation, and restores confidence. It helps hyperactivity. By calming and relaxing you, it helps you sleep soundly.

PRECAUTIONS

The essential oil of valerian is very potent. Use minute amounts only—1 drop of valerian in 1 ounce of carrier oil is sufficient. Large doses can produce headaches, mental agitation, and delusion. Do not use it during pregnancy. Headaches, muscle spasms, and heart palpitations can occur after prolonged use or large doses.

VETIVER

Tall and tufted, vetiver grass has long, narrow aromatic leaves and straight stems. This perennial member of the *Poaceae* family is related to citronella and lemongrass and grows up to six feet tall. Washed and dried vetiver roots are steam-distilled to produce an amber or dark-brown oil with a viscous texture. It smells smoky and woody, earthy and musty, like a damp forest after heavy rainfall. It also has sweet and spicy undertones. About 200 pounds of vetiver roots yields about 1 pound of oil. The older the root, the better the oil; the oil itself also improves with age.

Vetiver, *Vetiveria zizanoides, Vetiveria odorata,* or *Andropogon muricatus,* is native to India, Indonesia, and Sri Lanka. It grows wild in the tropical climates of Haiti, India, Java, and Tahiti. Today, China, the Comoro Islands, Indonesia, Japan, Malaysia, the Philippines, and Réunion Island, and countries in South America, western

Africa, and the West Indies cultivate vetiver commercially. Most of the vetiver oil used in aromatherapy comes from Java, Haiti, and Réunion. Many people consider vetiver oil from Réunion to be the best.

FOLKLORE AND HERBAL HERITAGE

Since antiquity, many civilizations have regarded vetiver as a fine fragrance. Its calming action earned it the name "oil of tranquility" in India and Sri Lanka. East Indian peoples constructed awnings, called *tatties,* and sunshades from vetiver grass, which is also known as *khus khus.* They hung these shades to keep homes cool, to deter insects, and, when wetted down, to emit an enticing aroma. Javanese servants waved ceremonial fans of woven vetiver to cool their rulers. Ancient Indians also used vetiver fans. When ships brought vetiver to Louisiana, Creole belles quickly adopted this practice.

In India and Russia, sachets commonly contained vetiver roots. Because vetiver repels moths, it is also known as "moth root." People in tropical climates weave the roots and leaves into thatched roofs and huts. In many areas of the world, farmers and conservationists plant vetiver to counteract soil erosion; the plant's root system extends deep into the earth. Barriers of vetiver grass can halt landslides.

Many perfumes have contained vetiver. One of these was the famous Mousseline des Indes, named for the scent of Indian muslin; the Indians protected the cloth from

insects with vetiver. Today, it adds an earthy, mossy note to approximately one-third of all Western perfumes and one-fifth of men's fragrances.

MEDICINAL USES

Vetiver oil stimulates the production of red blood cells, which transport oxygen throughout the body. This improves circulation and immunity. Vetiver oil relives the muscular aches, pains, spasms, and stiff joints of arthritis, rheumatism, sprains, and strains.

Vetiver oil calms nervousness, regulates appetite, and has proven helpful with anorexia nervosa. It is a natural tranquilizer and helps to calm hyperactivity and induce restful sleep. It also helps to balance female hormones and to tone the reproductive organs. Because of its ability to induce relaxation, it may help overcome sexual dysfunction that is caused by nerves or stress. As a glandular tonic, it adjusts imbalances of progesterone and estrogen, relieving symptoms of menopause and premenstrual syndrome (PMS).

BEAUTY BENEFITS

Vetiver oil balances the activity of the sebaceous glands, or oil glands, and helps to normalize oily skin and clear acne. It replenishes moisture in dry and dehydrated skin. Because it strengthens connective tissue of the skin, vetiver has a rejuvenating effect on the complexion, particularly mature skin. It helps heal cuts and wounds and soothes irritated and inflamed skin. When used regularly during pregnancy, vetiver oil reportedly prevents stretch marks. It also has natural deodorizing properties.

EMOTIONAL EFFECTS

Vetiver oil strengthens the central nervous system. It is emotionally calming and is helpful in overcoming depression, insomnia, and nervousness. Vetiver oil reduces anxiety, stress, and tension by calming the mind. It settles nerves and can revive a person who is suffering from emotional exhaustion. As a root oil, vetiver comes from the earth. It helps reestablish a connection to the earth, nature, the planet, and the universe by bestowing a sense of belonging. It integrates spirituality with materialism, restores balance and harmony, brings thoughts and actions into focus, and helps to stabilize mental and physical energy. It normalizes either extreme sensitivity or insensitivity. Some people use vetiver oil as an aphrodisiac.

VITEX

Pyramids of flowers thrust forth from fans of fragrant leaves. Vitex's sweet-scented blossoms range in hue from white to pink to lilac to deep blue. Its leaves are long, dark ovals with wavy edges. Small grayish fruits mature in autumn. Enclosed within are seeds. Vitex comes from the chaste tree, which is a beautiful and hardy deciduous tree that reaches heights of up to twenty-five feet. It is indigenous to western Asia and was introduced to Europe in the sixteenth century. Commercial crops come from Albania, Crete, Morocco, and Turkey.

Steam distillation of *Vitex agnus-castus,* a member of the *Verbenaceae* family, produces two essential oils. One is from the seed, the other from the leaf. Both are golden yellow. Their clean, penetrating scents are warm and woody, spicy and slightly sweet, with a hint of mint. Their properties vary slightly; the leaf oil produces more pronounced and positive effects.

FOLKLORE AND HERBAL HERITAGE

Origins of the names *chaste tree* and *Vitex agnus-castus* vary. In Latin, *vitex* comes from *viere,* which means "to bind," a reference to its flexible branches. *Agnus* means "lamb"; *castus* means "chaste." The Greek word *agnos* means "purity." Common names include Abraham's balm, chaste lamb tree, and safe tree.

Since antiquity, the chaste tree has been associated with women. The Greek goddess Hera, the wife of Zeus and the protector of marriages, supposedly sprang to life beneath a chaste tree. Ancient Greek women honored the goddess Demeter by spreading the leaves and berries on their beds during the feast of Thesmophoria. Vestal virgins in Rome carried boughs of chaste tree to declare their chastity.

More than two thousand years ago, Hippocrates recommended chaste tree berries for female complaints. He also suggested this remedy for relieving the pain of injuries, various inflammations, and enlargement of the spleen. The Roman scholar Pliny the Elder praised chaste tree as a most useful and versatile plant. In his medical manual *De Materia Medica,* the Greek physician Dioscorides wrote of the chaste tree's benefits for gynecological problems—to balance hormones, to ease inflammation of the womb, to relieve heavy menstrual flow and cramps, to release retained water, to resolve chronic menstrual troubles, and to encourage menstrual flow. Since then, chaste tree has enjoyed continuous use for easing female troubles, balancing hormones, and stimulating the flow of mother's milk.

Ancient Greeks believed that vitex was an anaphrodisiac. Monks reputedly sought out the seeds and berries when feeling weak of the flesh. In fact, one of its names is Monk's pepper tree. People also drank the tea to cleanse their intestines, soothe hemorrhoids, and relieve headache. The thirteenth-century Persian *Materia Medica* recommended chaste tree to treat insanity, madness, and epilepsy.

In medieval Europe, vitex continued to be a symbol of chastity. Novices entering convents or monasteries stepped upon and crushed the strewn chaste tree branches. In Europe, herbalists gave chaste tree tea to soothe joint and muscular aches and pains of rheumatism and arthritis. Those sick with colds or flu drank the tea. People ate the fruits to aid digestion. By the eighteenth century, the medical establishment recognized that chaste tree could not save the clergy from sexual seductions. Probably the herb balanced sexual desire more than extinguished it. In the nineteenth century, medicine used tincture of chaste tree berries to promote lactation and to reduce menstrual problems and irregularities. Basket makers wove the chaste twigs into containers. The small, spicy fruits were substituted for pepper and were called Indian spice and wild pepper.

MEDICINAL USES

Vitex is experiencing renewed popularity. For more than two thousand years, vitex has given women relief from menstrual difficulties, menopause, and other feminine complaints. The pituitary gland secretes progesterone and estrogen according to signals from the brain and other areas of the body. Chaste tree regulates and tones the female reproductive system through its action on the pituitary. Scientists have not isolated any one component within the plant that accounts for its remarkable effects on women; most likely the synergy of the components acting together is responsible for its actions.

By restoring balance of hormonal secretions, vitex can prevent many of the problems associated with premenstrual syndrome (PMS), including bloating, breast tenderness, depression, digestive difficulties, irritability, mood swings, nervousness, weight gain, and skin breakouts and disorders. It can also subdue many menstrual difficulties, such as backache, cramps, headaches, heavy or painful periods, and menstrual irregularity. Vitex restores ovarian function. It helps to bring the body back into hormonal balance after discontinuing birth-control pills.

During menopause, you can use vitex to soothe or avert many distressing symptoms, such as confusion, depression, hot flashes, irregularity, irritability, and nervousness. It can make the transition through menopause smoother. Vitex can help you avoid the guesswork of hormone replacement therapy (HRT), with which it often takes time, money, and patience to find the right medication in the right amount to relieve symptoms without creating severe side effects. Vitex offers a safe, natural way to balance your hormones at the source of their secretion—the pituitary gland. Instead of supplementing your body with synthetic hormones that can make symptoms worse and produce intolerable side effects, you can regulate hormone secretion so that you produce the perfect balance— for you—of estrogen and progesterone. Vitex offers a safe alterative to HRT, especially if the side effects of taking synthetic hormones exceed the discomfort of the original menopausal complaints.

Some researchers speculate that an imbalance or an overproduction of estrogen may lead to serious female disorders such as endometriosis, osteoporosis, and breast cancer. Women using vitex have reported positive changes in fibroid cysts and endometriosis.

For PMS or menopause, some women take 1 drop in a gelatin capsule orally once daily. Others prefer inhaling the pure oil, undiluted, directly from the bottle several times daily, or as needed, to avert menstrual cramps, hot flashes, depression, and anxiety. You can also prepare a body or massage oil and apply it topically.

Men too can benefit from vitex. Besides the obvious implications of restoring the emotional harmony, peace, and sense of stability in women in their lives who use vitex to regulate menstrual cycles and fluctuations in hormone levels, men can use vitex to allay sexual problems such as performance anxiety. Some men report that it helps prevent premature ejaculation. It may also help balance hormone levels in both men and women.

BEAUTY BENEFITS

Vitex can reduce breakouts of blemishes and acne due to its ability to balance hormones. It can exert an equalizing effect on skin problems caused by the overproduction of sebum, or oil, which is frequently due to hormonal imbalances. It may soothe the symptoms of seborrhea caused by overactivity of the oil glands as a direct response to hormonal imbalance.

EMOTIONAL EFFECTS

For women, vitex is calming, relaxing, and settling to the nerves, to the emotions, and to the spirit. By helping to bring your hormones back into balance, vitex helps you experience a new freedom to enjoy being female. It helps decrease depression, anxiety, and anguish brought on by hormonal irregularities, premenstrual syndrome, menstrual difficulties, and the transition of menopause.

In general, vitex can help in times of change to guide you through traumatic transitions into positive transformations. Because of its association with and assistance to females, vitex is a naturally nurturing oil. It can increase concentration and direct your focus. Sniff it directly from the bottle to avert anxiety or panic attacks.

YLANG YLANG

Tall and willowy, the majestic ylang ylang, or perfume, tree displays clusters of large star-shaped flowers on downward drooping branches. These unusual flowers range in color from white to pink to yellow to yellowish green. Their fragrance is fresh and floral, sweet and seductive, exciting and exotic. This refreshing scent is relaxing, almost intoxicating.

Shortly after sunrise in either early summer or autumn, workers gather ylang ylang blossoms. Immediately afterward, they begin the steam distillation process, which lasts several days. About 50 pounds of fresh-picked flowers yields 1 pound of ylang ylang oil.

Ylang ylang *(Cananga odorata,* var. *genuina),* is a subspecies of cananga *(Cananga odorata).* Both are members of the *Annonaceae* family, and both yield essential oils. Ylang ylang oil, however, is far superior to cananga oil. Also known as *poor man's jasmine,* ylang ylang flowers can produce six different grades of syrupy yellowish oil. Experts contend that the yellow flowers produce the best oil. Whole ylang ylang oil is most desirable for aromatherapy purposes. The perfume industry purchases some of the finest quality ylang ylang oil, which it includes in small amounts in some expensive scents. Cosmetic manufacturers utilize the lower grade ylang ylang oil or cananga oil.

Originally native to Southeast Asia and the Philippines, the "flower of flowers"— the Malay meaning of *ylang ylang*—now thrives throughout the tropics. Blossoms of trees growing in the wild produce little fragrance, but when the trees are carefully tended, their scent intensifies. Ylang ylang is cultivated commercially in the Comoro Islands, Haiti, Java, Sumatra, and Zanzibar.

FOLKLORE AND HERBAL HERITAGE

In tropical climates, leis strung with ylang ylang flowers were worn around the neck. In Indonesia, ylang ylang flowers covered the marriage beds of newlyweds. This tradition probably stems from its use as an aphrodisiac and sexual stimulant. For centuries, people in tropical cultures have scented coconut oil with ylang ylang for its beautifying benefits in skin treatments. They also smoothed it over their skin to soothe insect bites.

Tropical women—famous for their thick, shiny, lustrous hair—have used ylang ylang in hair preparations for hundreds of years. Ylang ylang reputedly helps control split ends. During the Victorian era, a hair treatment called Macassar oil contained ylang ylang. This preparation supposedly promoted hair growth by stimulating the scalp. In Samoa and Tonga, indigenous cultures used ylang ylang to treat colic, constipation, indigestion, and stomachaches. Throughout the tropics, many people have regulated their respiration and heart rates with ylang ylang.

MEDICINAL USES

In Europe, aromatherapists, massage therapists, and medical professionals prescribe ylang ylang to lower blood pressure, regulate respiration, and calm heart palpitations. They say that ylang ylang is soothing to the nervous system. Because it eases muscle spasms and relaxes tense muscles, it provides relief for backache, sciatica, and TMJ syndrome. In England, some people with epilepsy sniff ylang ylang oil to avert attacks or to bring seizures under control. Studies indicate that it may benefit certain cases of diabetes. Ylang ylang oil is often helpful in treating female disorders such as irregular periods, menstrual cramps, and premenstrual syndrome (PMS). It calms and comforts women going through menopause. It

also soothes the inflammation and irritation of psoriasis, eczema, and other types of dermatitis.

BEAUTY BENEFITS

Ylang ylang oil benefits any type of skin but is especially effective in treating oily skin because it balances oil production and reduces excessive oiliness. By fighting bacterial infection, it helps control acne and blemishes. Ylang ylang oil softens and smoothes skin and stimulates new cell growth. It reportedly can ward off wrinkles and premature aging because it relaxes facial muscles and releases facial tension that can contribute to lines, wrinkles, and sagging skin.

EMOTIONAL EFFECTS

European psychotherapists treat depression, emotional exhaustion, insomnia, and nervous tension with ylang ylang oil. It relaxes and calms excited emotional states. Ylang ylang oil subdues anxiety, stress, and stress-related disorders. It reduces worrying and tension and stabilizes moods. It minimizes aggressive behavior, anger, fear, and frustration, while fostering feelings of confidence, love, security, and serenity. It stimulates enthusiasm and can provide comfort during times of change. Ylang ylang oil encourages positive emotions and feelings, helping to improve harmony and confidence. It awakens an appreciation of self and others, as well as of the beauty of life. It helps you attract and recognize enjoyable experiences and pleasure in your everyday life. It inspires creativity, intuition, and understanding, and helps both men and women to enjoy their feminine qualities. Some European medical and psychological professionals recommend ylang ylang oil for sexual difficulties such as frigidity, impotence, and feelings of sexual inadequacy, especially when these problems stem from stress. Ylang ylang oil arouses sensuality, creates erotic and euphoric moods, and induces deep relaxation.

Part Three

WAYS TO USE AROMATHERAPY

Introduction

✳

You can *introduce aromatherapy and its many benefits into your life in a variety of ways—in baths, hair care, massages, personal fragrances, skin care, and many other forms. Aromatherapy can help you deal with emotional and physical problems, enhance the appearance of your skin and body, and freshen your home and office.*

This part of the book describes many different ways in which you can use aromatherapy. It will help you determine what might work best for your particular condition and for your lifestyle. Be willing to experiment. You'll have fun, and you'll reap many of the rewards that aromatherapy offers. The possibilities are limited only by your imagination and your willingness to explore the wide world of aromatherapy.

Essential Oil Guidelines at a Glance

To ensure that you obtain the best possible results from using essential oils, always keep in mind the guidelines below. These apply whether you are using the aromatherapy blends suggested in this book or experimenting with essential oils on your own.

- Use only pure essential oils.
- Less is plenty. When in doubt, use less, not more.
- Always dilute essential oils before applying them to your skin.
- When using an essential oil, open the bottle, dispense the oil, and close the lid quickly.
- Cap essential oil bottles tightly. Essential oils evaporate rapidly.
- Follow the directions for formulas exactly.
- Use glass bottles for undiluted essential oils.
- Put carrier oil or water into a plastic container before adding essential oils.
- When making a blend with essential oils, *gently* roll the bottle. Don't shake it.
- Mix up only small quantities of aromatherapy blends—the essential oils with the carrier oil—at any one time, since carrier oils can go rancid quickly. If you want to make bigger batches of the essential oil combinations only, you can, but be sure to use the same proportions of essential oils. For example, if you want to increase a formula by ten times, multiply the number of drops of each essential oil in the formula by ten. Thus, if the original formula states 3 drops of marjoram, 2 drops of chamomile, and 1 drop of thyme oil, you would use 30 drops of marjoram, 20 drops of chamomile, and 10 drops of thyme oil for the larger batch. Then, whenever you want to use the essential oils, you can add about 6 drops of the blend to 1 ounce of carrier oil. (Note that valerian oil is an exception to this rule—it is so powerful that 1 to 3 drops in a formula is adequate.)
- Inhale essential oils briefly, for a few seconds.
- Diffuse oils for only five to ten minutes at a time.
- Trust your instincts. If you dislike the smell of a certain oil, don't use it.
- Apply essential oils externally *only*.
- Discontinue using any oil that causes irritation, sensitivity, or an unpleasant reaction.
- Wash your hands immediately after using essential oils.
- Do not use essential oils near your eyes.

AIR FRESHENERS

Aromatherapy air fresheners can quickly fragrance your environment or create certain moods in your home or office. They can purify or cleanse the air in your home and remove unpleasant odors. They can also provide fast, effective relief for respiratory ailments or sinus congestion. Some aromatherapy air fresheners can help control germs and infections in sickrooms.

To make an aromatherapy air freshener, fill a spray bottle almost full with distilled water. Add 1 to 3 drops of the essential oil or oils of your choice for each ounce of water. Shake the bottle well to blend, and spray it around the room. Spray as often as you wish. Shake the bottle well before each use.

ATOMIZERS

An atomizer is a glass bottle with a metal sprayer that is operated by an attached rubber bulb. When you squeeze the bulb, it sends a fine cloud of essential oil through the sprayer and into the atmosphere. An atomizer provides a simple, convenient, and economical way to dispense room-freshening and mood-creating essential oils quickly into the atmosphere.

To use an atomizer, fill an atomizer bottle with the desired essential oil or mixture of oils. Mist your room, home, or office. You can use your atomizer as often as you wish. Any of the diffuser blends mentioned in Part Four will work fine in an atomizer.

BATHS

Plunging your body into a pool of warm water scented with soothing or energizing essential oils practically guarantees that you will step out feeling refreshed and rejuvenated. Surrendering your emotionally or physically depleted body and soul to an aromatherapy bath can restore and revitalize you. Let your worldly worries wash down the drain with the bathwater! You'll emerge feeling revived, ready to conquer your chores, dive into your deadlines, or simply slip between the sheets and sleep peacefully like a baby. Bathing regularly with essential oils helps to control stress, alleviate anxiety and tension, and ease muscular aches and pains.

To prepare an aromatherapy bath, add a total of 2 to 8 drops of an essential oil or oils to a bathtub filled with warm water. The amount of oil required depends on the essential oil you choose. Some oils, such as black pepper, eucalyptus, ginger, lemon, orange, peppermint, and thyme, can give the desired results with only 2 to 3 drops to a tub of water. If you are using a blend of several different oils, use no more than 8 drops total.

You can make your bathing experience even more enjoyable by running your diffuser, putting on some soothing music, and turning *off* the telephone before you sink into your aromatherapy bath.

If you are preparing a bath for an infant or child, first dilute the essential oil by blending 1 to 3 drops of essential oil in

1 ounce of carrier oil. Add 2 to 6 drops of the resulting diluted oil to the tub.

CLAY PACKS

Clay is a naturally detoxifying and cleansing substance that nourishes and softens skin. It contains many minerals, such as iron, magnesium, potassium, and zinc. It also can draw out impurities as it decreases swelling and inflammation. Clay improves circulation and promotes healing. Using clay packs can soothe sore muscles and aching joints, and relieve the swelling and inflammation of such conditions as arthritis, backache, carpal tunnel syndrome, muscular sprains and strains, sciatica, and TMJ syndrome. Clay packs can speed healing and help decrease congestion of asthma, colds, flu, sinusitis, and other respiratory problems. They can calm an upset stomach and ease cramps. They offer relief for acne, blemishes, insect bites, varicose veins, and skin disorders such as dermatitis, eczema, psoriasis, and seborrhea. You can find many different types of clay at herbal shops or health-food stores. Some favorites include bentonite, French green clay, fuller's earth, Kaolin, and Redmond clay.

To make a clay pack for a large area, in a large bowl, mix 1 cup of clay powder with approximately 1 cup of warm or hot water to form a smooth paste. Add 4 to 6 drops of an essential oil or blend of essential oils appropriate for the condition being treated. To make a clay pack for a small area, in a small bowl, combine 2 teaspoons of clay with about 1 teaspoon of warm or hot water. Add 1 or 2 drops of an essential oil. Spread the clay mixture over the area being treated and relax. You can cover it with a warm towel, if desired. When the clay dries, you can wash it off or soak in a tub of water to remove it.

COMPRESSES

Compresses are useful for relieving pain and reducing inflammation and swelling. They can also help cool fevers or eliminate chills. Both chronic and acute conditions respond to compresses.

Hot compresses relax muscles, reduce stiffness, ease aches and pains, and dilate blood vessels, increasing circulation to the treated area. Use hot compresses for chronic conditions and for abscesses, backaches, chills, earaches, and toothaches, as well as for flareups of arthritis or rheumatism.

Cold compresses reduce swelling and inflammation and cause blood vessels to contract, decreasing circulation to the treated area. Use cold compresses for acute conditions and fevers, headaches, inflamed and swollen conditions, and as first aid for sprains, tennis elbow, and other injuries.

To make a compress, pour 1 quart of either cold or hot water, depending on the condition you're treating, into a 2-quart glass bowl. Add 1 to 6 drops of an essential oil or an essential oil blend to the water. If you will be using the compress on an infant or child, add only 1 drop of essential oil. Soak a clean cloth in the water. Wring it out and apply the cloth to the affected area. You can wrap a towel or piece of plastic around the cloth to keep in the warmth or prevent the compress from dripping. If you are using a cold compress, you can apply an ice pack on top of the compress to make it more effective. Replace the compress with a fresh one every five to fifteen minutes, as needed.

DIFFUSERS AND LAMPS

A diffuser is a device that disperses minute molecules of essential oils throughout your room, home, or office. Most diffusers operate on electricity. They provide an almost effortless way of using aromatherapy. Simply add essential oils to the diffuser, plug it in, and within minutes you'll be breathing the fragrant aroma that is permeating your room. Use a diffuser to freshen the air, create a mood, fight infection from a cold or the flu, treat asthma or bronchitis, help you overcome emotional upsets, or simply enhance your well-being. Your choice of oils will determine the outcome.

To use most diffusers, you attach a bottle of essential oil, plug the diffuser in, and turn it on. Follow the directions that come with your diffuser. All of the diffuser blends mentioned in Part Four will work in any kind of diffuser.

Aromatherapy lamps have the same purpose as diffusers; they release minute molecules of essential oils into the air. A small bowl atop the lamp holds water and essential oils. Beneath the bowl is a heat source, either a candle or lightbulb that gently heats the water and essential oils and sends the aroma into the atmosphere.

To use an aromatherapy lamp, fill the bowl with water. Add 5 to 20 drops of an essential oil or essential oil blend. Turn on the electricity or light the candle and enjoy the sweet smell that wafts through your environment. The diffuser blends described in Part Four will work in lamps as well as in diffusers.

FACIAL STEAM BATHS

Facial steam baths are a delightful addition to your regular skin-care program. They are a wonderful way to deep-clean your pores and add moisture to your skin. They also increase the circulation to your face.

Facial steam baths are similar to steam inhalations, except that their purpose is to improve your complexion. Steaming your face once a week will help prevent blemishes and blackheads, keep your skin looking moist, and give your complexion a healthy glow.

To prepare a facial steam bath, pour about 1 quart of steaming water into a large (approximately 2-quart) glass bowl. Add 1 to 5 drops of an essential oil or combination of oils suitable for your skin type (see page 157). Hold your clean face over the bowl for five to ten minutes. To capture the steam, drape a towel over your head to create a "tent." Afterward, apply a cleanser, scrub, or mask to remove any impurities that the steaming released from your pores.

FOOT BATHS

A hot foot bath brings welcome relief to tired, aching feet. Foot baths are one of the best treatments for athlete's foot and foot odor. They improve circulation. They can also diminish the discomfort of a variety of non-foot-related ailments, such as colds and flu, cramps, insomnia, low blood pressure, poor circulation, respiratory problems, scant or late menstrual periods, and sinusitis. A cold foot bath can revive you on a sweltering summer day when you've begun to wilt. Aromatherapy foot baths also make a practical alternative for people who are ill or disabled, or who have difficulty getting into a full-sized bathtub.

To prepare an aromatherapy foot bath, add 1 to 6 drops of an essential oil or essential oil blend to a foot bath filled with water. If you are preparing a foot bath for a child, add only 1 or 2 drops of essential oil. Use hot or cold water, depending on the condition you're treating. If you do not have a foot bath, use a bowl or tub large enough to immerse the feet. Soak your feet for ten to fifteen minutes. Repeat the procedure as necessary.

HAIR CARE AND CREATING HAIR-CARE PRODUCTS

A healthy head of hair begins with a healthy scalp; essential oils can help improve the condition of your hair and scalp by stimulating circulation to your scalp. Aromatherapy hair-care treatments can make your hair shiny and healthy-looking.

Although commercial aromatherapy shampoos and conditioners flood the market, they probably contain very low levels of low-quality essential oils or no pure essential oils at all. In addition, mixing essential oils with synthetic chemicals of commercial cosmetics can create undesirable chemical changes in the essential oils, detracting from their therapeutic properties. The best way to assure that you're getting the essential oils you want at therapeutic levels is by making your own treatments.

The aromatherapy blends suggested under HAIR AND SCALP PROBLEMS in Part Four are easy to make and are effective. You can create your own scalp treatments to nourish your scalp and improve the condition of your hair.

The following are general guidelines to use for making your own customized hair-care products:

• *Hair-conditioning treatments.* Add 2 to 8 drops of an essential oil or blend of essential oils for your hair type or condition to 1 ounce of honey, clay, or vegetable oil such as coconut, hemp, olive, or jojoba oil. Mix well. Work the mixture into your hair and scalp and leave on for fifteen to thirty minutes. Shampoo as usual.

• *Scalp oil treatments.* Add 2 to 8 drops of an essential oil or blend of essential oils appropriate for your hair type or condition to 1 ounce of coconut, hemp, olive, or jojoba oil. Mix well. Massage enough of the mixture into your scalp and hair to saturate

TABLE 3.1 ESSENTIAL OILS FOR HAIR CARE

✳

This table lists essential oils that are known to be helpful for specific hair types or conditions. Use the recommendations here to help you choose which oil or oils you want to try in customized hair-care products. A detailed discussion of each of the individual essential oils listed here may be found in Part Two. Essential oils that are useful for more than one condition appear under each condition for which they are appropriate.

NORMAL HAIR	DRY HAIR	OILY HAIR	DANDRUFF	HAIR LOSS
Chamomile	Cedarwood	Bergamot	Cedarwood	Cedarwood
Lavender	Chamomile	Cedarwood	Clary sage	Clary sage
Thyme	Clary sage	Clary sage	Cypress	Rosemary
Ylang ylang	Lavender	Cypress	Lemon	Ylang ylang
	Rosemary	Juniper	Patchouli	
		Lavender	Pine	
		Lemon	Rosemary	
		Patchouli	Tea tree	
		Pine		
		Rosemary		
		Tea tree		
		Thyme		
		Ylang ylang		

them. Leave it on for fifteen to thirty minutes or overnight. Shampoo as usual. Scalp oil treatments are useful for nourishing dry hair or scalp, stimulating hair growth or preventing hair loss, controlling dandruff, and regulating seborrhea. You can also massage a few drops of a scalp oil treatment into your scalp or into the ends of clean wet hair instead of using a commercial hair conditioner.

• *Scalp tonics.* Add 2 to 8 drops of an essential oil or blend of essential oils appropriate for your hair type or condition to 1 ounce of apple cider vinegar, vodka, or pure grain alcohol. (*Do not* use isopropyl or rubbing alcohol.) Mix well. Massage the mixture into your scalp. You can make tonics to stimulate hair growth or prevent hair loss, to control dandruff or seborrhea, or to regulate oiliness.

To find out which essential oils are appropriate for your hair type or condition, consult Table 3.1.

HAND BATHS

Hand baths are a perfect way to slow down, relax, and treat almost any condition. They are great treatments for specific problems affecting the hands, such as arthritis, carpal tunnel syndrome, dermatitis, dry or chapped skin, fingernail fungus, muscle aches, rheumatism, sprains, tension, or tired hands that ache from overwork. Hand baths are a simple way to nurture yourself; there is something calming and settling about soaking your hands in a bath of water.

Cool hand baths can alleviate hot flashes, reduce fever, calm hyperactivity, and revive the body and mind from fatigue. Warm hand baths can warm a chill, relax a racing mind, and reduce symptoms of premenstrual syndrome (PMS).

To prepare an aromatherapy hand bath, add 1 to 3 drops of an essential oil or essential oil blend to a large bowl filled with 1 quart of water. Choose hot or cold water, depending on the condition you're treating. For a child, add only 1 or 2 drops of essential oil to the hand bath. Soak your hands for ten to fifteen minutes. To increase circulation and work out tension or soreness, wiggle your fingers back and forth. Repeat the procedure as necessary.

INHALANTS

Inhalants are essential oils that you breathe directly from the bottle. The aromatic molecules of the essential oils will waft up your nose, into your brain, and into your respiratory system. You'll feel a difference quickly.

Inhalants work well for asthma, allergies, colds and flu, emotional conditions, sinusitis, and stress. You can inhale any single oil or make an inhalant from any of the blends mentioned in Part Four. Diffuser blends will work as inhalants, too.

To make an inhalant, simply place your choice of essential oils in a small glass bottle that has an airtight cover. Blend the oils by gently turning the container upside down several times or rolling it between your hands. Do not shake vigorously. You can also use a single essential oil as an inhalant.

Depending on the condition you wish to treat, you can prepare an aromatherapy inhalant blend recommended in the appropriate entry in Part Four. Or, if no inhalant blend is suggested, choose two or three oils from the list of essential oils suggested for that condition and mix them together in a small bottle. To use the inhalant, simply open the bottle and inhale the aroma. You can also place 2 or 3 drops of the blend on a tissue or handkerchief and inhale it that way. You can carry an inhalant with you almost anywhere for a refreshing aromatherapy break.

Alternate nostril breathing is a technique that works especially well with inhalants. It balances your breathing, exercises both sides of your lungs, and stimulates both sides of your brain by directing your breath through one nostril at a time.

Sit upright in a comfortable position. Pay attention to your posture, uncross your legs and ankles, and do not slump. Inhale several times to clear your nostrils and become conscious of your breathing. Cover one nostril by gently capping it with the tip of a finger. Hold the bottle of essential oils below the open nostril. Slowly inhale the essential oils for a few seconds, to a count of eight. Hold in your breath for a few seconds, up to a count of eight. Move the bottle away from your nostrils. Exhale slowly to the count of eight. Change sides. Then repeat the entire procedure.

Variation 1: Inhale through one nostril and exhale through the other.

Variation 2: Inhale through one nostril to a count of four. While retaining the breath, continue inhaling through the other nostril to a count of four. Hold in both sides for a few seconds, up to a count of eight. Exhale slowly to the count of eight.

You can mentally direct your breath to the areas of your body that need healing energy. Imagine the energy of the essential oils infusing all your cells with balance and great health. Or you can simply relax and allow the energy to go where it will. Repeat throughout the day as needed.

Precautions: Do not breathe onto or exhale into the bottle. This can change the chemical composition of the oils and alter their therapeutic properties. Do not place the bottle on or inside your nostrils. Undiluted essential oils can burn or irritate skin. This can also contaminate the oils and compromise their quality and freshness.

MASSAGE

Incorporating essential oils into massage is a marvelous way to ease muscular aches and pains, subdue stress and tension, and treat a variety of conditions in a pleasant, relaxing way. Besides feeling great, massage can soothe the nervous system, reduce blood pressure, relax muscles, diminish swelling, and stimulate blood and lymphatic circulation. It also can release cellular wastes from your muscles, relax your breathing, and slow a racing pulse.

If you receive professional massages, take your aromatherapy massage oil blends for your therapist to use on you. You can also gain tremendous advantage from self-massage. Whether you massage deep into your own muscles or lightly spread the oils onto your skin, you will derive the benefits mentioned above.

To make your own massage and skin oils, add 3 to 8 drops of an essential oil or essential oil blend to 1 ounce of a carrier oil and blend well. Place several drops in your hand and apply the oil over your body as you massage. If you are preparing a blend for use on an infant or child, dilute 1 to 3 drops of essential oils in 1 ounce of carrier oil.

Use the massage movements described below whenever you give yourself a massage or apply skin oil over your body.

MASSAGING YOUR BODY

You can massage yourself every day when you apply your skin or massage oils. Massaging your body boosts your circulation, and the aromatherapy blends will help moisturize your skin and improve its appearance. Use either long, sweeping strokes or short, overlapping strokes. You can also make circular movements in an upward direction. You can knead an area, or you can tap it with your fingertips. When you massage your body, direct the strokes toward your heart (see Figure 3.1). Massage from your feet upward toward your head. Stroke your skin upward from your fingertips toward your heart. Make a clockwise circle over your abdomen.

In addition to giving yourself a whole-body massage, you can target specific areas of your body for aromatherapy massage treatment. If you are having a problem affecting one organ or system of the body, such as your lungs or respiratory system, you can massage an aromatherapy blend over the specific organ or along the entire system. Figure 3.2 will help you to see where the major organs and systems of the body are located.

For certain conditions, it can be beneficial to massage an aromatherapy blend over the affected organ or system of the body.

MASSAGING YOUR ABDOMEN

To give yourself an abdominal massage, move in a clockwise direction from your right side to your left. This follows the direction in which your large intestines eliminate wastes. Begin on your lower right

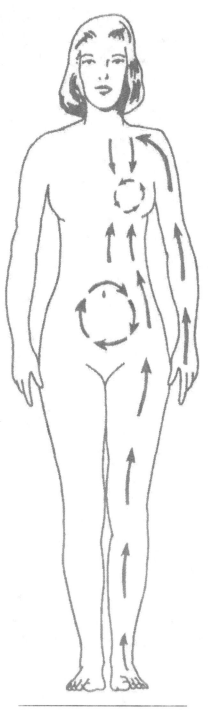

Figure 3.1 Massaging Your Body

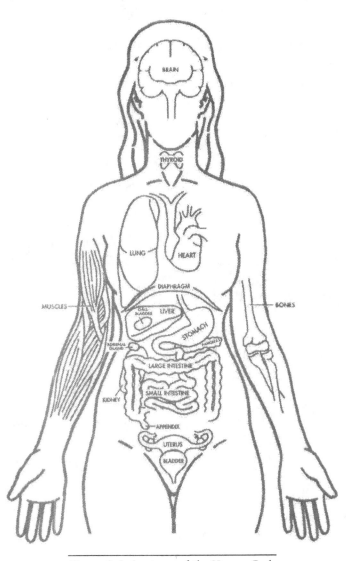

Figure 3.2 Anatomy of the Human Body

abdomen just above your upper right thigh. Stroke upward and across your abdomen above your navel. Continue downward to the left side of your abdomen above your left leg. You can continue in a circle, spiraling inward over your small intestines (see Figure 3.3).

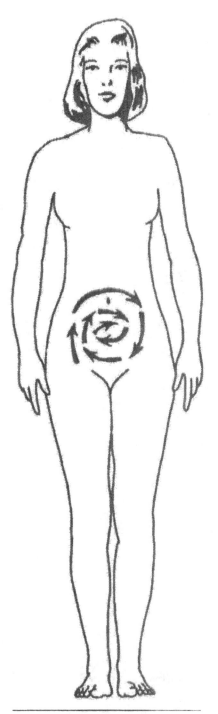

Figure 3.3 Massaging Your Abdomen

MASSAGING YOUR FACE

Massaging and touching your face properly can help counteract some of the effects of gravity and reduce facial tension. Facial massage also increases circulation to your skin and improves your complexion.

Always massage your skin gently, with upward motions, and use a facial oil to avoid stretching your skin. Figure 3.4 shows the basic direction of strokes for facial massage. Begin at the base of your neck and stroke upward toward your jawline. Make circles around your mouth. Stroke your cheeks diagonally: along your jawline; from the corner of your mouth to your ears; from the corner of your nose to your temples. Beginning on your upper eyelids, make a circle from the inner corners, across your lids, under your eyes, and finish near your tear ducts. Avoid getting oil in your eyes. Stroke your forehead upward into your hairline. Use these same movements any time you touch your facial skin.

MOUTHWASHES, GARGLES, AND GUM TREATMENTS

Aromatherapy oral hygiene products can help you maintain or improve the condition of your mouth and teeth. They fight bacteria and infections, strengthen your gums, and help protect against gum disease.

The aromatherapy blends suggested under GUM DISEASE in Part Four are easy to make and are effective oral hygiene products. If you wish to make your own mouthwash or gargle fresh each day, add

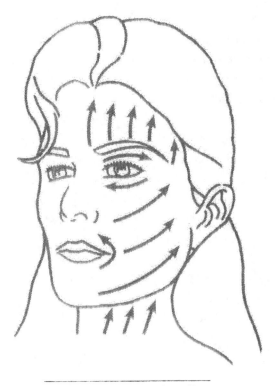

Figure 3.4 Massaging Your Face

1 or 2 drops of an essential oil to a 4-ounce glass of water and mix well. Gargle or swish the mixture around in your mouth. To blend your own gum treatment oil, add 2 to 6 drops of essential oils to ¼ ounce of a carrier oil and massage the mixture into your gums once or twice daily.

PERSONAL FRAGRANCES AND PERFUMES

You can easily create your own perfumes and fragrances with essential oils. Whatever your lifestyle, natural fragrances are a wonderful way of bringing aromatherapy into your daily life. Personal fragrances made with essential oils are not overpowering, as synthetic scents sometimes are. And unlike commercial fragrances, which are made almost exclusively of synthetic petrochemicals and can cause allergies and irritation, essential oils can be emotionally and physically therapeutic. These pleasing personal perfumes smell lovely, and they can enhance your physical and emotional well-being.

You can make fragrances as intense or subtle as you desire, depending on your choice of essential oils and the amount of each oil that you use.

The easiest way to create your own fragrance oils is to follow the formulas in this book, particularly the personal blends intended to influence the emotions that are listed under EMOTIONAL ISSUES in Part Four. You can also create your own blends by adding 2 to 10 drops of essential oils to ⅛ ounce of jojoba oil. Jojoba oil is the best carrier oil for fragrances; it does not become rancid, so it cannot spoil your perfume. To make cologne, add 1 to 10 drops of essential oils to 1 ounce of vodka or pure grain alcohol. Do not smell directly from the bottle. Apply to the skin and allow the alcohol to evaporate for thirty to sixty seconds. You will enjoy the aroma much more without the alcohol. Do not use isopropyl or rubbing alcohol with essential oils.

Never apply pure essential oils as fragrances directly to your skin. Always dilute them. Essential oils are highly concentrated and in their pure form can cause skin irritation.

SITZ BATHS

Sitz baths can relieve congestion, pain, and spasms that occur in the pelvic area. They can help with ailments of the lower abdominal area, the intestinal tract, the reproductive organs, and the urinary tract. Conditions that respond well to sitz baths include constipation, cystitis, hemorrhoids, menstrual cramps, poor circulation, scant or late menstrual periods, and prostate problems.

To prepare a sitz bath, add 5 to 10 drops of an essential oil or an essential oil blend to a sitz bath or a small tub filled with water. You can also fill your bathtub to hip level and prop your feet up on the sides of the tub so your hips are tilted upward. Sit hip-deep in the water for ten to thirty minutes. Slightly elevate your feet to enhance the effect of the treatment.

SKIN BRUSHING

Skin brushing increases circulation, helps the body to eliminate cellular wastes, and improves the appearance of the skin. You can dry-brush your skin, or you can first apply a few drops of an aromatherapy skin oil, body oil, massage oil, or skin-brushing oil. It is best to brush before bathing every day. Use a clean, firm natural-bristle brush.

Begin at your feet and stroke upward toward your heart (see Figure 3.5). Apply enough pressure to stimulate circulation, but not so much that it hurts you. Make circles around your knees and at the top of your thighs, where lymphatic tissue is located. Brush your abdomen in a circle that follows the direction of your intestines: Start from your lower right abdomen and move upward and across your abdomen above your navel; then continue downward along your left side. Circle around your breast or chest. Brush upward from your hands to your shoulders. Make circles around your shoulder joint, another site of lymphatic tissue. From the base of your neck, stroke downward to your heart. On

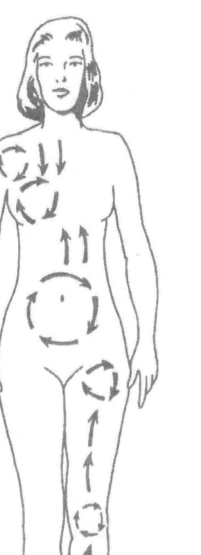

Figure 3.5 Brushing Your Skin

your back, stroke up and down along your spine.

SKIN CARE AND CREATING SKIN-CARE PRODUCTS

Skin care is one of the most popular applications of aromatherapy. With the increasing awareness of the benefits of good skin care, along with competition to get ahead in the workplace, both men and women today want to look their absolute best. In addition, the desire to feel more self-confident and to stay physically fit is prompting people to take better care of their skin.

Many essential oils can improve the condition of your skin by increasing circulation to the surface. Good circulation will impart a healthy, youthful glow to your complexion. Some essential oils have cell-regenerating properties that can give your skin a more youthful appearance. They also have a positive impact on your emotions that will show up on your skin. Essential oils have minute molecules that can easily penetrate your pores and can affect the condition of your skin from the inside out.

You can buy commercial aromatherapy skin-care products. However, I highly recommend that you make your own. Most ready-made aromatherapy products contain very low levels of essential oils, and some companies use synthetic oils instead of pure essential oils. The aromatherapy blends suggested under SKIN PROBLEMS AND SKIN CARE in Part Four are easy to make and are effective.

To determine the essential oils appropriate for your skin type or condition, consult Table 3.2. Following are some general guidelines for how to choose and blend ingredients to make your own custom natural cosmetics with essential oils.

• *Cleansers.* For cleansers, choose a base of clay (bentonite, French green clay, fuller's earth, or Redmond clay), oil (hazelnut, hemp, jojoba, olive, safflower, sesame, or sunflower oil), honey (raw and unfiltered), or yogurt (unsweetened and plain).

To 1 teaspoon of clay, honey, or yogurt, add 1 drop of essential oil. Blend with water as needed and massage into your skin.

To make an oil cleanser, you can add 3 to 6 drops of essential oil to 1 ounce of carrier oil. Blend well. Massage about ½ to 1 teaspoon into your skin. Blot off with a clean towel or splash off with water for a very moisturizing effect.

• *Facial toners.* Lavender, orange blossom, or rose hydrosols make the best toners. Or you can make essential oil water by adding 1 to 3 drops of an essential oil or oils of your choice to 8 ounces of water.

• *Facial scrubs.* You can use almost any kind of flour, finely ground seeds, finely ground nuts, or a combination of your choice. Some suitable choices are almond meal, buckwheat flour, cornmeal (blue is finer, yellow is coarser), flaxseed meal, garbanzo flour, hemp flour, oat flour or oatmeal, sunflower meal, or whole-wheat flour. You can blend a combination of the grains together and store in a clean, dry bottle or jar. Before each application, place ½ to 1 teaspoon of grains in the palm of your hand. Combine with enough water to make a paste. Add 1 or 2 drops of essential oil and mix well. Massage into your skin. Rinse thoroughly. For dry skin, add several drops of carrier oil to the scrub blend.

• *Moisturizers.* By applying your aromatherapy facial oil to moist or wet skin, you can create your own moisturizer—free of preservatives, colorings, fragrance, and dozens of other ingredients common in commercial moisture creams and lotions. You can adjust the oiliness and lubricating qualities of the oil by the proportions of oil and water you use. For dry skin, add more oil. For oilier skin, choose jojoba oil and use more water.

Prepare a blend of 1 ounce of your favorite carrier oil or oils, such as borage, hazelnut, hemp, jojoba, olive, sesame, or sunflower, ahead of time. Add a total of 3 to 8 drops of essential oils of your choice. Blend well.

After cleansing your skin, put several drops of your facial oil into the palm of your wet hand. Add a few drops of distilled water, hydrosol, or aromatherapy facial toner. Blend and apply to wet skin. Spray with water or add a few more drops of water and massage into your skin. For dry skin, splash your face with water, add a few drops of facial oil, splash your face again, then

TABLE 3.2 ESSENTIAL OILS FOR SKIN CARE

This table lists essential oils that are known to be helpful for specific skin types or conditions. Use the recommendations here to help you choose which oil or oils you want to try in customized skin-care products. A detailed discussion of each of the individual essential oils listed here may be found in Part Two. Essential oils that are useful for more than one condition appear under each condition for which they are appropriate.

NORMAL SKIN	DRY SKIN	OILY SKIN	MATURE SKIN	SENSITIVE SKIN
Cedarwood	Benzoin	Cedarwood	Elemi	Chamomile
Clary sage	Bergamot	Clary sage	Frankincense	Frankincense
Elemi	Cedarwood	Cypress	Geranium	Jasmine
Frankincense	Clary sage	Elemi	Helichrysum	Neroli
Geranium	Elemi	Frankincense	Jasmine	Rose
Jasmine	Fennel	Geranium	Lemon	Rosewood
Lavender	Frankincense	Jasmine	Myrrh	Sandalwood
Neroli	Geranium	Juniper	Neroli	
Palmarosa	Jasmine	Lemon	Palmarosa	
Patchouli	Lavender	Neroli	Rose	
Rose	Myrrh	Orange	Rosemary	
Rosemary	Neroli	Palmarosa	Sandalwood	
Rosewood	Palmarosa	Patchouli	Vetiver	
Sandalwood	Patchouli	Peppermint		
Vetiver	Rose	Rosemary		
	Rosemary	Rosewood		
	Rosewood	Sandalwood		
	Sandalwood	Tea tree		
	Vetiver	Thyme		
		Vetiver		
		Ylang ylang		

massage the oil into your wet skin. Don't dry your face. Instead, apply more facial oil as described above.

• *Facial masks.* Make your own facial masks from natural ingredients free of any chemicals, colorings, or preservatives. Clays, flours, honey, yogurt, or any combination of these ingredients will nourish and invigorate your skin while relaxing your mind. You can blend custom facial mask powder containing your choice of clays and flours such as garbanzo, oat, rice flour, or any other flour that has a fine texture. When you are ready to make a mask, put about ½ to 1 teaspoon of the powder blend into the palm of your hand. Add water, honey, yogurt, carrier oil, or any combination of these to form a paste. Add 1 or 2 drops of essential oil and blend. Apply to clean skin. Lie down and relax for fifteen minutes. Rinse. Moisturize as suggested above.

STEAM INHALATIONS

When you breathe in essential oils, they are immediately taken into your respiratory system. From there, they can travel throughout your body. Aromatherapy steam inhalations can bring relief for respiratory ailments, anxiety, colds, the flu, headaches, sinusitis, sore throats, and stress. You can also use an aromatherapy steam inhalation simply for relaxation or pleasure.

To prepare a steam inhalation, place a large (approximately 2-quart) glass or ceramic bowl on a protected tabletop. Pour about 1 quart of steaming water into the bowl. Add 1 to 6 drops of an essential oil or essential oil blend. If you are preparing an inhalation for an infant or child, add only 1 drop of essential oil. Sit in a comfortable position and hold your head over the bowl and breathe in the vapor for five to ten minutes. If possible, capture the steam by draping a towel over your head and the bowl, creating a "tent." Keep your face far enough from the bowl so that the steam does not irritate or burn your skin (if you are using the inhalation on a child, be particularly careful about this). If necessary, allow the water to cool for a few minutes. Repeat as necessary.

Part Four

COMMON CONDITIONS THAT CAN BE TREATED WITH AROMATHERAPY

Introduction

✳

Long before man-made medicines lined the shelves of pharmacies, supermarkets, and bathroom cabinets, people sought relief from their physical and mental ailments with botanicals. Healing plants helped earth's earliest inhabitants maintain health and well-being, fight illness and disease, and live in balance and harmony with the earth. The first known physicians were priests and perfumers who prepared aromatic oils, unguents, and ointments infused from healing plants to nurture both body and soul. Since ancient times, herbalists, physicians, and healers have shared an evolving knowledge of plants from one generation to the next through herbal folklore.

For thousands of years, botanicals were the only kind of healing medicines available. Up until the beginning of the twentieth century, many European homes had their own "still rooms" for making essential oils and aromatic waters. Many people created their own perfumes and medicines with essential oils. Apothecaries, or pharmacies, sold medicines made from essential oils and other botanicals.

As recently as the 1940s, the American medical community still officially recognized the germ-killing effects of many essential oils. Physicians treated gonorrhea with sandalwood oil. Thyme oil was prescribed to treat hookworm. Camphor, eucalyptus, and clove oils were administered as anesthetics; benzoin, eucalyptus, and peppermint oils were used to treat respiratory ailments; citronella oil was used to repel insects; and geraniol, a major component of such essential oils as geranium and palmarosa, was the key ingredient in an agricultural insecticide.

Essential oils were frequently employed to mask the unpalatable tastes of many medicines. Through World Wars I and II, the first-aid kits that soldiers carried into battle contained essential oils such as lavender and tea tree for disinfecting and treating wounds.

With the advent of modern chemistry and modern medicine, physicians and pharmaceutical companies relegate most essential oils to the shelves of perfumery laboratories. However, even today many pharmacists and medical professionals recognize the therapeutic value of some essential oils. *Martindale: The Extra Pharmacopoeia* (Pharmaceutical Press, 1993) details the modern-day usage of many essential oils, including anise, bay, bergamot, cajuput, caraway, cassia, cinnamon, citronella, clove, coriander, dill, eucalyptus, fennel, geranium, juniper, lavender, lemon, lemongrass, mace, neroli, niaouli, nutmeg, orange, peppermint, pine, rose, rosemary, rue, sassafras, spearmint, and thyme. It states, for example, that eucalyptus helps to ease nasal congestion and coughs and is helpful for respiratory tract disorders. Rosemary dispels gas and is popular in hair lotions and liniments. Thyme helps in the treatment of respiratory tract disorders because it acts as an expectorant and eases coughs. It also helps dispel gas.

The food and beverage industries employ a variety of essential oils to flavor many foods we find on the shelves of stores nationwide. Bergamot, black pepper, cardamom, cinnamon, clove, coriander, eucalyptus, ginger, juniper, lemon, lime, mandarin, nutmeg, orange, patchouli, peppermint, pimento berry, pimento leaf, spearmint, and tangerine are a few of the essential oils we ingest internally, often without even knowing it.

For more than five thousand years, inhabitants of the earth have enjoyed the pleasure, sustenance, and health that botanicals bring by their presence. People have long revered and respected the healing properties of plants. For thousands of years, inhabitants of earth have lived more or less in harmony with nature. Yet, in little over a century, people in industrialized countries have virtually forgotten the alliance with and mutual reliance on the plant world and nature. Our familiarity with plants is slipping away from our lives, even as entire species of plants are slipping away forever from the planet. Nowadays many people are suspicious of plants and natural remedies. Some rely almost exclusively on man-made chemicals to cure their ailments.

Is it mere coincidence that, in the years since synthetic substances have supplanted botanicals as healing remedies and as food sources, human health has declined? Diseases proliferate, particularly among infants and children. We seem increasingly willing to accept birth defects, drug addiction, genetic abnormalities, personality disorders, environmental illnesses, contaminated water, polluted air, and littered landscapes as acceptable risks—the price society seems willing to pay for technology and advancement. These risks are the end result of living out of harmony with nature, with one another, and with our inner selves. When we relinquish our responsibilities to personal health and the health of the planet, we lose touch with what matters. Until we restore balance in our lives, disease, depression, and pollution will dominate. Until we take responsibility for our actions—including the actions of inaction and silence that permit politicians and corporate giants to determine the fate of humankind and the future of the planet—we cannot expect to find health, peace, and happiness.

Health is a state of balance, and illness indicates a state of imbalance. If we can restore balance, healing will take place. Plants have the power to guide our bodies and minds back to balance through their extensive properties and their beautiful aromas. Aromatherapy offers you new options for taking care of yourself and your health. Instead of running to the medicine cabinet for an aspirin to quell a headache, you can inhale the fragrant aroma of lavender or peppermint oil, or apply the essential oil to painful areas. Instead of clutching a bottle of antacid, you can massage your abdomen with an aromatherapy blend of chamomile, fennel, and peppermint oil. Instead of taking painkillers for a toothache, you can dab a drop of tea tree or chamomile oil onto your gums. Aromatherapy gives you greater freedom to take care of your health in a natural way as you learn to resume responsibility for your health and look beyond the symptoms to the causes of your complaints.

Each section in this part of the book is devoted to a common condition that can benefit from aromatherapy, either as a treatment or as a preventive measure. Following a description of the usual causes and typical symptoms of the condition, a section on Helpful Treatments outlines some alternative treatments such as nutrition, exercise, and relaxation that you can employ with aromatherapy. Although this book focuses on aromatherapy, a combination of different treatments usually provides the best results. Each section also contains a list of essential oils that are helpful in treating the condition, as well as suggestions for ways to use aromatherapy.

A section on Aromatherapy Blends includes one or more formulas that you can prepare to treat each particular condition. These blends are easy to make and easy to use; simply follow the directions. You will notice that most of the suggested aromatherapy treatments in this book involve combinations of several essential oils. Combining different essential oils produces a synergistic effect; each oil supports and supplements the actions of the others. Finally, when appropriate, each section concludes with a section on Cautions that discusses any reasons for special care or concern when using essential oil to treat that particular condition.

These formulas represent guidelines. They are adaptable. If you do not have a particular essential oil suggested in an aromatherapy blend, you can feel free to substitute another essential oil from the list. Another way you can benefit is to use fresh or dried herbs if you do not have the essential oils. Brew a cup of tea such as chamomile, eucalyptus, fennel, ginger, lavender, lemon, peppermint, rose petal, St. John's wort, valerian, or vitex (chaste tree berry), or brew a blend of your choice. Cut up culinary herbs such as basil, coriander, cilantro, fennel, ginger, bay leaves, marjoram, oregano, rosemary, and/or thyme and put them on your salad or in your salad dressing. You can also take herbal tinctures of the herb. Herb and health-food stores sell botanicals as bulk herbs, capsules, and tinctures.

Once you become more familiar with the essential oils, you may wish to experiment with creating your own blends. I suggest that you start by looking at the essential oils mentioned in the section for the condition you want to treat. Then reread the sections on each of those essential oils in Part Two. Select the three or four oils that seem most appropriate. Next, decide which method or methods best suits your lifestyle. (Consult Part Three: Ways to Use Aromatherapy for complete instructions on mixing blends for each method.)

Essential oils are very versatile. Each one is helpful for a variety of conditions. If you have multiple health issues, you may be able to treat more than one condition simultaneously. Read the section on each condition. Note any essential oils that all conditions have in common. Choose three or four of those essential oils to create a blend using one of the methods described in Part Three: Ways to Use Aromatherapy. Follow the instructions to create your custom blend.

I recommend mixing small quantities of the aromatherapy blends—the essential oils with the carrier oil—since carrier oils can go rancid quickly. When mixing aromatherapy blends, please follow the instructions regarding the amounts of essential oils and carrier oils. Essential oils are extremely concentrated, and using higher levels of essential oils or applying them to your body undiluted could irritate your skin. Also, be sure to use only pure essential oils, not synthetic imitations, for all your aromatherapy blends. Synthetics are made from petroleum byproducts, and they simply do not have the therapeutic properties of pure essential oils. Worse, they may even be harmful when absorbed through the skin. In many cases, they can create new problems and contribute to the very conditions you wish to treat.

I hope you will find the aromatherapy blends as much fun to make and use—and as helpful—as have the many people who have used them successfully to treat these common conditions. I urge you to experiment with the blends and, in doing so, to discover the wide world of natural remedies. Plants possess the power to help us balance our lives and heal our bodies, minds, and spirits. We can unleash their amazing curative abilities. Good health is our choice.

ACNE

Acne occurs when the sebaceous glands—the oil-producing glands that lubricate the skin—secrete too much sebum, or oil. Normally, sebum flows from the sebaceous glands to the surface of the skin. When dead skin cells accumulate inside the pores, they can clog the pores and prevent the normal flow of sebum. As a result, otherwise harmless bacteria that live beneath the surface of the skin and in the pores can multiply. This overgrowth of bacteria, together with the blocked sebum, causes pimples to form.

The skin mirrors internal health, and blemishes or acne may indicate internal problems. Acne sometimes signals a general toxic condition within the body. When the kidneys, lungs, and intestines cannot eliminate all the body's wastes, the skin must filter out the overload.

Other factors can make the skin more prone to develop pimples. These include allergies; cosmetic ingredients, most notably coloring, fragrances, preservatives, and sunscreens; dehydration; a diet high in fats, preservatives, sugar, and pesticide and herbicide residues; emotional problems; environmental pollution; too much exposure to the sun; heredity; hormones; oral contraceptives; poor hygiene; stress; and weakened immunity.

Skin care can be a major contributing factor. Cosmetics, especially ones that contain colors, dyes, fragrances, and preservatives, can cause breakouts. Sunscreens generally are harsh chemicals that can irritate skin and aggravate acne. In addition, waterproof sunscreens also clog pores. Hair-care products can contribute, too. Both facial cosmetics and hair products rub off on your pillow or clothing and then get on your face. A dirty pillowcase can cause breakouts. Dirty telephone receivers can trigger blemishes, particularly around the mouth and along the cheeks.

Nothing good can come from picking at pimples. It aggravates them so they look worse and last longer. It can also spread infection to other areas, thereby encouraging more blemishes.

HELPFUL TREATMENTS

A nutritious diet rich in fresh vegetables and whole grains, an adequate intake of water, plenty of fresh air and exercise, and aromatherapy skin care can help clear acne. If you suspect you have a weak immune system, you may wish to consult a nutritionist to help you boost it with dietary changes.

Make positive lifestyle changes such as reducing stress, relaxing more often, and nurturing yourself. Be conscious of all objects or fabrics that come into contact with your skin, especially your hands; make certain they are clean. Eliminate products with perfume, dyes, sunscreens, and fragrances. Unrefined sesame oil makes a suitable sunscreen and usually will not break out skin. (*See* SUNBURN.)

Aromatherapy also can help you increase your immunity, in addition to helping you reduce stress. (*See* STRESS *and* WEAKENED IMMUNE SYSTEM.)

Essential oils recommended for acne include anti-inflammatory oils, which reduce painful irritation and swelling; balancing oils, which normalize oil production, often through their hormone-regulating activity as they improve the condition of the skin; and astringent oils, which help control oiliness. Anti-inflammatory essential oils that are effective against acne include benzoin, bergamot, chamomile, clary sage, elemi, eucalyptus, fennel, frankincense, geranium, helichrysum, juniper, lavender, myrrh, neroli, niaouli, orange, oregano, patchouli, peppermint, pine, rose, rosemary, rosewood, St. John's wort, sandalwood, spruce, thyme, vetiver, and ylang ylang.

Bergamot, clary sage, cypress, elemi, eucalyptus, frankincense, geranium, helichrysum, jasmine, lavender, lemon, orange, palmarosa, pine, rose, rosewood, sandalwood, spruce, vetiver, vitex, and ylang ylang oils exert a balancing effect on the oil glands. Recommended astringent oils are basil, cedarwood, clary sage, cypress, elemi, frankincense, geranium, juniper, lavender, lemon, niaouli, orange, palmarosa, patchouli, peppermint, pine, rosewood, sandalwood, tea tree, thyme, vetiver, vitex, and ylang ylang. Recent tests in Australia showed that tea tree oil was as effective in clearing acne as benzoyl peroxide, the most common over-the-counter acne medication. And benzoyl peroxide causes numerous side effects, such as a burning sensation, dryness, flakiness, irritation, and redness, whereas tea tree oil does not.

If you have acne, resist the temptation to squeeze or pick at blemishes; this aggravates them and makes them last longer. It also leads to infection and subsequent scarring. Instead, apply one of the treatments below to your blemishes. When blemishes are left alone and treated with essential oils, which fight the bacteria that cause pimples, they can go away within a few days—without scarring skin.

Proper skin care is crucial for clearing acne. Keeping your skin clean and your pores unclogged and reducing oil secretions can help clear up your complexion. Cleanse your skin twice a day, use a facial scrub several times a week, and spot-treat blemishes with essential oils to help control breakouts. In addition, apply a facial mask one or more times a week. This will help minimize oiliness and clear plugged pores. As you eliminate toxins from your system with diet, change your skin-care routine to eliminate commercial cosmetics, and follow the program below, your face will clear up. The blends below are designed specifically for acne, to be used as follows:

• Twice a day, cleanse your skin with Clay Cleanser. Clay is very cleansing and healing for blemished skin. Follow this with an application of Skin-Clearing Toner, then Oily Skin Treatment.
• Dab Spot Treatment or Blemish Blend on individual blemishes several times a day, as needed, to clear them quickly, often overnight. Apply as often as every few minutes when you first feel the blemish.
• At least twice a week, massage Grainy Scrub into your skin to discourage blackheads and blemishes. If desired, use daily.
• At least once a week, apply Clearing Mask to regulate oiliness and to remove dead skin cells and impurities that can block pores and contribute to blemishes.
• Once a week, steam your face with Acne-Clearing Facial Steam to loosen sebum and bacteria that clog pores. Follow with Clay Cleanser, Grainy Scrub, or Clearing Mask.
• Men can use Blemish-Banishing Aftershave to prevent blemishes and infected ingrown hairs.

AROMATHERAPY BLENDS

You can prepare the aromatherapy blends below using pure essential oils. For a more detailed explanation of how to put together and use these blends, see Part Three: Ways to Use Aromatherapy. To review general guidelines for using essential oils, see page 142.

CLAY CLEANSER

1 teaspoon clay powder
1 teaspoon honey or water
1 drop geranium oil
1 drop lavender oil
1 drop tea tree oil

Mix all the ingredients into a paste in your palm. Massage the paste into your skin until it feels clean. Rinse. Repeat if necessary.

SKIN-CLEARING TONER

8 ounces distilled water
1 drop elemi oil
1 drop palmarosa oil
1 drop rosewood oil

Place the water in a clean bottle, add the essential oils, and turn the bottle upside down several times to blend. Saturate a cotton ball with toner and apply it to your skin after cleansing. Blend the mixture again before each use.

OILY SKIN TREATMENT

2 ounces jojoba oil

3 drops lavender oil

2 drops patchouli oil

2 drops tea tree oil

2 drops ylang ylang oil

1 drop geranium oil

1 drop rosewood oil

1 drop vetiver oil

Place the jojoba oil in a clean container, add the essential oils, and turn the container upside down several times or roll it between your hands to blend. Apply 1 or 2 drops to your skin as a moisturizer. Jojoba oil is very similar in composition to your skin's own natural oils and helps to balance oil production. It does not aggravate acne.

SPOT TREATMENT

½ ounce jojoba oil

8 drops lavender oil

4 drops tea tree oil

3 drops cypress oil

2 drops helichrysum oil

Place the jojoba oil in a clean container and add the essential oils. Turn the container upside down a few times or roll it between your hands to blend. Apply a dab of Spot Treatment directly to each blemish several times daily.

BLEMISH BLEND

1 ounce pure grain alcohol or vodka

4 drops cypress oil

4 drops eucalyptus oil

4 drops niaouli oil

2 drops geranium oil

2 drops helichrysum oil

2 drops tea tree oil

Place the alcohol in a clean container, add the essential oils, and turn the container upside down a few times or roll it between your hands to blend. Dab a bit of the mixture on each blemish several times daily. Blend well before each use. Do not smell directly from the bottle. Do not use isopropyl alcohol with essential oils.

GRAINY SCRUB

½ teaspoon blue cornmeal

½ teaspoon oat flour

1 drop bergamot oil

1 drop clary sage oil

½ to 1 teaspoon honey or water

Combine the blue cornmeal, oat flour, bergamot, and clary sage oils in your palm. Add enough honey or water to form a paste. Massage the paste into clean skin for one to two minutes. Add water as needed to keep the scrub moist. Rinse.

CLEARING MASK
1 teaspoon clay
1 teaspoon (approximately) honey or water
1 drop helichrysum oil
1 drop rosemary oil

Place all the ingredients in your palm and blend together well. Apply the mask to clean skin and leave it on for ten minutes. Rinse thoroughly.

ACNE-CLEARING FACIAL STEAM
1 quart steaming water
1 drop clary sage
1 drop lemon oil
1 drop palmarosa oil

Pour the water into a 2-quart glass bowl. Drop the oils into the water and gently disperse them. Lean your clean face over the bowl and drape a towel over both your head and the bowl to capture the steam. Steam your face for five minutes. Cleanse your skin afterward with Clay Cleanser or Grainy Scrub.

BLEMISH-BANISHING AFTERSHAVE
8 ounces distilled water
2 drops sandalwood oil
1 drop cedarwood oil
1 drop vetiver oil

Add the water to a clean bottle, drop in the essential oils, and turn upside down several times to combine. Splash the mixture on your skin after shaving. Blend well before each use.

ANXIETY

Anxiety produces an uneasy feeling or a warning to become aware of threats to your well-being. Everyone fears or worries about something sometime. But when your fears or apprehensions dominate or interfere with your life, you experience anxiety. The most extreme manifestation of anxiety is an anxiety attack. Your heart pounds rapidly in your chest. Breathing becomes difficult. An awful gnawing sensation in your stomach nauseates you. Your head may pound as panic sets in.

Anxiety can become the focal point of your life and, paradoxically, prevent you from dealing with the precise problems that are prompting it. Anxiety shows up in your health, on your skin, and in your attitude. Chronic anxiety can weaken your immune system, making you more susceptible to illness or disease.

Many factors can contribute to or aggravate anxiety. Some of the most common are the consumption of caffeine and other stimulants, chemical sensitivities, childhood trauma, emotional difficulties, environmental pollutants, heredity, lifestyle factors such as problems at work or in relationships, nutritional deficiencies, physical illness, poor diet, and stress, especially chronic stress.

Cigarette smoking; the use of alcohol; taking prescription, over-the-counter, or recreational drugs; the consumption of too much salt or sugar, junk food, and food additives; and exposure to pesticides, household or industrial chemicals, or synthetic fragrances contribute to anxiety attacks in many people. Monosodium glutamate (MSG), an additive that is found in many processed food products and is often added to Chinese and fast food, can also trigger anxietylike symptoms in susceptible people.

HELPFUL TREATMENTS

Evaluate your situation. Determine what is causing your anxiety and decide what you can do to eliminate the problems or alter your environment. If you feel that you cannot change the situation that is the focus of your anxiety, decide what you can do to change your attitude and your way of handling or responding to problems. Remember, chronic anxiety takes its toll on both physical and emotional health. Talking to a qualified counselor may help you to manage your anxiety. If your anxiety has led to health problems, consult your health-care professional.

If you suffer from anxiety, you should eliminate or reduce your intake of caffeine, which is present not only in coffee and tea but often also in candy, chocolate, cocoa, medications, nutritional supplements, soft drinks, and sports beverages. Read product labels carefully. Avoid additive-laden and processed foods. Keep track of your reactions to the foods you eat and substances in your environment. Avoid anything that triggers anxiety. Apricots, asparagus, avocados, bananas, broccoli, brown rice, dried fruits, figs, garlic, green leafy vegetables, legumes and beans, raw nuts and seeds, whole grains, and yogurt are rich sources of calcium, magnesium, and potassium and can help restore nerve health and reduce anxiety.

Relaxation and stress reduction are important parts of any program to overcome anxiety. Aromatherapy can relax you, strengthen your emotional stamina, and tone your nervous system, allowing you to deal better with anxiety-provoking situations. Essential oils such as basil, benzoin, bergamot, cedarwood, chamomile, clary sage, coriander, frankincense, geranium, jasmine, juniper, marjoram, melissa, neroli, orange, patchouli, rose, rosewood, St. John's wort, tea tree, thyme, valerian, vetiver, vitex, and ylang ylang help reduce anxiety. During trying times, disperse Anxiety Diffuser Blend throughout your home or office. Bathe in Anxiety Bath Blend once or twice daily to avert or control anxiety. Carry Quick-Fix Anxiety Inhalant with you to inhale directly from the bottle as needed to remain calm.

AROMATHERAPY BLENDS

You can prepare the aromatherapy blends below using pure essential oils. For a more detailed explanation of how to put together and use these blends, see Part Three: Ways to Use Aromatherapy. To review general guidelines for using essential oils, see page 142.

ANXIETY DIFFUSER BLEND

12 drops clary sage oil
10 drops bergamot oil
8 drops geranium oil
8 drops juniper oil
6 drops patchouli oil
5 drops orange oil

Drop the essential oils into a small glass bottle and gently turn the bottle upside down a few times or roll it between your hands to blend. Add some of the mixture to your diffuser or lamp bowl. Run your diffuser or lamp as necessary to prevent or reduce anxiety.

ANXIETY BATH BLEND

2 drops frankincense oil
2 drops geranium oil
2 drops rosewood oil
1 drop lavender oil

Disperse the essential oils in a bathtub filled with warm water. Enjoy a calming soak for twenty to thirty minutes.

QUICK-FIX ANXIETY INHALANT

3 drops benzoin resin
2 drops geranium oil
2 drops rosewood oil
2 drops ylang ylang oil
1 drop frankincense oil
1 drop vetiver oil

Drop the essential oils into a small glass bottle with an airtight cover and blend. In-

hale directly from the bottle to avert or alleviate an anxiety attack. Repeat as often as needed.

APPETITE DISTURBANCES

Some people experience a loss of appetite; others have difficulty curbing theirs. When considering disturbances of appetite, it is important to remember that, while hunger is a physical sensation, appetite is a psychological one. The hypothalamus area of the brain, which controls appetite, is closely connected with the emotions.

Alcohol, cigarettes, drugs, allergies, depression, emotional upset, illness, nutritional deficiencies, stress, and weather among other things can affect appetite. Sometimes simply seeing, smelling, or talking about a favorite food can stimulate your appetite, even if you've just eaten. Conversely, the sight of an unappealing or disliked food can decrease your appetite, even when you're hungry. In times of stress, anxiety, tension, or emotional upset, some people tend to react by overindulging in food, while others stop eating entirely.

HELPFUL TREATMENTS

If you experience a notable change in appetite, whether a loss of appetite or excessive appetite, you should first consult a health-care practitioner or nutritionist to rule out any underlying physical illness or nutritional deficiencies. Whether you wish to stimulate or curb your appetite, changing the way you eat may help. If you want to increase your appetite, more frequent small meals of healthy and nutritious foods may be more appetizing than two or three larger ones. Avoid fast food and processed foods, which offer little appeal or nutritional value. Instead, concentrate on eating a diet that contains lots of fresh vegetables, fruits, and whole grains, which look, smell, and taste more tempting; are nutritionally safer choices; and are more apt to satisfy hunger and your energy requirements.

If you want to suppress your appetite, you should also change your diet to one that focuses on fresh, healthy foods. Eating fresh vegetables and whole grains as your primary foods will help you to feel full while furnishing your body with necessary nutrients. When your nutritional needs are met, you won't get as hungry between meals. Modern diets offer roller-coaster rides for both bodies and emotions. By contrast, initiating healthful and permanent changes in diet and lifestyle makes more sense, is less dangerous, and delivers steady results that last. Instead of counting calories, make your calories count. Choosing healthy and nutritious foods will guide you toward a healthy body.

Aromatherapy can help to regulate appetite. Essential oils that come from culinary herbs, including basil, black pepper, clary sage, coriander, fennel, ginger, laurel, marjoram, oregano, peppermint, rosemary, and thyme, are particularly good for stimulating appetite. Several other oils, including bergamot, chamomile, juniper, myrrh, pal-marosa, and orange, also arouse the appetite. Aromatherapy can help if loss of appetite is linked to stress or depression, because it can work directly on those problems. Aromatherapy may also help some people with eating disorders such as anorexia nervosa. Used in conjunction with medical and psychological attention, essential oils may help a person with anorexia to regain appetite and self-esteem. To increase appetite, breathe in Appetite-Stimulating Inhalant, beginning thirty minutes to one hour before mealtime. Repeat as necessary. Massage Appetite-Stimulating Stomach Rub over your entire abdominal area several times a day.

Some people wish to suppress their appetites, usually for the purpose of losing weight. Bergamot, fennel, juniper, patchouli, and vetiver can decrease or regulate the desire for food, according to the body's needs. To tame your appetite, breathe in Appetite-Suppressing Inhalant when you crave food between meals. Massage Appetite-Suppressing Stomach Rub over your entire abdominal area as many times a day as necessary to curb your appetite.

AROMATHERAPY BLENDS
TO STIMULATE APPETITE

You can prepare the aromatherapy blends below using pure essential oils. For a more detailed explanation of how to put together and use these blends, *see* Part Three: Ways to Use Aromatherapy. To review general guidelines for using essential oils, see page 142.

APPETITE-STIMULATING INHALANT
8 drops clary sage oil
6 drops coriander oil
4 drops black pepper oil
3 drops ginger oil
2 drops laurel oil
1 drop peppermint oil

Drop the essential oils into a small glass bottle with an airtight cover and gently turn the bottle upside down a few times or roll it between your hands to blend. Inhale directly from the container as necessary.

APPETITE-STIMULATING STOMACH RUB
2 ounces carrier oil
2 drops basil oil
2 drops orange oil
2 drops thyme oil
1 drop coriander oil
1 drop oregano oil
1 drop rosemary oil

Place the carrier oil in a clean container, add the essential oils, and blend well. Massage the mixture over your stomach and abdominal area as needed.

AROMATHERAPY BLENDS TO SUPPRESS APPETITE
You can prepare the aromatherapy blends below using pure essential oils. For a more detailed explanation of how to put together

and use these blends, *see* Part Three: Ways to Use Aromatherapy. To review general guidelines for using essential oils, see page 142.

APPETITE-SUPPRESSING INHALANT
10 drops bergamot oil
5 drops fennel oil
5 drops patchouli oil

Drop the essential oils into a small glass bottle with an airtight cover. Gently turn the bottle over a few times or roll it between your hands to blend. Inhale directly from the container as necessary.

APPETITE-SUPPRESSING STOMACH RUB
2 ounces carrier oil
8 drops fennel oil
4 drops juniper oil
3 drops patchouli oil

Place the carrier oil in a clean container, add the essential oils, and blend. Massage the mixture over your stomach and abdominal area several times daily, as needed.

ARTHRITIS
Arthritis, which literally means "joint inflammation," may appear in the joints of the elbows, fingers, hips, knees, neck, shoulders, toes, or wrists, or along the spine. Medically, arthritis constitutes a general category that includes more than 100 different joint disorders with symptoms ranging from mild aches and pains, stiffness, and

swelling to severe, crippling pain and deformities. Osteoarthritis and rheumatoid arthritis are the most common forms.

Osteoarthritis, or degenerative joint disease, involves wear and tear on the joints due to use and aging. The cartilage at the end of the bones becomes rough, and the ligaments, muscles, and tendons weaken. Bones begin to grind against each other during movement. Symptoms of osteoarthritis include stiffness, soreness, and pain in the joints of the feet, toes, thumbs, and weight-bearing bones. A number of different factors including heredity, physical stress, and injuries can increase a person's chances of developing osteoarthritis.

Rheumatoid arthritis affects both the bones and the surrounding tissue. It is an autoimmune disease, which means that the immune system begins attacking the body's own tissues. Rheumatoid arthritis often destroys the bone surface, the cartilage, and the tissues surrounding the joint. Fluids accumulate and inflame the joints. The small joints of the ankles, feet, hands, knees, and wrists are most often affected, although rheumatoid arthritis can attack any joint in the body. It causes pain, stiffness, swelling, and sometimes disabling deformities.

The exact cause or causes of most cases of rheumatoid arthritis are unknown. Researchers suspect that abnormal bowel function, food allergies, heredity, infections, nutritional deficiencies, and weakened immunity contribute. Another possibility is increased intestinal permeability, which allows bacterial toxins or tiny particles of undigested food to leak from the intestines into the bloodstream, where they can initiate an immune response. Foods that can trigger or aggravate arthritis in susceptible people include alcohol, corn, dairy products, sugar, and wheat. Members of the nightshade family—which includes potatoes, eggplant, peppers, tomatoes, and tobacco—may also promote joint inflammation and interfere with joint repair in some people.

HELPFUL TREATMENTS

Determine what factors are contributing to arthritis. Good nutrition can play a big role in controlling this disorder. A nutritionist or health-care professional can detect and help you correct any nutritional deficiencies. A low-fat, low-sugar diet centered on fresh vegetables and whole grains may provide relief. Some people find that avoiding citrus fruits, dairy products, processed and refined foods, red meat, salt, and sugar, as well as vegetables in the nightshade family, diminishes inflammation. Iron supplements can exacerbate arthritis, while flaxseed oil and garlic may bring relief. Physical therapy and exercise can maintain and restore muscle strength and, in some cases, can decrease symptoms.

Aromatherapy complements other treatments for arthritis. Essential oils that benefit people with arthritis include basil, benzoin, black pepper, cedarwood, chamomile, coriander, elemi, eucalyptus, fennel, ginger, helichrysum, juniper, laurel, lemon, marjoram, myrrh, neroli, niaouli, pine, rosemary, St. John's wort, thyme, valerian, and vetiver. These oils can ease pain and discomfort, reduce swelling, and relieve sore muscles. Carrier oils that benefit arthritis and rheumatism when massaged into affected areas include borage, calophyllum inophyllum, flaxseed, hemp, and sesame oils.

Soak in Arthritis Bath Blend daily to relieve pain and discomfort. Apply Arthritis Massage Blend over your entire body for a detoxifying and pain-relieving effect. Massage Deep Relief Arthritis Oil into your joints and muscles as often as necessary to relieve pain and reduce swelling.

AROMATHERAPY BLENDS

You can prepare the aromatherapy blends below using pure essential oils. For a more detailed explanation of how to put together and use these blends, see Part Three: Ways to Use Aromatherapy. To review general guidelines for using essential oils, see page 142.

ARTHRITIS BATH BLEND

3 drops lemon oil
2 drops helichrysum oil
1 drop laurel oil

Drop the oils into a bathtub filled with warm water and gently disperse them. Enjoy a leisurely soak for twenty to thirty minutes. Repeat as necessary.

ARTHRITIS MASSAGE BLEND

1 ounce flaxseed oil
1 ounce hemp oil
4 drops chamomile oil
4 drops helichrysum oil
3 drops coriander oil
2 drops benzoin resin
1 drop black pepper oil
1 drop ginger oil

Place the carrier oils in a clean container, add the essential oils, and gently turn the container upside down several times or roll it between your hands to blend. Massage the mixture into your joints and muscles as necessary.

DEEP RELIEF ARTHRITIS OIL

1 ounce flaxseed oil
1 ounce sesame oil
4 drops vetiver oil
3 drops helichrysum oil
3 drops St. John's wort oil
2 drops cedarwood oil
2 drops marjoram oil
1 drop valerian oil

In a clean container, blend the essential oils with the carrier oils. Apply the mixture to your joints and muscles as needed.

ASTHMA AND BRONCHITIS

An asthma attack occurs when the muscles around the bronchi, the two main breathing tubes that lead from the windpipe to the lungs, go into spasms. The bronchial tubes narrow and breathing becomes difficult. Sometimes inflammation also swells the lining of these air tubes, restricting breathing. Mucous secretions may increase then block the bronchi. As a result, air cannot pass into or out of the lungs as easily as it normally does. Carbon dioxide becomes trapped in the lungs and cannot be exhaled; fresh oxygen cannot be inhaled. Coughing and wheezing may result from a desperate attempt to breathe.

A wide variety of factors can trigger or contribute to an asthma attack, including airborne and food allergies, especially allergies to dairy products, wheat, fermented foods, and yeast- or mold-containing foods; chemical sensitivities; exposure to cigarette smoke; changes in climate, humidity, and/or temperature; a diet high in dairy products, fried foods, and sugar; subnormal functioning of the adrenal glands; hypoglycemia; infections; poor circulation; reactions to food additives and preservatives; and stress. Aspirin, emotional upset, sinusitis, exercise, exposure to chemical irritants, food colorings, monosodium glutamate, newsprint, sulfites, or synthetic fragrances may aggravate symptoms or trigger attacks.

Bronchitis is a condition in which the bronchial walls become inflamed, and thick, sticky mucus accumulates in the bronchi. In some cases, bronchial spasms accompany inflammation. The swelling and mucus block the exchange of oxygen and carbon dioxide in the lungs. Breathing becomes

difficult, and coughing results as the body attempts to expel the mucus. At first the cough is a dry cough, but after several days it usually produces mucus.

Bronchitis most often occurs as part of an upper respiratory infection such as a cold. Exposure to cigarette smoke (whether by smoking or inhaling secondhand smoke) and other irritants, such as environmental pollutants and noxious chemicals, can contribute to or predispose a person to developing bronchitis. Poor nutrition and fatigue can play a role.

HELPFUL TREATMENTS

If you have asthma or are prone to bronchitis, avoid exposure to cigarette smoke. If you smoke, quit. Practice deep-breathing exercises, engage in mild aerobic exercise such as walking or swimming, do yoga, and eat a healthy diet. Avoid contact with noxious chemicals. Determine which foods or food ingredients trigger acute attacks, and eliminate them from your diet. Rest is an important healing factor. Doctors advise against suppressing the cough, because coughing clears mucus from the lungs and restores breathing. Drink plenty of water to thin secretions and make them easier to cough out.

Whether you are suffering from asthma or bronchitis, aromatherapy can help you breathe more easily by clearing congestion, reducing inflammation, and releasing excess mucus. Essential oils that can calm or prevent asthma attacks and can relieve bouts of bronchitis include basil, benzoin, cedarwood, clary sage, cypress, elemi, eucalyptus, frankincense, helichrysum, juniper, laurel, lavender, lemon, marjoram, melissa, myrrh, niaouli, orange, oregano, peppermint, pine, rose, rosemary, sandalwood, spruce, tea tree, and thyme. Essential oils that can soothe coughs are basil, benzoin, black pepper, cedarwood, clary sage, elemi, eucalyptus, fennel, frankincense, ginger, helichrysum, jasmine, juniper, lavender, lemon, marjoram, melissa, myrrh, niaouli, orange, oregano, pine, rose, rosemary, rosewood, sandalwood, tea tree, and thyme.

To relieve respiratory congestion or improve your breathing, breathe in Respiratory Relief Steam Inhalation as necessary. Apply Respiratory Rub or Breathe Easier Blend to your chest, back, and throat. Use your diffuser or lamp to circulate All-Purpose Diffuser Breathing Blend through your room, home, or office. To ward off an asthma attack, breathe in Asthma Inhalant directly from the bottle as needed. Ease the pain of coughing by massaging Chest Rub for Coughs over your chest, back, and throat.

AROMATHERAPY BLENDS

You can prepare the aromatherapy blends below using pure essential oils. For a more detailed explanation of how to put together and use these blends, see Part Three: Ways to Use Aromatherapy. To review general guidelines for using essential oils, see page 142.

RESPIRATORY RELIEF STEAM INHALATION
1 quart steaming water
1 drop cypress oil
1 drop eucalyptus oil
1 drop oregano oil

Pour the water into a 2-quart glass bowl and add the essential oils. Lean your face over the bowl and drape a towel over both your head and the bowl to capture the steam. Inhale the steam for five minutes. Repeat as necessary.

RESPIRATORY RUB
1 ounce jojoba oil
3 drops elemi oil
2 drops pine oil
2 drops tea tree oil
1 drop thyme oil

Place the jojoba oil in a clean container, add the essential oils, and gently turn the container upside down a few times or roll it between your hands to blend. Massage the mixture over your chest and back as needed to aid breathing and to clear excess mucus.

BREATHE EASIER BLEND
1 ounce carrier oil
3 drops eucalyptus oil
2 drops ginger oil
2 drops niaouli oil
1 drop rosemary oil

In a clean container, add the essential oils to the carrier oil and blend. Apply the mixture to your chest, throat, and back. Repeat as necessary.

ALL-PURPOSE DIFFUSER BREATHING BLEND
12 drops eucalyptus oil
10 drops lemon oil
8 drops laurel oil
8 drops thyme oil
6 drops cypress oil
6 drops myrrh oil
4 drops frankincense oil
4 drops spruce oil

Drop the essential oils into a small glass bottle. Gently turn the bottle upside down a few times or roll it between your hands to blend. Add some of the mixture to your diffuser, lamp bowl, or atomizer. Run your diffuser, lamp, or atomizer as necessary to ease breathing.

ASTHMA INHALANT
8 drops eucalyptus oil
6 drops spruce oil
4 drops marjoram oil
4 drops pine oil
2 drops cypress oil
2 drops niaouli oil

Add all the ingredients to a small glass bottle with an airtight cover and blend well. Inhale directly from the bottle as necessary to prevent or minimize asthma attacks.

CHEST RUB FOR COUGHS
2 ounces carrier oil
3 drops cedarwood oil
3 drops ginger oil
2 drops cypress oil
2 drops thyme oil
1 drop tea tree oil

Place the carrier oil in a clean container, add the essential oils, and blend. Massage the oil over your chest, neck, and throat as necessary.

CAUTIONS
People with asthma should exercise caution when using essential oils. Certain oils may trigger an asthma attack in susceptible individuals. If you have asthma, consult with your medical practitioner before using any essential oils.

ATHLETE'S FOOT
More than 30 percent of all Americans suffer from athlete's foot, or *tinea pedis,* at some time in their lives. This highly contagious fungal infection most commonly occurs between the toes and on the soles of the feet.

Fungi thrive in dark and damp places with little light or air. The warm, moist area between the toes, enclosed in nylons or synthetic-fiber socks and shoes most of the time, provides a perfect breeding ground for these microbes. The dead skin cells that accumulate between your toes sustain them. Athlete's foot causes the skin to itch, flake, and burn, and it becomes irritated and inflamed.

HELPFUL TREATMENTS

Good hygiene is vital. Keeping your feet clean and dry is crucial for eliminating athlete's foot. Whenever possible, go barefoot or wear open sandals to allow air to circulate between your toes. Select socks made entirely or primarily of cotton. Change socks and shoes several times a day. Freshen your shoes, particularly athletic shoes, by wiping them out with a clean cloth sprinkled with a drop of niaouli or tea tree oil. Since fungi hide in public showers and locker rooms, always wear shoes in public showers, gyms, and locker rooms.

Essential oils such as cedarwood, coriander, elemi, eucalyptus, helichrysum, laurel, lavender, myrrh, niaouli patchouli, spruce, tea tree, and thyme fight athlete's foot by destroying fungi. These oils also relieve the uncomfortable burning, flaking, inflammation, and itching. Twice a day, give your feet a soak in Tea Tree Oil Foot Bath or Athlete's Foot Bath. Many people claim that adding apple cider vinegar to the water makes the bath more effective. Afterward, apply Athlete's Foot Relief Oil. Once your athlete's foot is under control, weekly treatment can avert further attacks.

AROMATHERAPY BLENDS

You can prepare the aromatherapy blends below using pure essential oils. For a more detailed explanation of how to put together and use these blends, see Part Three: Ways to Use Aromatherapy. To review general guidelines for using essential oils, see page 142.

TEA TREE OIL FOOT BATH

3 drops tea tree oil

Add the tea tree oil to a small tub or foot bath filled with warm water. Soak your feet for ten to twenty minutes. Dry thoroughly, especially between the toes, and apply Athlete's Foot Relief Oil.

ATHLETE'S FOOT BATH

¼ cup apple cider vinegar (optional)
2 drops tea tree oil
1 drop myrrh oil
1 drop patchouli oil

Add the oils to a small tub or foot bath filled with warm water. Soak your feet for ten to twenty minutes. Dry your feet well and apply Athlete's Foot Relief Oil.

ATHLETE'S FOOT RELIEF OIL

2 ounces carrier oil
5 drops tea tree oil
4 drops eucalyptus oil
2 drops laurel oil
2 drops myrrh oil

Place the carrier oil in a clean container, add the essential oils, and turn the container upside down a few times or roll it between your hands to blend. Apply a few drops of the mixture directly to the affected areas, making sure your feet are clean and dry first. Use this blend before putting on your shoes.

ATTENTION DEFICIT DISORDER

See HYPERACTIVITY AND ATTENTION DEFICIT DISORDER.

BACKACHE AND BACK PROBLEMS

More than 80 percent of adults experience backaches. Most back problems result from poor posture and misuse of the spine and the spinal muscles while lifting, sitting, sleeping, standing, and walking. Muscle strain typically develops gradually over time.

Backaches cause pain and discomfort. As the body attempts to compensate for the pain, it exaggerates the misuse of the muscles and spine. This creates even more pain and improper use. A vicious cycle continues. Often, people in pain seek relief through surgery or simply resign themselves to a limited, sedentary life.

Poor posture changes the curvature of the spine, stresses the muscles and ligaments that support the spine, and leads to back problems and pain. Chronic poor posture contributes significantly to this suffering, as your body constantly seeks to compensate for misuse of muscles and misalignment of your spine. Carrying extra weight compounds the problem. Even a few extra pounds put enough additional stress on your spine to cause pain. People in modern Western countries tend to lead sedentary lives, sitting for long hours in chairs and on sofas that promote bad posture. Slouching while sitting compounds the problem—particularly on the lower back. Failure to exercise regularly leaves muscles lax. Then a binge of physical activity can overwork the muscles and sprain or strain them. Sprains are injuries to ligaments that hold bone to bone, while strains are small tears in the muscle.

Lazy abdominal muscles can contribute to back pain, particularly lower back pain. Dehydration—particularly chronic dehydration, which allows toxins to accumulate in the muscles—intensifies pain. Emotional upsets and stress can increase muscle tension and pain. Inflammation and swelling in the muscles, tendons, bones, or ligaments of the abdomen can trigger back pain. Other factors in back pain include abnormalities in the spinal curve, arthritis, bone disease, calcium deficiency, constipation, disorders or infections of the reproductive organs, intestinal problems, rheumatism, spinal misalignment, and urinary tract problems. Some women experience back pain during menopause, menstruation, or pregnancy. Carrying a heavy shoulder bag or briefcase on one side can create muscle imbalances that cause pain. Wearing high-heeled or improperly fitting shoes amplifies the problem. Sleeping on a soft or lumpy mattress is enough to create back pain.

HELPFUL TREATMENTS

Assess your lifestyle to determine what is creating and contributing to the problem and what steps you can take to diminish or eliminate those factors. When pain first strikes, drink two glasses of water to eliminate dehydration as the culprit. In addition to correcting dehydration, drinking water disperses acidic wastes to prevent their accumulation in your muscles. Flaxseed and hemp oils, added to the diet and/or applied to the affected areas, offer relief for muscle and joint pain and inflammation.

Become aware of your posture while you sit, stand, lift objects, walk, and sleep. Reprogramming your muscles to assume proper posture can resolve many problems. (See Proper Posture on page 183 and follow the guidelines for reprogramming your movements.) Isolate your abdominal muscles and strengthen them by gently contracting the muscles around your navel. These muscles support your lower back, and as they become stronger, pain will diminish.

Initially, sitting, standing, or walking correctly may make your muscles ache because you are using them differently. But as you persevere through this adjustment period, your body will be stronger and function better.

Reduce stress. If you are overweight, shed the extra pounds. Walk regularly. Swimming and yoga are other forms of exercise that can help improve your posture and strengthen your muscles without placing too much stress on your spine. Depending upon the severity of your problem, you may choose to wear a back brace as a temporary means of increasing your awareness of how you are using your spine and muscles. Don't allow your muscles to get lazy with the brace, however. Consider consulting with a physical therapist or an orthopedist (bone specialist) for pointers on improving your posture.

Physicians and physical therapists recommend managing back strains and sprains with bed rest, warm baths, anti-inflammatory treatments, compresses, and massage. Aromatherapy can supplement these therapies. Essential oils can relax you, soothe away stress and tension, and provide pain relief as they reduce inflammation in the tender tissues around your joints and in your muscles. Essential oils that help reduce pain of both muscles and joints are chamomile, coriander, cypress, eucalyptus, lavender, laurel, oregano, pine, spruce, rosemary, valerian, and vetiver. Anti-inflammatory oils include chamomile, cypress, eucalyptus, geranium, helichrysum, juniper, oregano, peppermint, spruce, and thyme.

Soak regularly in Back Relaxing Bath. Adding Dead Sea salts, Epsom salts, or sea salt provides additional relief. Apply Muscle Relaxation Massage Oil on affected areas to relax muscles, reduce inflammation, and minimize pain. Put a Clay Back Pack on your back and rest. You can apply a Compress for Back Pain either together with the Clay Back Pack or separately.

AROMATHERAPY BLENDS

You can prepare the aromatherapy blends below using pure essential oils. For a more detailed explanation of how to put together and use these blends, see Part Three: Ways to Use Aromatherapy. To review general guidelines for using essential oils, see page 142.

BACK RELAXING BATH

2 drops laurel oil
1 drop chamomile oil
1 drop helichrysum oil
1 cup Dead Sea salts (optional)

Disperse the essential oils, and the Dead Sea salts, if desired, in a bathtub filled with warm water. Soak for twenty minutes once daily to relax back muscles.

MUSCLE RELAXATION MASSAGE OIL

1 ounce hemp oil
½ ounce flaxseed oil
3 drops helichrysum oil
2 drops chamomile oil
2 drops St. John's wort oil
1 drop valerian oil

In a clean container, add the essential oils to the carrier oils and blend. Massage into sore muscles, especially around the spine, as needed.

CLAY BACK PACK

1 cup clay
1 cup hot water (approximately)
3 drops cypress oil
2 drops spruce oil
1 drop peppermint oil

In a bowl, mix the clay with enough of the hot water to form a smooth paste. Add the essential oils and blend. Spread over your back. Cover with a warm towel or a compress. Relax for twenty to thirty minutes. Rinse off or soak in a bath.

COMPRESS FOR BACK PAIN

1 quart cold water
2 drops eucalyptus oil
1 drop helichrysum oil
1 drop thyme oil

Pour the water into a 2-quart glass bowl, add the essential oils, and blend. Saturate a clean cloth in the water and apply it to the affected area as needed.

BLOOD PRESSURE PROBLEMS

See HIGH BLOOD PRESSURE AND LOW BLOOD PRESSURE.

BRONCHITIS

See ASTHMA AND BRONCHITIS.

BRUISES

See CUTS AND BRUISES.

Proper Posture

Maintaining proper posture is very important for preventing or eliminating back pain. Poor posture can restrict blood circulation, lymph flow, and nerve activity and can thereby contribute to numerous ailments. If you have practiced poor posture for a very long time, you will probably need to reprogram your muscles so that you can use them correctly. Following are guidelines to help you learn and practice correct posture while standing, sitting, sleeping, and lifting objects.

STANDING

Stand upright, with your shoulders back. Gently flex your abdominal muscles to hold your stomach flat. Keep your chin parallel to the floor. Curve the small of your back slightly, and keep your pelvis straight.

Wear low, comfortable shoes. The flatter your shoes, the less pressure they put on your back.

SITTING

Sit balanced on your buttocks with your weight equally distributed on the back of your upper thighs. Place your feet firmly on the floor or evenly elevated with your knees higher than your hips. Don't curve your tailbone under you, and don't cross your legs or ankles, as this impairs circulation. Choose chairs that support your back and encourage upright posture. Take breaks frequently to walk around and stretch your spine.

SLEEPING

Sleep on a firm mattress. A board beneath the mattress adds support. Lying on your side, with your knees bent at a right angle to your body, in a fetal position, reduces stress on your spine. Support your neck with a small cervical pillow. If you prefer to sleep on your back, place one supportive pillow beneath your neck and another under your knees.

LIFTING OBJECTS

Instead of bending over at the waist, bend at your knees in front of the object to be lifted, keeping your back straight. Pick up the object and rise slowly, allowing your thigh muscles to do the work. Push large objects ahead of you instead of lifting or pulling them.

CANDIDIASIS

Candida albicans is a single-celled fungus that is one of many microorganisms normally found in the intestines, the colon, and the genitourinary tract. Ideally, the body maintains a healthy balance among all of these microorganisms. If this balance is upset, candida (also often called yeast) may thrive and even spread to other parts of the body, causing the condition known as candidiasis.

Antibiotics are one major contributing factor in candidiasis; they kill not only the bacteria that cause infections but also beneficial bacteria, which are a natural means of keeping candida under control. Other factors that can upset the body's natural balance include birth control pills, anti-inflammatory drugs, immunosuppressant drugs, and cortisone; a diet high in sugar, refined carbohydrates, and yeast-laden foods; food allergies; pregnancy; stress; and hormonal imbalances. Sugar is a major culprit, because yeast thrives on sugar. The category of sugar includes refined white sugar as well as brown sugar, corn syrup, fructose, honey, maple syrup, and sucrose. Other foods and food ingredients that can contribute to or aggravate candidiasis are alcohol; dairy products, particularly from animals that are fed huge doses of antibiotics; fresh or dried fruits and fruit juices; grains such as barley, oats, rye, and wheat; and certain yeast-containing foods such as breads and nutritional yeast.

Animal products are an increasing threat. Livestock farmers, particularly factory farmers who crowd thousands of animals into unsanitary and cramped warehouses, rely heavily upon antibiotics to keep animals alive and upon hormones to promote rapid growth. Each year, they give them increasing volumes of antibiotics, hormones, and other medicines, as the microbes become more resistant to them. These drugs survive in the flesh sold as meat and concentrate in dairy products and poultry eggs. In addition, the hormones in growth-hormone serums used to "bulk up" animals wreak havoc on human hormones and the intestinal flora.

Two common manifestations of candida infection occur: in the mouth, where it is called oral thrush, and in the vagina, where it is called vaginitis or a yeast infection. (*See also* VAGINITIS.) However, systemic candidiasis is often hard to pin down, because it can cause or contribute to a host of different physical symptoms, including acne, arthritis, asthma, athlete's foot, blurred vision, chemical sensitivity, chronic fatigue, clumsiness, constipation, cystitis, diabetes, diaper rash, diarrhea, dizziness, eczema, endometriosis, headaches, hyperactivity, hypoglycemia, hypothyroidism, indigestion, lethargy, loss of libido, menstrual difficulties or irregularity, muscular aches and pains, premenstrual syndrome, respiratory ailments, sinusitis, skin disorders, sore throat, and even cravings for sugar. In addition, many mental or emotional symptoms may appear, among them anxiety, depression, difficulty coping, impaired memory, irritability, lack of confidence, low self-esteem, mood swings, and poor concentration.

A candida infection may surface on the

skin around the mouth, on the throat, and in the corners of the ears, eyes, mouth, and nose. It appears as a dry, scaly, weeping rash or tiny cuts or cracks in the skin. It itches and burns, and it may be painful and become inflamed.

HELPFUL TREATMENTS

Many alternative health-care practitioners have designed programs to combat or control candida. These long-term treatments emphasize making changes in lifestyle and diet to minimize symptoms and eliminate, or at least control, the causes. Successful treatment includes reestablishing the proper balance of intestinal bacteria, usually by taking acidophilus and digestive enzymes; avoiding foods and other substances that trigger symptoms; and strengthening the immune system. Eliminate all types of sugar as well as other foods that contribute to candidiasis. A diet to control candida centers on fresh vegetables; fresh grains such as brown rice, barley, millet, and quinoa; plus at least eight to ten glasses of water daily to help flush out wastes.

Aromatherapy alone cannot eliminate candida, but in conjunction with lifestyle changes, an elimination diet, and a positive attitude, aromatherapy can speed your recovery. The essential oils of benzoin, chamomile, clary sage, elemi, eucalyptus, geranium, juniper, lavender, marjoram, myrrh, niaouli, oregano, patchouli, rosemary, tea tree, and thyme are helpful in treating candidiasis.

Regular use of Candida Bath Treatment and Candida Immune-Boosting Body Oil will help to fight candida, strengthen immunity, and soothe stress. You can bathe in Candida Bath Treatment once or twice daily and apply Candida Immune-Boosting Body Oil to your entire body once or twice daily, as necessary. If a candida infection appears on your face, keep your skin clean and avoid wearing makeup. Apply Candida Facial Oil to the affected areas several times daily, as needed.

AROMATHERAPY BLENDS

You can prepare the aromatherapy blends below using pure essential oils. For a more detailed explanation of how to put together and use these blends, see Part Three: Ways to Use Aromatherapy. To review general guidelines for using essential oils, see page 142.

CANDIDA BATH TREATMENT

4 drops tea tree oil
2 drops eucalyptus oil
1 drop patchouli oil

Once or twice daily, add these oils to a bathtub filled with warm water. Soak for twenty minutes.

CANDIDA IMMUNE-BOOSTING BODY OIL

4 ounces carrier oil
8 drops spruce oil
6 drops laurel oil
4 drops geranium oil

3 drops elemi oil
3 drops thyme oil
2 drops patchouli oil

Place the carrier oil in a clean container, add the essential oils, and gently turn the container upside down a few times or roll it between your hands to blend. Massage the mixture onto your skin daily until symptoms cease.

Note: Geranium oil can lower your blood sugar level. Use it with caution (or omit it) if you have hypoglycemia (low blood sugar).

Candida Facial Oil
1 ounce jojoba oil
3 drops clary sage oil
2 drops geranium oil
2 drops myrrh oil
1 drop patchouli oil

Place the jojoba oil in a clean container, add the essential oils, and blend. Apply several drops of the mixture to soothe skin and relieve irritation. Apply to the affected areas as needed, until symptoms subside.

CAPILLARIES, BROKEN

Broken capillaries usually appear on dry, delicate, or mature skin that is thin and fragile. Sometimes called thread veins, spider veins, or couperose skin, the condition occurs when cells in the capillary walls become weak and lose their elasticity. Nor-mally, capillaries, like all blood vessels, expand and contract in rhythmic fashion to move blood through the circulatory system. When capillaries lose their elasticity after dilation, they cannot return to their previous size. They then collapse and the skin turns red.

Broken capillaries most commonly appear on the face, but they can also occur elsewhere on the body. Numerous factors may cause or contribute to the development of broken capillaries, including the use of abrasive cleansers and facial scrubs; the consumption of alcohol, caffeine, and/or certain drugs; exposure to cold weather, harsh winds, or extreme changes in temperature; the use of certain cosmetics; forceful massage; overexposure to the sun; rough handling of the skin; and the consumption of spicy food and stimulants.

HELPFUL TREATMENTS
If you have broken capillaries, avoid alcohol, extremes of temperature, facial steaming and saunas, harsh or irritating cosmetics, spicy food, and stimulants such as caffeine and other stimulant drugs. Always protect your skin in cold or windy weather. Touch your skin gently. Bioflavonoid supplements may reduce redness and strengthen capillaries.

Aromatherapy treatment can achieve good results with commitment over time. Certain essential oils, including chamomile, cypress, geranium, lemon, neroli, palmarosa, peppermint, rose, and rosemary help restore elasticity to blood vessels and diminish the redness on the surface of the skin. Some carrier oils, such as borage, calophyllum inophyllum, evening primrose, hazelnut, and rose hip seed oils, enhance the effectiveness of aromatherapy blends with their own abilities to help reduce broken capillaries.

Apply Facial Oil for Broken Capillaries or Floral Facial Oil for Broken Capillaries to the affected area every day. Since several months can pass before you see results, continue treatment and don't despair. Use the oil blends to maintain results. For broken capillaries on your body, use Capillary-Conditioning Body Oil daily.

AROMATHERAPY BLENDS

You can prepare the aromatherapy blends below using pure essential oils. For a more detailed explanation of how to put together and use these blends, see Part Three: Ways to Use Aromatherapy. To review general guidelines for using essential oils, see page 142.

FACIAL OIL FOR BROKEN CAPILLARIES

1 ounce jojoba oil
½ ounce rose hip seed oil
10 drops borage oil
4 drops cypress oil
3 drops lemon oil
2 drops palmarosa oil

Mix the jojoba and rose hip seed oils together in a clean container, add the essential oils, and gently turn the container upside down a few times or roll it between your hands to blend. Apply the mixture to the affected area once or twice a day.

FLORAL FACIAL OIL
FOR BROKEN CAPILLARIES

½ ounce hazelnut oil
¼ ounce rose hip seed oil
10 drops borage oil
3 drops neroli oil
3 drops rose oil
2 drops geranium oil

Mix the carrier oils together in a clean container, add the essential oils, and blend well. Apply the oil to the affected areas daily.

CAPILLARY-CONDITIONING BODY OIL

1½ ounces sunflower oil
½ ounce rose hip seed oil
20 drops borage oil
5 drops geranium oil
3 drops lemon oil
3 drops rosemary oil
2 drops cypress oil
2 drops palmarosa oil

Mix the carrier oils together in a clean container, add the essential oils, and gently turn the container upside down a few times to blend. Massage the oil over the affected areas daily.

Note: Geranium oil can lower your blood sugar level. Use it with caution (or omit it) if you have hypoglycemia (low blood sugar).

CARPAL TUNNEL SYNDROME

The carpal tunnel is a small channel that surrounds the median nerve as it passes from the arm through the wrist and into the hand, fingers, and thumb. This nerve controls the thumb muscles and gives sensation to the thumb, palm, and the first three fingers. When tendons in the tunnel swell, it blocks circulation and nerve activity within the tunnel. As the tissue around the median nerve in the wrist becomes compressed or damaged, the hand tingles and may feel numb as if it is falling asleep. Carpal tunnel syndrome (CTS) can become painful and a nuisance as your muscles weaken, your strength lessens, and your dexterity decreases.

CTS often occurs as a repetitive motion disorder. People in professions requiring rapid, repetitious movements that flex or extend the wrist, particularly with quick use of the fingers, frequently suffer from CTS. It is an occupational hazard of assembly-line workers, athletes, bookkeepers, cashiers, musicians, computer operators, taxi and truck drivers, writers, and operators of machinery, such as jackhammers and chainsaws, that vibrates the wrists. Even hobbies such as beading, crocheting, hand sewing, knitting, and needlework can cause or contribute to CTS. Arthritis, diabetes mellitus, hypothyroidism, overweight, Raynaud's disease, tendinitis, and medications that promote fluid retention can exaggerate CTS. Symptoms may worsen at night and interfere with sleep. Lying on your hands can cut off circulation, numb them, and intensify pain.

Bloating and water retention during menopause, menstruation, or pregnancy, or as a symptom of premenstrual syndrome (PMS) can exacerbate CTS. Inflammation resulting from infection or injury, improper or prolonged use, or bone spurs can exert pressure on the carpal tunnel. Iron supplements and foods with a high sodium or oxalic-acid content may aggravate joint pain and swelling, as can cool and damp climates.

HELPFUL TREATMENTS

Some cases of carpal tunnel syndrome improve if you simply rest the hand or vary its movements frequently during the day. Shaking your wrists will bring temporary relief by stimulating circulation to the area. Long-term relief may require retraining in the way you use your hands. For example, grasp objects with your entire hand instead of your fingers only, and whenever possible, employ hand tools to avoid forcibly flexing your wrists. Finding new ways to move your hands and wrists often solves current problems and prevents recurrences. Wearing a wrist brace, splint, or athletic bandage wrapped around the wrist restricts movement while you learn more efficient ways to use your hands. Improving your overall posture helps to improve overall circulation. (See Proper Posture on page 183.)

Many cases of CTS respond to treatment with vitamin B_6, which has the ability to reduce inflammation. Eliminate asparagus, beets and beet greens, eggs, fish, parsley, rhubarb, sorrel, spinach, Swiss chard, and members of the cabbage family from your diet. These foods contain oxalic acid and can aggravate joint problems. Salty foods and sodium promote water retention and can increase inflammation. Some people report relief from either eating fresh papaya and pineapple, which contain enzymes that can reduce swelling, or placing the fruit on the affected area. Flaxseed oil, taken internally and applied externally, helps to reduce pain and inflammation as it replenishes essential fatty acids. If you are overweight, reducing your weight may help to ease the pain and inflammation.

If you work at a computer, place the screen about two feet away from you and below your eye level. Use armrests or wrist pads to support and relieve pressure on your wrists. Take breaks frequently. Rotate and shake out your wrists often. Stimulate circulation to your wrists by moving your arms at the shoulder and elbow joints.

Aromatherapy can provide relief for CTS by reducing inflammation, relieving stress, easing pain, and relaxing your mind and body. Essential oils such as cedarwood, chamomile, helichrysum, laurel, marjoram, oregano, pine, and spruce offer relief for CTS.

Soak your hands in Carpal Tunnel Syndrome Hand Bath every day to reduce inflammation and relax your muscles. Gently and gracefully move your hands through the water while soaking. You can also wave your hands through the water during regular baths. Apply Carpal Tunnel Massage Oil to your wrists and hands daily as needed to relieve pain and reduce inflammation. Carrier oils such as calophyllum inophyllum, flaxseed, and hemp oils help reduce inflammation.

AROMATHERAPY BLENDS

You can prepare the aromatherapy blends below using pure essential oils. For a more detailed explanation of how to put together and use these blends, see Part Three: Ways to Use Aromatherapy. To review general guidelines for using essential oils, see page 142.

CARPAL TUNNEL SYNDROME HAND BATH

1 drop chamomile oil
1 drop helichrysum oil
1 drop spruce oil

Add the oils to a large bowl filled with warm water. Soak your hands for ten to twenty minutes. Move your hands and wrists back and forth in the water to gently massage the affected areas.

CARPAL TUNNEL MASSAGE OIL

1 ounce flaxseed oil
1 ounce hemp oil
4 drops chamomile oil
4 drops helichrysum oil
3 drops marjoram oil
2 drops laurel oil

In a clean container, add the essential oils to the carrier oils and blend. Massage over the wrist and hand daily, as needed.

CELLULITE

Approximately 90 percent of all females over the age of eighteen have cellulite, those unsightly fatty deposits also known as "orange-peel skin." Cellulite is more than ordinary fat; it is a combination of fat, cellular wastes, and water that forms a gellike mass and traps in the connective tissue below the skin's surface. It causes visible ripples, bumps, and bulges. Cellulite usually appears on the hips and thighs but can also show up on the arms, abdomen, and upper back.

Such factors as bad diet, constipation, poor posture, a sedentary lifestyle, sluggish blood circulation, and sluggish lymphatic circulation allow cellular wastes to accumulate. Hormonal imbalances may also contribute to cellulite; these can occur as a result of an internal metabolic problem or some external factor, such as the use of oral contraceptives, which disrupt hormonal balance. Stress can also be involved, because it taxes the body, impairing circulation and obstructing elimination. Dietary culprits can include alcohol, caffeine, carbonated sodas, dairy products, fatty and fried foods, meats and animal products, pesticide residues, preservatives, processed foods, salt, and sugar. In addition to being high in fat, most meat, poultry, and dairy products come from animals raised on growth hormone and antibiotics. These drugs remain as residues in the foods and can contribute greatly to cellulite. Inadequate water intake also contributes to sluggish circulation and inhibits the elimination of wastes.

HELPFUL TREATMENTS

To conquer cellulite, first identify the factors that are causing your condition; take necessary steps to minimize or eliminate them. This will probably mean drinking more water, exercising regularly, improving your posture, modifying your diet, practicing deep breathing, and reducing stress. A diet that focuses on fresh vegetables and fruits, whole grains, and lots of water will help cleanse your body. Movement—bicycling, dancing, swimming, walking, yoga, or anything else that gets circulation pumping to your extremities—will benefit you and help your body eliminate cellulite wastes. Reprogramming your posture to eliminate exaggerated lower back or lumbar curves will boost circulation to your lower body. Breathing deeply will improve circulation, delivering more oxygen and nutrients to your cells and promptly removing wastes.

Eliminating cellulite takes time. After all, it took several years or even decades for it to accumulate in your body. Essential oils that help combat cellulite include basil, black pepper, cedarwood, clary sage, cypress, fennel, geranium, juniper, lemon, orange, oregano, patchouli, rosemary, spruce, thyme, and vitex. Aromatherapy baths and body oils help counteract cellulite by improving circulation, encouraging the elimination of wastes, and restoring hormonal balance. Seaweed or algae powder, added to the bath, is especially effective for eliminating toxins.

Skin brushing boosts circulation to the surface of the skin. Apply Skin-Brushing Blend and brush your body before taking the Cellulite Bath. Afterward, apply Cellulite Skin Oil to all affected areas. Repeat this regimen daily for the best results. Once you achieve the desired effect, continue brushing daily, and use a Cellulite Bath and Cellulite Skin Oil once or twice weekly to maintain results.

AROMATHERAPY BLENDS

You can prepare the aromatherapy blends below using pure essential oils. For a more detailed explanation of how to put together and use these blends, see Part Three: Ways to Use Aromatherapy. To review general guidelines for using essential oils, see page 142.

SKIN-BRUSHING BLEND
2 ounces carrier oil
4 drops lemon oil
4 drops orange oil
3 drops cypress oil
2 drops coriander oil
2 drops ginger oil

Place the carrier oil in a clean container and add the essential oils. Gently turn the container upside down a few times or roll it between your hands to blend. Massage a few drops of the mixture onto the areas with cellulite, then dry-brush your skin.

CELLULITE BATH
¼ cup algae or seaweed powder (optional)
3 drops lemon oil
1 drop cypress oil
1 drop fennel oil
1 drop rosemary oil

Add the algae or seaweed powder, if desired, to a bathtub filled with warm water. Drop the essential oils into the tub and disperse well. Soak in the bath for twenty to thirty minutes.

CELLULITE SKIN OIL
4 ounces carrier oil
4 drops lemon oil
4 drops orange oil
4 drops patchouli oil
3 drops cedarwood oil
2 drops clary sage oil

Place the carrier oil in a clean container, add the essential oils, and blend. Apply the mixture to the affected areas after bathing or showering.

CHRONIC FATIGUE SYNDROME

Chronic fatigue syndrome (CFS) is a chronic, debilitating illness, usually lasting several years or longer. Some researchers believe that infection with the Epstein-Barr virus, which is a member of the herpes family of viruses and the same virus that produces infectious mononucleosis, may cause or contribute to it. Other herpes viruses include herpes simplex viruses (which cause cold sores and genital herpes) and varicella zoster (which causes herpes zoster, or shingles, and chickenpox).

The physical symptoms of CFS vary. They include lethargy or incapacitating fatigue, fever, swollen glands, cough, diarrhea, digestive and intestinal problems, dizziness, fever, headaches, outbreaks of herpes or fever blisters, hot flashes (unrelated to menopause), insomnia, joint pain, menstrual problems, muscular aches and pains, nausea, recurrent sore throat, respiratory ailments, ringing in the ears, skin rashes, sweating or flushing (unrelated to physical exertion), swelling or dark circles around the eyes, tingling or numbness in different parts of the body, and weight loss. Mental and emotional symptoms, including anxiety, confusion, depression, difficulty concentrating, emotional stress, lack of interest in pleasurable activities, low self-esteem, temporary memory loss, mood swings, panic attacks, thoughts of suicide, and unexplained feelings of sadness or guilt may appear.

The Epstein-Barr virus can be spread by kissing, sharing food, and other forms of intimate contact, including sexual intercourse. Once infected with the virus, a person remains infected for life, although symptoms may diminish or disappear when the virus goes dormant. However, any weakening of the immune system can reactivate the latent virus.

Most people who suffer from CFS have weakened immune systems; many have a history of mononucleosis. Other factors associated with CFS include anemia; emotional imbalances; exposure to environmental pollutants and cigarette smoke; hypoglycemia; hypothyroidism; infections; intestinal parasites; long-term antibiotic, cortisone, or steroid drug therapy; mental or physical stress; mercury poisoning from silver or amalgam dental fillings; overuse of prescription, over-the-counter, or recreational drugs; and reactions to vaccinations.

HELPFUL TREATMENTS

Treatment for CFS usually consists of a detoxification program, elimination of contributing factors, stress reduction, measures to strengthen the immune system, a healthy diet deriving vitamins and minerals from fresh fruits and vegetables and herbal supplements. Many medical specialists consider stress reduction as important as nutritional therapy in fighting this syndrome.

A number of essential oils can help with CFS by reducing stress, boosting immunity, and eliminating toxins. These include basil, bergamot, chamomile, clary sage, coriander, geranium, ginger, laurel, lavender, lemon, marjoram, niaouli, orange, oregano, peppermint, rosemary, spruce, tea tree, and thyme. If you suffer from CFS, bathe in Energizing Bath Blend daily. Apply Therapeutic Body Oil for CFS over your entire body once or twice daily, and inhale Stimulating Inhalant for CFS as needed to energize you.

AROMATHERAPY BLENDS

You can prepare the aromatherapy blends below using pure essential oils. For a more detailed explanation of how to put together and use these blends, see Part Three: Ways to Use Aromatherapy. To review general guidelines for using essential oils, see page 142.

ENERGIZING BATH BLEND

2 drops orange oil
2 drops thyme oil
1 drop oregano oil
1 drop tea tree oil

Drop the essential oils into a bathtub filled with warm water. Soak in the bath for fifteen to twenty minutes.

THERAPEUTIC BODY OIL FOR CFS

2 ounces carrier oil
6 drops geranium oil
3 drops oregano oil
2 drops basil oil
2 drops coriander oil
2 drops thyme oil

Place the carrier oil in a clean container and add the essential oils. Gently turn the container upside down several times or roll it between your hands to blend. Massage the mixture onto your skin daily.

STIMULATING INHALANT FOR CFS

8 drops spruce oil
6 drops geranium oil
5 drops coriander oil
4 drops bergamot oil
4 drops lemon oil

Drop the essential oils into a small glass bottle with an airtight cover and blend. Inhale directly from the bottle as needed.

Note: Geranium oil can lower your blood sugar level. Use it with caution (or omit it from the above blends) if you have hypoglycemia (low blood sugar).

CIRCULATION, POOR

The circulation of blood throughout the body delivers nutrients and oxygen to every cell in the body, laying the foundation for good health. Circulation also transports wastes from cells to the skin, kidneys, and intestines for elimination. Poor or sluggish circulation detracts from health, allows wastes to build within the body, and can contribute to many illnesses and diseases.

Sluggish circulation can result from clogged arteries, constipation, excess weight, illness, incorrect posture, lack of exercise, low blood pressure, poor diet, a sedentary lifestyle, or your body's inability to eliminate toxins properly. Symptoms may include cold feet and hands, difficulty concentrating, dizziness, dull-looking skin, fatigue, a high cholesterol level, poor memory, shortness of breath, and varicose veins.

HELPFUL TREATMENTS

Daily exercise, such as doing aerobics, taking a brisk walk, or doing yoga will stimulate circulation. If you are overweight, losing the excess weight will help. Eat a healthy diet concentrating on fresh vegetables and fruits, whole grains, and legumes. Drink eight to ten glasses of water daily. Massaging and brushing your skin will encourage circulation to extremities and to the surface of the skin. Applied to the skin, sesame oil increases circulation. Stimulating a sluggish lymph system will boost blood circulation. (*See* LYMPHATIC SYSTEM, SLUGGISH/SWOLLEN LYMPH GLANDS.)

Many essential oils stimulate circulation, including basil, benzoin, black pepper, cedarwood, coriander, cypress, eucalyptus, fennel, geranium, ginger, juniper, laurel, lavender, lemon, marjoram, myrrh, neroli, orange, oregano, palmarosa, peppermint, pine, rose, rosemary, thyme, vetiver, and ylang ylang. Apply a few drops of Circulation-Boosting Body-Brushing Oil to your body and brush your skin every morning to invigorate your circulation. Then take a Circulation-Boosting Bath. Apply Circulation-Boosting Body Oil once or twice daily to your entire body, especially to your extremities.

As your circulation improves, your blood cells will bring more nutrients into the tissues and take away wastes more efficiently. Your health will begin to improve at the cellular level, and your entire body will function better.

AROMATHERAPY BLENDS

You can prepare the aromatherapy blends below using pure essential oils. For a more detailed explanation of how to put together and use these blends, see Part Three: Ways to Use Aromatherapy. To review general guidelines for using essential oils, see page 142.

CIRCULATION-BOOSTING
BODY-BRUSHING OIL

2 ounces sesame oil

4 drops rosemary oil

3 drops lemon oil

2 drops laurel oil

2 drops thyme oil

1 drop basil oil

1 drop black pepper oil

1 drop ginger oil

Blend all the ingredients together well in a clean container. Apply a few drops to your skin and brush.

CIRCULATION-BOOSTING BATH

2 drops cypress oil
2 drops orange oil
2 drops peppermint oil
2 drops pine oil

Add the essential oils to a bathtub filled with warm water. Soak in the bath for twenty to thirty minutes.

CIRCULATION-BOOSTING BODY OIL

2 ounces sesame oil

6 drops rosemary oil

4 drops lemon oil

2 drops geranium oil

2 drops myrrh oil

1 drop ginger oil

1 drop vetiver oil

Add the essential oils to the carrier oil and blend. Apply the oil to your skin as needed to stimulate circulation.

Note: Rosemary and peppermint oils are extremely stimulating. If you plan to use any of the above blends before going to sleep, you may wish to omit these oils from the formula so that they do not interfere with your rest.

COLD SORES

See HERPES VIRUS.

COLDS AND FLU

Congestion, coughs, fatigue, fever, chills, grogginess, headache, runny nose, sore throat, swollen glands, and watery or burning eyes can signal an approaching cold. Many different viruses cause colds. Colds are the most common communicable diseases, spreading easily from person to person.

Symptoms of the flu are similar to those of a cold but usually include a higher temperature and an all-over feeling of aching in joints and muscles. The runny nose, sore throat, and watery eyes that are characteristic of a cold may or may not be present with the flu. Like colds, the flu is a highly contagious viral illness that spreads rapidly from one person to another. Because the structure of the flu virus changes every two or three years or so, the disease normally occurs in epidemics when a new type of flu virus appears.

Colds and flu will most likely strike when immunity is low as a result of inadequate rest, overwork, poor nutrition, or stress. Under these conditions, your body's defenses may be too weak to fight off invading viruses.

HELPFUL TREATMENTS

Since there is no cure for the common cold or for the flu, assisting the body in fighting the infection is the best course of action. Sleeping and resting, drinking lots of liquids, and avoiding sugar and sweets will help your immune system to recuperate. Taking supplements of vitamin C, beta-carotene, and zinc can help. The herbs echinacea, goldenseal, and licorice root are helpful in fighting viruses and strengthening immunity.

Essential oils can help fight colds and flu in two ways. First, they can ward off illness or hasten recovery by boosting immunity. Second, they can ease many of the discomforts of colds and the flu when used in baths, chest rubs, compresses, and inhalants, as well as in the diffuser. Essential oils that can help are basil, benzoin, bergamot, black pepper, cedarwood, coriander, clary sage, elemi, eucalyptus, fennel, frankincense, ginger, helichrysum, juniper, laurel, lemon, marjoram, myrrh, niaouli, orange, oregano, palmarosa, pine, rosemary, rosewood, St. John's wort, tea tree, and thyme.

At the first sign of a cold or the flu, take a Cold- and Flu-Fighting Bath. Then prepare an Inhalant for Colds and Flu and use it in a steam inhalation or inhale it directly from the bottle. Massage Cold and Flu Chest Rub onto your chest, throat, and back. Then get in bed! If you have a fever or chills, you can apply a Compress for Fever or Chills (choose cool water for fever, hot water for chills). Drink lots of liquids, particularly water, to flush out wastes. Disperse Cold-Combating Diffuser Blend throughout your room. Repeat this entire treatment once or twice daily for several days or until symptoms subside.

AROMATHERAPY BLENDS

You can prepare the aromatherapy blends below using pure essential oils. For a more detailed explanation of how to put together and use these blends, see Part Three: Ways to Use Aromatherapy. To review general guidelines for using essential oils, see page 142.

COLD- AND FLU-FIGHTING BATH

2 drops tea tree oil

1 drop myrrh oil

1 drop niaouli oil

1 drop oregano oil

1 drop thyme oil

Disperse the essential oils in a bathtub filled with warm water. Soak in the bath for

twenty to thirty minutes, taking care not to become chilled. Repeat as necessary.

INHALANT FOR COLDS AND FLU

8 drops bergamot oil

4 drops elemi oil

3 drops ginger oil

3 drops laurel oil

2 drops basil oil

2 drops black pepper oil

2 drops eucalyptus oil

Add all the oils to a small glass bottle with an airtight cover and blend well. You can inhale the mixture directly from the bottle, apply 2 drops to a tissue, or add 3 drops to a bowl of steaming water and lean your face over the bowl for five minutes while inhaling the steam.

COLD AND FLU CHEST RUB

2 ounces carrier oil

3 drops pine oil

2 drops eucalyptus oil

2 drops frankincense oil

1 drop ginger oil

1 drop oregano oil

1 drop thyme oil

Place the carrier oil in a clean container, add the essential oils, and blend. Massage the oil over your chest and back several times daily until your symptoms subside.

COMPRESS FOR FEVER OR CHILLS

1 quart hot or cool water
2 drops orange oil
2 drops pine oil
1 drop ginger oil

Pour the water into a 2-quart glass bowl (use cool water for fever, hot water for chills) and add the essential oils to the water. Soak a clean cloth in the water and apply it to your chest or forehead as needed.

COLD-COMBATING DIFFUSER BLEND

12 drops lemon oil
12 drops orange oil
10 drops eucalyptus oil
10 drops oregano oil
10 drops pine oil
6 drops basil oil
6 drops niaouli oil
4 drops ginger oil

Add the essential oils to a small glass bottle with an airtight cover. Turn the bottle upside down several times or roll it between your hands to blend the oils, and add some of the mixture to your diffuser. Run the diffuser as necessary.

CONSTIPATION

Constipation, a condition in which bowel movements decrease in frequency, is a common digestive complaint. Dehydration, poor diet, a sedentary lifestyle, and stress can contribute to constipation.

The average American diet lacks sufficient amounts of fiber, the indigestible portion of plant foods that binds with wastes in the intestines to eliminate the wastes. Instead, most Americans eat a diet loaded with chemical additives, fats, pesticide residues, preservatives, salt, and sugar, which are difficult to digest, difficult to assimilate, and difficult to eliminate. Such a diet burdens the digestive tract with wastes that often linger in the body. Particles of waste lodge on the intestinal walls, making complete elimination difficult or impossible.

A sedentary lifestyle can contribute to constipation because it does not give the body enough stimulation to keep everything moving properly. Stress overloads the body, preventing it from functioning normally. Insufficient water intake interferes with the body's ability to flush out wastes.

HELPFUL TREATMENTS

Eating a diet that focuses on fresh vegetables, fruits, and whole grains will provide necessary dietary fiber; drinking lots of water (at least 64 ounces a day) will help flush out wastes. Regular exercise, such as walking, swimming, or yoga, stimulates circulation, digestion, and elimination. Finding ways to manage stress is also important. (*See* STRESS.)

Essential oils can help by improving digestion, increasing peristalsis (the rhythmic contractions of intestinal muscles that push wastes out of the body), and encouraging the elimination of wastes. Essential oils can also reduce stress. Basil, black pepper, chamomile, coriander, fennel, ginger, lemon, marjoram, orange, pine, rose, rosemary, and ylang ylang are essential oils that can help overcome constipation. If you suffer from constipation, massage Constipation Abdominal Rub over your abdomen every morning and every evening to encourage regular bowel movements.

AROMATHERAPY BLENDS

You can prepare the aromatherapy blends below using pure essential oils. For a more detailed explanation of how to put together and use these blends, see Part Three: Ways to Use Aromatherapy. To review general guidelines for using essential oils, see page 142.

CONSTIPATION ABDOMINAL RUB

4 ounces carrier oil
8 drops fennel oil
6 drops orange oil
4 drops coriander oil
4 drops lemon oil
2 drops ginger oil

Place the carrier oil in a clean container, add the essential oils, and gently turn the container upside down a few times or roll it between your hands to blend. Twice a day, massage the oil over your abdominal area, moving clockwise from right to left.

CUTS AND BRUISES

Cuts and bruises usually result from injuries to or incisions into the skin. Most superficial cuts and wounds require little treatment

and will heal naturally. Immediately after the skin is broken, the blood begins clotting to stop the bleeding. A scab forms, protecting the underlying tissue and allowing the skin to regenerate and repair itself.

Skin acts as a barrier to prevent foreign matter and microorganisms from invading the body; therefore, any break in the skin increases the possibility of infection. Cuts and wounds also can lead to scarring if they are extensive or if they are not cleansed and treated properly. Seek medical attention for any wound from a rusty metal object or a deep puncture, or that bleeds heavily.

Bruising occurs when an injury damages tiny blood vessels under the skin. Black, blue, and purple discoloration occurs as blood leaks from the damaged blood vessels into the surrounding tissues. As the blood is absorbed, the bruise will fade and heal naturally. People who suffer from anemia, obesity, or nutritional deficiencies may bruise more easily than others. A variety of medications, including anti-inflammatory drugs, anticoagulants, painkillers, steroids, and some antibiotics, can also increase susceptibility to bruising.

HELPFUL TREATMENTS

Thoroughly cleanse and treat cuts and wounds immediately to reduce pain, speed healing, and minimize scarring. Essential oils that can help prevent infection and speed healing of cuts and wounds are benzoin, bergamot, clary sage, cypress, elemi, eucalyptus, frankincense, geranium, helichrysum, juniper, lavender, lemon, melissa, myrrh, oregano, palmarosa, patchouli, pine, rose, rosemary, rosewood, St. John's wort, sandalwood, tea tree, thyme, valerian, and vetiver. Essential oils that diminish scarring include benzoin, frankincense, geranium, lemon, palmarosa, patchouli, and rosewood. Neroli oil reputedly will prevent scarring if applied to the cut or wound regularly. Certain carrier oils enhance healing of injuries that break the skin. Calophyllum inophyllum, flaxseed, rose hip seed, sesame, and wheat germ oils promote healing while reducing scarring.

To speed the healing of an injury that breaks the skin, apply Cut- and Wound-Healing Oil to the injured area several times daily. To prevent or lessen scarring, once the wound has healed, massage Scar Massage Oil onto the affected area once or twice daily, until the scar fades.

Everyone gets bruises from time to time. If you bruise easily or frequently, however, you may wish to consult a healthcare professional to check for a vitamin C or vitamin K deficiency or an underlying health problem. Essential oils to use on bruises include chamomile, geranium, ginger, helichrysum, juniper, laurel, lavender, marjoram, St. John's wort, and thyme. Immediately after an injury, apply ice or a cold Muscle Strain Compress to the area. Rub Bruise-Diminishing Blend over the bruised area two or more times daily to speed healing and stimulate blood flow through the bruised area. Carrier oils that diminish in-

flammation of bruising include almond, borage, calophyllum inophyllum, evening primrose, flaxseed, and hemp oils.

AROMATHERAPY BLENDS

You can prepare the aromatherapy blends below using pure essential oils. For a more detailed explanation of how to put together and use these blends, see Part Three: Ways to Use Aromatherapy. To review general guidelines for using essential oils, see page 142.

CUT- AND WOUND-HEALING OIL

½ ounce flaxseed oil
10 drops calophyllum inophyllum oil
6 drops tea tree oil
4 drops frankincense oil
3 drops cypress oil
3 drops helichrysum oil
2 drops St. John's wort oil
1 drop myrrh oil

Place the carrier oils in a clean container, add the essential oils, and blend. After thoroughly cleansing a cut or wound, apply this mixture to the affected area. Repeat the application several times daily, as needed.

SCAR MASSAGE OIL

1½ ounces sunflower oil
½ ounce flaxseed oil
10 drops wheat germ oil
4 drops neroli oil
3 drops patchouli oil
2 drops geranium oil

2 drops rosewood oil
1 drop benzoin resin
1 drop frankincense oil

Mix the carrier oils together in a clean container. Add the essential oils and gently turn the container upside down a few times to blend all the ingredients together. Until the wound closes and heals over, apply the oil to the skin surrounding the wound. Once it heals, you can apply it on the entire area to prevent or minimize the appearance of scars.

MUSCLE STRAIN COMPRESS
1 quart cold water
2 drops chamomile oil
1 drop ginger oil
1 drop St. John's wort oil

Pour the water into a 2-quart glass bowl and add the essential oils. Saturate a clean cloth in the water and apply it to the affected area for at least ten minutes. Do this immediately after an injury and repeat the treatment often for the first twenty-four hours thereafter.

BRUISE-DIMINISHING BLEND
1 ounce hemp oil
½ ounce borage oil
½ ounce flaxseed oil
3 drops geranium oil
3 drops helichrysum oil
3 drops laurel oil

2 drops chamomile oil
2 drops St. John's wort

In a clean container, add the essential oils to the carrier oils and blend. Apply the mixture to the bruised area several times daily.

CYSTITIS

Cystitis is an infection or inflammation of the bladder. When bacteria from outside invade the urethra, the passageway that carries urine from the bladder for elimination, cystitis can occur. Typical symptoms of cystitis are frequent or painful urination, a burning sensation during urinating, and a nearly constant urge to urinate. Urine may leak involuntarily—a sign of incontinence. (*See* INCONTINENCE.) These symptoms are occasionally accompanied by back pain, blood or mucus in the urine, fever, nausea, or vomiting. Failure to treat cystitis promptly can allow the infection to spread to the kidneys, causing permanent damage.

Bladder infections affect women more often than men, because the female urethra is shorter and located very near the anus; bacteria often migrate from the anal area to the urethra. However, during intercourse, women may transmit bacteria that can lead to cystitis or urethritis in men. Women who are pregnant and people of either sex who have weakened immune systems are more likely than others to get cystitis. A number of external factors can lead to cystitis: poor personal hygiene and the use of such products as scented toilet tissue, deodorant tampons or sanitary pads, diaphragms, spermicidal creams, colored and/or fragranced condoms, feminine hygiene sprays, perfumed bath oils, bubble baths, and soaps. Holding on to urine despite the urge to void the bladder, engaging in sexual intercourse (especially if a diaphragm or a scented sexual preparation is used), and wearing tight-fitting clothing or synthetic underwear that hinders circulation can contribute to cystitis. Some women who take oral contraceptives are susceptible to urinary tract infections.

HELPFUL TREATMENTS

To discourage cystitis, eliminate any possible underlying factors. Always empty your bladder when it first signals you. Drink eight to ten glasses of water daily. Avoid wearing tight-fitting clothes like pantyhose, girdles, and jeans, and choose underwear made of natural fibers. Cranberries contain a substance that prevents bacteria from clinging to the interior surface of the bladder and the urinary tract. Drinking several glasses of unsweetened cranberry juice daily can speed recovery and prevent future infections.

Hygiene is important for both preventing and treating cystitis. Women should keep the vaginal area clean by wiping from front to back after bowel movements. Urinating after bathing and before and after in-

tercourse also reduces the risk of bacterial infection, for women as well as men. A man with recurring urinary tract infections can protect himself with a condom to reduce the risk of bacterial infection during sexual intercourse.

Aromatherapy can minimize the discomfort of cystitis and speed recovery. Aromatherapy may also prevent recurring bouts of cystitis. Essential oils such as benzoin, bergamot, cedarwood, cypress, elemi, eucalyptus, frankincense, juniper, niaouli, pine, sandalwood, tea tree, and thyme help to relieve cystitis. Benzoin, eucalyptus, niaouli, oregano, sandalwood, tea tree, and thyme oils are especially effective against bacterial infection. In addition, benzoin, cedarwood, chamomile, cypress, eucalyptus, juniper, pine, sandalwood, and thyme oils are diuretics and increase urination, which cleanses the bladder. This is helpful if cystitis makes urination difficult. If you develop cystitis, immerse yourself in a Sitz Bath for Cystitis once or twice a day until your symptoms subside. Apply Cystitis Massage Oil to your abdomen, lower back, pubic area, and pelvic region several times daily.

AROMATHERAPY BLENDS

You can prepare the aromatherapy blends below using pure essential oils. For a more detailed explanation of how to put together and use these blends, see Part Three: Ways to Use Aromatherapy. To review general guidelines for using essential oils, see page 142.

SITZ BATH FOR CYSTITIS
2 drops tea tree oil
1 drop bergamot oil
1 drop cypress oil
1 drop thyme oil

Add the oils to a shallow tub filled with warm water. Sit hip-deep in the tub for fifteen minutes. Repeat once or twice each day until your symptoms subside.

CYSTITIS MASSAGE OIL
1 ounce carrier oil
3 drops sandalwood oil
2 drops cedarwood oil
2 drops niaouli oil
1 drop chamomile oil
1 drop frankincense oil

Add all the ingredients to a clean container and blend. Massage the mixture over your abdomen, lower back, and pelvic area. Repeat several times daily until symptoms cease.

DEPRESSION

Although many people use the word *depression* to describe passing feelings of sadness, true depression is actually an illness classified as a mood disorder. The many faces of depression may show up as anger, anxiety, confusion, diminished sex drive, fatigue, feelings of worthlessness, hyperactivity, insomnia, irritability, lethargy, loss of interest in usual activities, loss of appetite or overeating, mood swings, poor concentration, thoughts of suicide, and weight loss or weight gain.

The cause or causes of depression are not well understood but may be associated with the activity of nerve cells that receive norepinephrine or serotonin as neurotransmitters. A deficiency or inefficiency, or perhaps the ineffectiveness of these brain chemicals, could contribute to depression. Life events and circumstances such as loss of a loved one, a job, or reputation may be related to the onset of depression, but such events are likely to cause the condition only in susceptible people. Many cases of depression occur without any traumatic incident.

A multitude of physical conditions can lead to or exacerbate symptoms of depression. These include allergies, overconsumption of caffeine or alcohol, candidiasis, certain drugs, chemical sensitivities, chronic fatigue syndrome, cigarette smoking, digestive disorders, endometriosis, exposure to environmental pollutants, high sugar intake, hormonal imbalances, hypoglycemia, illness, nutritional deficiencies, poor diet, stress, and thyroid disorders.

Decreased daylight during winter contributes to a type of depression called seasonal affective disorder syndrome (SAD). Clinical psychologists have observed an increase in depression during wintertime with shorter days and fewer hours of sunlight. One theory is that the eyes don't receive enough natural sunlight. SAD can also affect people who sleep during the day and are awake at night.

HELPFUL TREATMENTS

If you are experiencing symptoms of depression, you should consider seeking psychological counseling to help discover the causes of your depression. If necessary, consult your health-care professional to rule out any physical problems or nutritional deficiencies.

Changing your diet and correcting nutritional deficiencies can often have a positive impact on the way you feel. Eliminate all junk food, refined foods, and sugar, as well as most fats, from your diet. Focus on eating whole grains, fresh vegetables, and other complex carbohydrates. Regular physical exercise has also been shown to diminish depression. Keep as involved and active as possible. Reducing stress often helps to decrease depression, as does writing about your problems and emotions.

Aromatherapy can help to alter your moods. The aroma of certain essential oils can stimulate the production of neurotransmitters within your brain that regulate your behavior and moods. If you want to be more calm and relaxed, use benzoin, chamomile, clary sage, frankincense, geranium, jasmine, lavender, melissa, neroli, patchouli, rose, rosewood, St. John's wort, sandalwood, spruce, valerian, vetiver, vitex, and ylang ylang oils. If you're feeling lethargic or sluggish, stimulate your stamina with

basil, bergamot, geranium, helichrysum, jasmine, lavender, lemon, neroli, orange, patchouli, peppermint, rose, rosemary, and spruce oils. For the quickest relief, simply open a bottle of one of the above oils and sniff it full strength. Borage, flaxseed, and sesame oils can decrease depression when massaged onto to the skin.

Depending on how your depression manifests itself, choose either Sedating Anti-Depression Bath or Stimulating Anti-Depression Bath every day. Afterward, apply either Calming Anti-Depression Massage Oil or Energizing Anti-Depression Massage Oil, again depending on your needs. Several times a day, apply either Relaxing Personal Fragrance or Uplifting Personal Perfume or inhale it directly from the bottle. You can also disperse Anti-Depression Diffuser Blend throughout your home or office during the day as needed.

AROMATHERAPY BLENDS

You can prepare the aromatherapy blends below using pure essential oils. For a more detailed explanation of how to put together and use these blends, see Part Three: Ways to Use Aromatherapy. To review general guidelines for using essential oils, see page 142.

SEDATING ANTI-DEPRESSION BATH

2 drops chamomile oil
1 drop clary sage oil
1 drop valerian oil
1 drop ylang ylang oil

Add the oils to a bathtub filled with warm water. Soak in the bath for twenty minutes before bedtime. Follow with Calming Anti-Depression Massage Oil.

STIMULATING ANTI-DEPRESSION BATH
3 drops rosemary oil
2 drops geranium oil
2 drops spruce oil

Add the oils to a bathtub filled with warm water and soak for twenty minutes. Follow with an application of Energizing Anti-Depression Massage Oil.

CALMING ANTI-DEPRESSION MASSAGE OIL
1 ounce sesame oil
4 drops sandalwood oil
2 drops German chamomile oil
1 drop benzoin resin
1 drop jasmine absolute or enfleurage
1 drop St. John's wort oil
1 drop ylang ylang oil

Place the carrier oil in a clean container and add the essential oils. Gently turn the container upside down several times or roll it between your hands to blend. Massage the oil over your body daily, as necessary.

ENERGIZING ANTI-DEPRESSION MASSAGE OIL
1 ounce sesame oil
3 drops orange oil

2 drops spruce oil
1 drop peppermint oil

Place the carrier oil in a clean container, add the essential oils, and blend. Massage the mixture into your skin daily.

RELAXING PERSONAL FRAGRANCE
⅛ ounce jojoba oil
4 drops sandalwood oil
3 drops melissa oil
2 drops jasmine absolute or enfleurage
2 drops ylang ylang oil
1 drop clary sage oil
1 drop vetiver oil

In a clean container, add the essential oils to the jojoba oil and gently turn the container over several times or roll it between your hands to blend. Dab the mixture on your pulse points or inhale the fragrance directly from the bottle as needed.

UPLIFTING PERSONAL PERFUME
⅛ ounce jojoba oil
4 drops bergamot oil
3 drops geranium oil
3 drops spruce oil
2 drops rosewood oil

Place the jojoba oil in a clean container and add the essential oils. Gently turn the container upside down several times or roll it between your hands to blend the oils. Apply the blend to your pulse points as a perfume. You can also inhale it directly from the bottle. Use it as needed.

ANTI-DEPRESSION DIFFUSER BLEND

20 drops lavender oil

15 drops geranium oil

8 drops orange oil

6 drops clary sage oil

6 drops spruce oil

4 drops rosewood oil

3 drops frankincense oil

2 drops ylang ylang oil

Drop the essential oils into a small glass bottle with an airtight cover and blend. Add some of the mixture to your diffuser as necessary.

DERMATITIS

Dermatitis is a broad category of skin disorders characterized by inflammation and, usually, itching. Many cases of dermatitis occur when the skin comes into contact with a substance that causes an allergic reaction. There are also forms of dermatitis that can result from a deficiency of essential fatty acids, a high-acid diet, overuse of drugs, stress, or the presence of too many refined foods or saturated fats in the diet.

Of the many kinds of dermatitis, the most common is contact dermatitis. Contact dermatitis occurs as a reaction to one or more of a variety of chemicals or other environmental elements when the offending substance comes into contact with an individual who is sensitive. Skin becomes irritated and inflamed, with itching and redness. It may be dry and flaky. Some of the things that most frequently produce contact dermatitis are antiperspirants and deodorants, cleaning products, fabric dyes, cosmetics, detergents, fragrances, hair coloring and permanent solutions, leather-processing chemicals, plants, rubber compounds, solvents, and certain metals, especially nickel, which may be present in jewelry, bra closures, wristwatches, and zippers. Eczema is another type of dermatitis that causes patches of skin to become dry and red, frequently with cracking, crusting, and weeping or watery blistered areas. (*See also* ECZEMA.)

HELPFUL TREATMENTS

If you suffer from dermatitis, pinpointing the cause or causes of the problem and then eliminating or minimizing your exposure to them is the first step toward alleviating the symptoms. Aromatherapy can help ease or eliminate symptoms as well. Essential oils such as benzoin, cedarwood, chamomile, clary sage, elemi, geranium, helichrysum, jasmine, juniper, lavender, lemon, neroli, orange, patchouli, peppermint, rose, rosemary, rosewood, sandalwood, tea tree, thyme, and ylang ylang soothe irritated skin, reduce inflammation, prevent dryness and itching, and subdue stress.

To ease irritation and inflammation and to combat dryness, bathe in Dermatitis-Soothing Bath once a day or several times a week, depending on the severity of your condition. Apply a Cool Compress for

Dermatitis to the affected areas to soothe hot, inflamed skin. Massage Dermatitis Skin Oil into your skin several times daily, as needed. Carrier oils that help relieve dermatitis include borage, evening primrose, hazelnut, hemp, jojoba, and wheat germ oils.

Many cases of dermatitis improve after bathing the skin in Dead Sea salts, seaweed or algae powder, or apple cider vinegar. The addition of essential oils will make the bath even more effective.

Aromatherapy Blends

You can prepare the aromatherapy blends below using pure essential oils. For a more detailed explanation of how to put together and use these blends, see Part Three: Ways to Use Aromatherapy. To review general guidelines for using essential oils, see page 142.

Dermatitis-Soothing Bath

½ cup apple cider vinegar (optional)
3 drops chamomile oil
3 drops lavender oil
2 drops cedarwood oil
1 drop elemi oil
1 drop helichrysum oil

Add all the essential oils to a bathtub filled with warm water and apple cider vinegar, if desired. Soak in the bath for twenty minutes.

Cool Compress for Dermatitis

1 quart cool water
1 drop cedarwood oil

1 drop patchouli oil
1 drop sandalwood oil

Pour the water into a 2-quart glass bowl and add the essential oils. Soak a clean cloth in the water and apply it to the affected areas as needed.

Dermatitis Skin Oil

1 ounce jojoba oil
½ ounce hazelnut oil
2 drops chamomile oil
2 drops lavender oil
1 drop neroli oil
1 drop rose oil
1 drop ylang ylang oil

Place the carrier oils in a clean container, add the essential oils, and gently turn the container upside down a few times or roll it between your hands to blend. Apply the oil to your skin as needed.

DIARRHEA

Frequent, watery bowel movements accompanied by abdominal pain and cramping are characteristic of diarrhea. Diarrhea is one way in which the body can rapidly rid itself of toxins and foreign substances. It may result from a bacterial or viral infection, food allergies, food poisoning, the consumption of caffeine or impure water, emotional upset, poor or inadequate digestion of food, reactions to drugs, spastic colon, or stress.

HELPFUL TREATMENTS

Diarrhea is usually a sign that the body is attempting to cleanse itself. When you experience a bout of diarrhea, drink plenty of pure water to prevent dehydration and to help your body flush out toxins. Avoid eating anything until symptoms start to subside. If you are traveling in a foreign country and are unsure about the water, drink only bottled water while avoiding any "hidden" sources of the local water, such as ice, raw fruits and vegetables washed in local water, and tap water used for brushing your teeth.

Aromatherapy can relieve some of the discomforts of diarrhea. Black pepper, chamomile, coriander, ginger, lavender, and peppermint oils relieve stomach spasms; myrrh, niaouli, oregano, patchouli, tea tree, and thyme oils fight infection caused by bacteria and other microbial infections. Cypress oil helps to restore balance when the body is excreting excessive amounts of fluids. Calming oils such as chamomile, geranium, orange, neroli, and sandalwood are soothing, both physically and emotionally, and are useful when stress or nerves are factors.

If you are suffering from diarrhea, massage All-Purpose Diarrhea Diminisher over your abdomen and lower back several times daily until symptoms subside.

AROMATHERAPY BLENDS

You can prepare the aromatherapy blends below using pure essential oils. For a more detailed explanation of how to put together and use these blends, see Part Three: Ways to Use Aromatherapy. To review general guidelines for using essential oils, see page 142.

ALL-PURPOSE DIARRHEA DIMINISHER

2 ounces carrier oil
6 drops cypress oil
4 drops lemon oil
4 drops niaouli oil
2 drops coriander oil
2 drops peppermint oil

Place the carrier oil in a clean container, add the essential oils, and gently turn the container upside down a few times or roll it between your hands to blend. Massage the mixture over your abdominal area and lower back as necessary.

DIGESTIVE DISORDERS

See CONSTIPATION; DIARRHEA; INDIGESTION.

EARACHE

An earache can produce a dull ache, sharp stabbing pains, ringing, or throbbing in the ear. Earaches that result from bacterial infection often occur when fluid builds up in the eustachian tube, which connects the middle ear with the nasal cavity and throat and equalizes pressure on both sides of the eardrum. The eustachian tube also permits excess secretions to drain away from the ear. When the eustachian tube does not drain properly, these secretions build up in the middle ear, pressure in the ear rises, and you may experience pain in the ear. In addition, microorganisms may migrate from the nose and throat to the ear by means of the eustachian tube, causing infection. If pressure rises sufficiently, the eardrum may rupture. Symptoms of a ruptured eardrum include dizziness, ringing in ears, bleeding from the ear, a sudden increase or decrease in pain, or loss of hearing. These signs indicate a need for prompt medical attention.

Respiratory allergies, respiratory infections, food allergies, impacted earwax, and middle ear infections are the most common causes of earaches. Swimming or bathing in contaminated, chlorinated, or unclean water can contribute to an ear infection that results in earache. Sometimes a rapid change in air pressure (such as occurs with changes in altitude or decompression of an airplane's cabin), during diving, or from exposure to cold climates and winds can prompt an earache. Loud noises like explosions, gunshots, and overly loud music, especially when listened to through headphones, can create ringing in the ears and may affect hearing permanently. Earache, inner ear infections, or hearing loss may signal diseases of the heart or arteries.

A major cause of low-level hearing loss is the buildup of earwax beyond what is normal. Earwax lubricates the ear canal and traps bacteria, dust, and foreign matter. Normally it works its way out of the ear, taking along any foreign particles.

Earaches and ear infections are the most common complaint of infants and young children treated in medical clinics. People who spend time in environments with cigarette smoke are more susceptible to earaches and ear infections.

Chronic ear infections and hearing loss may affect behavior, mood, and personality, and can lead to depression and withdrawal that are often mistaken for antisocial behavior. In older people, the confusion, inattention, and indifference caused by hearing loss may be incorrectly attributed to senility.

Helpful Treatments

If you have an earache, you should see a medical practitioner as soon as possible, as it may signal a problem requiring a doctor's treatment. Keep ears clean and avoid the buildup of earwax.

A weakened immune system, chronic respiratory infections, and food allergies are all factors that can contribute to frequent earaches. If you suffer from recurring earaches, an elimination diet or food diary can help to isolate any foods causing allergies. Start by eliminating the most common offenders: dairy products, eggs, wheat, corn, citrus fruits, peanuts, and peanut butter.

Aromatherapy can help by decreasing discomfort and strengthening your immune system. It can fight infection, soothing symptoms of respiratory ailments. Basil, chamomile, eucalyptus, geranium, lavender, niaouli, oregano, rosemary, sandalwood, tea tree, and thyme oils are essential oils that can ease the pain of earaches. Massage Earache Oil Blend on and around your ears. Then apply an Earache Compress or Earache Clay Pack over your ears.

AROMATHERAPY BLENDS

You can prepare the aromatherapy blends below using pure essential oils. For a more detailed explanation of how to put together and use these blends, see Part Three: Ways to Use Aromatherapy. To review general guidelines for using essential oils, see page 142.

EARACHE OIL BLEND

1 ounce olive oil
3 drops niaouli oil
2 drops eucalyptus oil
1 drop oregano oil

Place the carrier oil in a clean container, add the essential oils, and gently turn the container upside down several times or roll it between your hands to blend. Massage the mixture over your ears as needed.

EARACHE COMPRESS

1 quart hot water
2 drops chamomile oil
1 drop basil oil
1 drop lavender oil
1 drop sandalwood oil

Pour the water into a 2-quart glass bowl and disperse the essential oils in the water. Soak a clean cloth in the water and apply it to your ear for fifteen minutes. Repeat as necessary.

EARACHE CLAY PACK

½ cup clay
½ cup water (approximately)
1 drop oregano oil
1 drop tea tree oil
1 drop thyme oil

In a small bowl, blend all ingredients to form a smooth paste. Put cotton dipped in Earache Oil Blend inside the ear to prevent the pack from entering the ear. Spread on the skin around the ear. Leave on for 30 to 60 minutes. Repeat several times daily.

ECZEMA

Eczema is a type of dermatitis that appears as dry patches of skin with cracking, crusting, redness, and swelling, often with weeping sores or watery blisters. The skin becomes hot, inflamed, and itchy.

Many different factors can cause or contribute to eczema in susceptible individuals. Stress can cause or aggravate eczema, as can exposure to cleaning compounds, colognes, cosmetics, detergents, household chemicals, soaps, and synthetic perfumes. Food allergies can often trigger an outbreak of eczema. Corn, dairy products, tomatoes, vinegar, and wheat are among the foods that most frequently cause the allergies that show up as skin problems. Acidic, hot, or spicy foods can also activate skin rashes in some people. Deficiencies of nutrients, such as essential fatty acids, can contribute to eczema as well.

HELPFUL TREATMENTS

The best approach for clearing or controlling eczema and most other skin disorders is to follow a healthy diet, minimize stress, and avoid synthetically fragranced cosmetics, perfumes, and other products, as well as all harsh chemicals. Keep track of your outbreaks to find out what may be provoking your skin sensitivities; then avoid those things. Flaxseed oil, applied externally or taken internally, often eases symptoms of eczema. One cup of apple cider vinegar, cornstarch, or finely ground oatmeal added to a bath can soothe itchiness and soften skin.

Aromatherapy can help relieve eczema by decreasing stress, calming inflammation, and healing the skin. Bathing the skin in Dead Sea salts and seaweed or algae powder eases many symptoms. Essential oils that help eczema are benzoin, bergamot, chamomile, clary sage, elemi, geranium, helichrysum, jasmine, lavender, lemon, myrrh, neroli, niaouli, orange, oregano, patchouli, peppermint, pine, rose, rosemary, rosewood, sandalwood, spruce, tea tree, thyme, and ylang ylang.

To help control eczema, bathe in Eczema-Calming Bath daily. Apply a Skin-Cooling Compress to the affected areas for additional relief. Several times each day, apply Eczema Body Oil or Eczema Facial Oil to the affected areas to reduce inflammation and irritation and to promote healing.

AROMATHERAPY BLENDS

You can prepare the aromatherapy blends below using pure essential oils. For a more detailed explanation of how to put together and use these blends, see Part Three: Ways to Use Aromatherapy. To review general guidelines for using essential oils, see page 142.

ECZEMA-CALMING BATH

1 cup cornstarch (optional)
2 drops chamomile oil
2 drops geranium oil
1 drop elemi oil

Disperse all the ingredients in a bathtub filled with warm water. Enjoy a leisurely thirty-minute soak.

SKIN-COOLING COMPRESS

1 quart cool water
2 drops chamomile oil
1 drop helichrysum oil
1 drop lavender oil

Pour the water into a 2-quart glass bowl, add the essential oils, and blend. Soak a clean cotton cloth in the water. Apply the cloth to the affected area as needed.

ECZEMA BODY OIL

1 ounce hemp oil
½ ounce flaxseed oil
2 drops geranium oil
1 drop benzoin resin
1 drop elemi oil
1 drop ylang ylang oil

Mix the carrier oils together in a clean container and add the essential oils. Gently turn the container upside down several times or roll it between your hands to blend all the ingredients together. Apply the oil to the affected areas as necessary.

Note: Geranium oil can lower your blood sugar level. Use it with caution (or omit it) if you have hypoglycemia (low blood sugar).

ECZEMA FACIAL OIL

1 ounce jojoba or flaxseed oil
2 drops neroli oil
1 drop helichrysum oil
1 drop myrrh oil
1 drop sandalwood oil

Place the carrier oil in a clean container, add the essential oils, and blend well. Apply the mixture to your face as necessary.

EMOTIONAL ISSUES

Everyone experiences emotional challenges from time to time. Emotions may manifest in many ways and have a multitude of causes. Some emotions, like grief and sadness, are normal responses to unavoidable circumstances. Others may be more within your control. Emotions like anger and impatience are often destructive and usually serve little or no purpose, except perhaps to signal the need to change some aspect of your life, such as your work, your relationships, or your manner of relating to yourself or to the people in your life. On the other hand, desirable feelings such as love, joy, and confidence have a positive impact and help to improve the quality of your life and the lives of other people.

Expressing emotions is natural and healthy. Yet many people deal with their emotions, especially negative ones, by repressing them. They prefer to become engrossed with such things as work, food, alcohol, or drugs—often to the point of obsession—in an attempt not to feel any unpleasant feelings. Other people withdraw into themselves, denying their feelings entirely. Unexpressed feelings and repressed emotions can often contribute to poor health, weakened immunity, and physical illness.

Chemical sensitivities, environmental pollutants, food additives and preservatives, nutritional deficiencies, and a poor diet can activate or aggravate certain emotional problems. Heredity and past experience often are factors. Physical illness or disease can lead to emotional and psychological problems; conversely, emotional and psychological issues can lead to physical illness.

HELPFUL TREATMENTS

If you find yourself facing constant challenges with your emotions, or if you are having trouble handling them, consider psychotherapy or counseling. An adept counselor can help you understand your feelings and discover new ways of effectively dealing with your problems. Often talking or writing about your problems reduces the emotional hold they have on you. Though not always easy, you—and you alone—can change your emotional state and responses.

Essential oils have amazing abilities to soothe emotional upsets, to help guide you through trying times, and to speed recovery from emotional distress. Aromatherapy can help you work on releasing undesirable emotions, as well as on developing or increasing desirable ones. Many European physicians, psychologists, and psychiatrists regularly prescribe essential oils as part of the treatment for their patients. Aromatherapy combines well with other therapies.

Essential oils can help you create a positive emotional environment, manage your emotions, change the way you feel, and improve the quality of your life. Throughout history, people in many different cultures have found comfort for their emotional problems with essential oils.

Aromatherapy can help you cope with challenging circumstances in your life by providing support during difficult times, by lifting your spirits, and by helping you improve or maintain an optimistic outlook. Take an emotional inventory. Which emotions and feelings would you like to subdue or eliminate? Which ones would you like to develop or enhance? Look at the Aromatherapy Blends for Undesirable Emotions and the Aromatherapy Blends for Positive Emotions in this section to choose the blends and methods that will work best for you and suit your lifestyle. Included are

recommendations for personal blends, baths, and diffusers or lamps. Use the following general instructions for preparing and using these aromatherapy treatments:

• *Personal blends.* In a clean container, add a total of up to 12 drops of any single oil or combination of oils of your choice to ⅛ ounce of jojoba oil, or mix one of the recommended blends. Mix the oils by gently turning the container upside down several times or by rolling it between your hands. Do not shake the mixture forcefully. Apply the blend as a fragrance or simply inhale it directly from the bottle, as needed.
• *Baths.* Add a total of 3 to 8 drops of any single oil or combination of oils you choose, or one of the blends suggested in this section, to a bathtub filled with warm water. Soak in the bath for twenty minutes. Repeat as needed.
• *Diffuser or lamp blends.* Choose any of the single oils mentioned, a combination of two or more of those oils, or one of the recommended blends. Drop the essential oils into a small glass bottle with an airtight cover and combine. Add the blend to your diffuser or lamp. For a diffuser, follow the manufacturer's directions. For a lamp, place 10 to 20 drops of a single oil or blend in the lamp bowl. Run the diffuser or lamp as needed.

AROMATHERAPY BLENDS FOR UNDESIRABLE EMOTIONS

Essential oils can help you overcome or rise above emotions that are no longer benefiting you. For any undesirable emotions you wish to change, use the oils suggested, either individually or in any combination you choose, or make one of the recommended blends.

Aggression

Essential oils that combat aggression include bergamot, cedarwood, chamomile, geranium, juniper, lemon, marjoram, rosemary, sandalwood, and ylang ylang. For instructions on using these essential oils, see page 212. Or use one or more of the aromatherapy blends that follow.

ANTI-AGGRESSION PERSONAL BLEND

⅛ ounce jojoba oil
4 drops bergamot oil
3 drops ylang ylang oil
2 drops cedarwood oil
2 drops sandalwood oil
1 drop lemon oil

Add the essential oils to the jojoba oil and blend. Wear as a fragrance or inhale directly from the bottle, as needed.

Note: Bergamot and lemon oils increase sensitivity to the sun. Omit them from your formula if you plan to expose your skin to sunlight.

NIGHTTIME BATH FOR EASING AGGRESSION

3 drops chamomile oil
3 drops marjoram oil
2 drops ylang ylang oil

Disperse the essential oils in a bathtub filled with warm water. Soak in the bath for twenty minutes before going to bed.

AGGRESSION-DIMINISHING DIFFUSER BLEND

20 drops lemon oil
15 drops geranium oil
10 drops bergamot oil
5 drops ylang ylang oil

Drop the essential oils into a small glass container with an airtight cover and combine. Add some of the blend to your diffuser or lamp as necessary.

Anger

Essential oils that subdue feelings of anger are benzoin, bergamot, cedarwood, chamomile, eucalyptus, helichrysum, jasmine, juniper, lavender, marjoram, neroli, peppermint, rose, rosemary, valerian, vitex, and ylang ylang. For instructions on using these essential oils, see page 212. Or use one or more of the aromatherapy blends that follow.

CALMING PERSONAL BLEND

⅛ ounce jojoba oil
3 drops chamomile oil

2 drops ylang ylang oil
1 drop jasmine absolute or enfleurage
1 drop rose oil

Add the essential oils to the jojoba oil and blend. Wear as a fragrance or inhale directly from the bottle as needed.

BATH BLEND FOR RELEASING ANGER
3 drops ylang ylang oil
2 drops marjoram oil

Disperse the essential oils in a bathtub filled with warm water. Soak in the bath for twenty minutes. Repeat as needed.

DIFFUSER BLEND FOR DIMINISHING ANGER
20 drops peppermint oil
18 drops rosemary oil
10 drops bergamot oil
6 drops cedarwood oil

Drop the essential oils into a small glass container with an airtight cover and combine. Add some of the blend to your diffuser or lamp as necessary.

Disappointment
Essential oils recommended for easing disappointment are jasmine, melissa, and rose. For instructions on using these essential oils, see page 212. Or use one or more of the aromatherapy blends that follow.

PERSONAL BLEND FOR DECREASING DISAPPOINTMENT
⅛ ounce jojoba oil
4 drops jasmine absolute or enfleurage
4 drops rose oil
2 drops melissa oil

Add the essential oils to the jojoba oil and blend. Wear as a fragrance or inhale directly from the bottle as needed.

BATH BLEND FOR DEALING WITH DISAPPOINTMENT
2 drops rose oil
1 drop melissa oil

Disperse the essential oils in a bathtub filled with warm water. Soak in the bath for twenty minutes. Repeat as needed.

Fear
Essential oils recommended for easing feelings of fear are basil, bergamot, cedarwood, clary sage, coriander, cypress, fennel, geranium, ginger, jasmine, lavender, lemon, orange, patchouli, sandalwood, thyme, and ylang ylang. For instructions on using these essential oils, see page 212. Or use one or more of the aromatherapy blends that follow.

FEAR-LESS PERSONAL BLEND
⅛ ounce jojoba oil
4 drops sandalwood oil
2 drops coriander oil
1 drop ginger oil
1 drop orange oil

Add the essential oils to the jojoba oil and blend. Wear as a fragrance or inhale directly from the bottle as needed.

FEAR-FREE BATH BLEND

3 drops clary sage oil
3 drops geranium oil
2 drops cedarwood oil

Disperse the essential oils in a bathtub filled with warm water. Soak in the bath for twenty minutes. Repeat as needed.

DIFFUSER BLEND FOR COMBATING FEAR

20 drops bergamot oil
20 drops clary sage oil
5 drops cypress oil
5 drops ginger oil
3 drops fennel oil

Drop the essential oils into a small glass container with an airtight cover and combine. Add some of the blend to your diffuser or lamp as necessary.

Grief

Essential oils recommended for dealing with grief are bergamot, chamomile, cypress, jasmine, marjoram, melissa, myrrh, neroli, and rose. For instructions on using these essential oils, see page 212. Or use one or more of the aromatherapy blends that follow.

GRIEF-RELIEF PERSONAL BLEND

⅛ ounce jojoba oil
4 drops neroli oil

2 drops melissa oil
2 drops myrrh oil
1 drop rose oil

Add the essential oils to the jojoba oil and blend. Wear as a fragrance or inhale directly from the bottle as needed.

BATH BLEND FOR GETTING THROUGH GRIEF

3 drops cypress oil
2 drops bergamot oil
1 drop marjoram oil

Disperse the essential oils in a bathtub filled with warm water. Soak in the bath for twenty minutes. Repeat as needed.

GRIEF-RELEASE DIFFUSER BLEND

25 drops bergamot oil
15 drops chamomile oil
5 drops cypress oil
5 drops marjoram oil

Drop the essential oils into a small glass container with an airtight cover and combine. Add some of the blend to your diffuser or lamp as necessary.

Hysteria

Essential oils recommended for combating hysteria are chamomile, clary sage, lavender, neroli, niaouli, orange, peppermint, tea tree, valerian, vetiver, and ylang ylang. For instructions on using these essential oils, see page 212. Or use one or more of the aromatherapy blends that follow.

Tranquil Personal Blend
⅛ ounce jojoba oil
4 drops chamomile oil
4 drops neroli oil
1 drop clary sage oil
1 drop valerian oil

Add the essential oils to the jojoba oil and blend. Wear as a fragrance or inhale directly from the bottle as needed.

Hysteria-Calming Bath Blend
4 drops lavender oil
2 drops orange oil
1 drop tea tree oil

Disperse the essential oils in a bathtub filled with warm water. Soak in the bath for twenty minutes. Repeat as needed.

Note: Orange oil may increase sensitivity to the sun. Omit it from your formula if you plan to expose your skin to sunlight.

Impatience/Irritability
Essential oils recommended for reducing impatience or irritability are benzoin, chamomile, clary sage, coriander, frankincense, geranium, helichrysum, lavender, oregano, St. John's wort, and sandalwood. For instructions on using these essential oils, see page 212. Or use the following aromatherapy blend.

Impatience/Irritability Eliminator Personal Blend
⅛ ounce jojoba oil
4 drops lavender oil

3 drops geranium oil
2 drops clary sage oil
1 drop frankincense oil

Add the essential oils to the jojoba oil and blend. Wear as a fragrance or inhale directly from the bottle as needed.

Indecision/Indifference
Essential oils recommended for overcoming indecision or indifference are basil, clary sage, cypress, jasmine, patchouli, and peppermint. For instructions on using these essential oils, see page 212. Or use one or more of the aromatherapy blends that follow.

Personal Decisiveness Blend
⅛ ounce jojoba oil
4 drops clary sage oil
2 drops jasmine absolute or enfleurage
1 drop patchouli oil

Add the essential oils to the jojoba oil and blend. Wear as a fragrance or inhale directly from the bottle as needed.

Bath Blend for Overcoming Indifference
3 drops cypress oil
2 drops basil oil
1 drop peppermint oil

Disperse the essential oils in a bathtub filled with warm water. Soak in the bath for twenty minutes. Repeat as needed.

DECISION-MAKING DIFFUSER BLEND
20 drops clary sage oil
10 drops basil oil
8 drops cypress oil
4 drops peppermint oil

Drop the essential oils into a small glass container with an airtight cover and combine. Add some of the blend to your diffuser or lamp as necessary.

Jealousy/Resentment
Essential oils recommended for dealing with feelings of jealousy and resentment are bergamot, cypress, helichrysum, jasmine, palmarosa, and rose. For instructions on using these essential oils, see page 212. Or use the following aromatherapy blend.

PERSONAL BLEND FOR OVERCOMING JEALOUSY
⅛ ounce jojoba oil
4 drops jasmine absolute or enfleurage
4 drops rose oil
2 drops palmarosa oil

Add the essential oils to the jojoba oil and blend. Wear as a fragrance or inhale directly from the bottle as needed.

Loneliness
Essential oils recommended for comforting loneliness are benzoin, marjoram, and myrrh. For instructions on using these essential oils, see page 212. Or use the following aromatherapy blend.

LONELINESS-EASING BATH
4 drops marjoram oil
2 drops benzoin resin
2 drops myrrh oil

Disperse the essential oils in a bathtub filled with warm water. Soak in the bath for twenty minutes. Repeat as needed.

Mental/Emotional Fatigue
Essential oils recommended for combating mental or emotional fatigue include basil, clary sage, coriander, elemi, ginger, helichrysum, jasmine, juniper, laurel, marjoram, orange, palmarosa, patchouli, peppermint, rosemary, St. John's wort, spruce, thyme, valerian, vetiver, and ylang ylang. For instructions on using these essential oils, see page 212. Or use one or more of the aromatherapy blends that follow.

STIMULATING PERSONAL BLEND
⅛ ounce jojoba oil
3 drops elemi oil
2 drops clary sage oil
2 drops pine oil
1 drop palmarosa oil
1 drop vetiver oil

Add the essential oils to the jojoba oil and blend. Wear as a fragrance or inhale directly from the bottle as needed.

STIMULATING MORNING BATH
2 drops basil oil
2 drops rosemary oil

1 drop juniper oil
1 drop peppermint oil

Disperse the essential oils in a bathtub filled with warm water. Soak in the bath for twenty minutes. Repeat as needed.

Mind-Activating Diffuser Blend
10 drops spruce oil
8 drops coriander oil
8 drops patchouli oil
5 drops ginger oil

Drop the essential oils into a small glass container with an airtight cover and combine. Add some of the blend to your diffuser or lamp as necessary.

Nervousness
Essential oils recommended for reducing nervousness are basil, benzoin, cedarwood, chamomile, clary sage, coriander, elemi, fennel, frankincense, ginger, jasmine, laurel, lavender, marjoram, melissa, neroli, orange, oregano, palmarosa, patchouli, peppermint, pine, rose, rosemary, St. John's wort, sandalwood, thyme, valerian, vetiver, and ylang ylang. Essential oils that act as nervous system tonics, which restore and strengthen the nervous system as a preventive measure, are basil, bergamot, black pepper, cedarwood, chamomile, clary sage, coriander, lemon, melissa, neroli, orange, oregano, peppermint, pine, rosemary, St. John's wort, spruce, thyme, and valerian. For instruc- tions on using these essential oils, see page 212. Or use one or more of the aromatherapy blends that follow.

Nerve-Settling Personal Blend
⅛ ounce jojoba oil
4 drops clary sage oil
3 drops spruce oil
2 drops laurel oil
1 drop benzoin resin

Add the essential oils to the jojoba oil and blend. Wear as a fragrance or inhale directly from the bottle as needed.

Nerve-Calming Bath
3 drops elemi oil
2 drops palmarosa oil
1 drop vetiver oil

Disperse the essential oils in a bathtub filled with warm water. Soak in the bath for twenty minutes. Repeat as needed.

Nerve Tonic Personal Blend
⅛ ounce jojoba oil
4 drops frankincense oil
3 drops clary sage oil
2 drops melissa oil
1 drop valerian oil
1 drop vetiver oil

Add the essential oils to the jojoba oil and blend. Wear as a fragrance or inhale directly from the bottle as needed.

NIGHTTIME NERVE TONIC BATH

3 drops chamomile oil

2 drops pine oil

1 drop cedarwood oil

1 drop marjoram oil

Disperse the essential oils in a bathtub filled with warm water. Soak in the bath for twenty minutes. Repeat as needed.

TANGY NERVE TONIC DIFFUSER BLEND

25 drops bergamot oil

20 drops lemon oil

15 drops orange oil

8 drops ylang ylang oil

2 drops black pepper oil

1 drop peppermint oil

Drop the essential oils into a small glass container with an airtight cover and combine. Add some of the blend to your diffuser or lamp as necessary.

Panic

Essential oils recommended for alleviating panic are bergamot, chamomile, clary sage, frankincense, geranium, jasmine, juniper, lavender, marjoram, melissa, neroli, patchouli, rose, rosewood, St. John's wort, tea tree, valerian, vitex, and ylang ylang. For instructions on using these essential oils, see page 212. Or use one or more of the aromatherapy blends that follow.

FLORAL PANIC-PREVENTING PERSONAL BLEND

⅛ ounce jojoba oil

4 drops geranium oil

2 drops lavender oil

2 drops melissa oil

1 drop jasmine absolute or enfleurage

1 drop neroli oil

1 drop ylang ylang oil

Add the essential oils to the jojoba oil and blend. Wear as a fragrance or inhale directly from the bottle as needed.

PANIC-SOOTHING BATH BLEND

2 drops clary sage oil

2 drops geranium oil

1 drop frankincense oil

1 drop marjoram oil

Disperse the essential oils in a bathtub filled with warm water. Soak in the bath for twenty minutes. Repeat as needed.

PANIC-STOPPING DIFFUSER BLEND

20 drops rosewood oil

15 drops lavender oil

12 drops clary sage oil

8 drops geranium oil

5 drops ylang ylang oil

Drop the essential oils into a small glass container with an airtight cover and combine. Add some of the blend to your diffuser or lamp as necessary.

Sadness

Essential oils recommended to help lift feelings of sadness are basil, benzoin, bergamot, jasmine, laurel, marjoram, melissa, orange, rose, rosewood, spruce, and ylang ylang. For instructions on using these essential oils, see page 212. Or use the following aromatherapy blend.

SO LONG SADNESS PERSONAL BLEND

⅛ ounce jojoba oil
6 drops rosewood oil
2 drops spruce oil
1 drop laurel oil
1 drop rose oil

Add the essential oils to the jojoba oil and blend. Wear as a fragrance or inhale directly from the bottle as needed.

Shock

Essential oils recommended for easing feelings of shock are cedarwood, coriander, lavender, melissa, neroli, rose, tea tree, and valerian. For instructions on using these essential oils, see page 212. Or use one or more of the aromatherapy blends that follow.

SHOCK-SOOTHING PERSONAL BLEND

⅛ ounce jojoba oil
2 drops melissa oil
2 drops neroli oil
1 drop rose oil
1 drop valerian oil

Add the essential oils to the jojoba oil and blend. Wear as a fragrance or inhale directly from the bottle as needed.

SHOCK ABSORBER BATH THERAPY

4 drops coriander oil
2 drops tea tree oil
1 drop melissa oil

Disperse the essential oils in a bathtub filled with warm water. Soak in the bath for twenty minutes. Repeat as needed.

Shyness

The best essential oil for overcoming shyness is jasmine. For instructions on using it in a bath, diffuser, or lamp, see page 212. Or use the following aromatherapy blend.

SHYNESS PERSONAL BLEND

⅛ ounce jojoba oil
6 drops jasmine absolute or enfleurage

Add the jasmine to the jojoba oil and blend. Wear as a fragrance or inhale directly from the bottle as needed.

Tension

Essential oils recommended for easing tension are basil, benzoin, cedarwood, chamomile, clary sage, coriander, cypress, frankincense, geranium, ginger, jasmine, lavender, lemon, marjoram, melissa, neroli, orange, palmarosa, peppermint, rose, rosewood, sandalwood, valerian, vetiver, and ylang ylang. For instructions on using these essential oils, see page 212. Or use one or more of the aromatherapy blends that follow.

TENSION-TAMER PERSONAL BLEND

⅛ ounce jojoba oil
3 drops sandalwood oil
2 drops neroli oil
2 drops rosewood oil
1 drop frankincense oil
1 drop valerian oil
1 drop ylang ylang oil

Add the essential oils to the jojoba oil and blend. Wear as a fragrance or inhale directly from the bottle as needed.

TENSION-EASING BATH BLEND

3 drops lavender oil
2 drops marjoram oil
2 drops rosewood oil
1 drop coriander oil

Disperse the essential oils in a bathtub filled with warm water. Soak in the bath for twenty minutes. Repeat as needed.

TENSION-RELEASE DIFFUSER BLEND

15 drops lavender oil
10 drops clary sage oil
8 drops rosewood oil
4 drops geranium oil
2 drops ylang ylang oil

Drop the essential oils into a small glass container with an airtight cover and combine. Add some of the blend to your diffuser or lamp as necessary.

AROMATHERAPY BLENDS FOR POSITIVE EMOTIONS

Essential oils can have a positive influence on your mental state by helping to restore equilibrium to your emotions and balance in your life. For any positive feelings, emotions, or mental conditions you wish to develop or deepen, use the suggested essential oils, either singly or in any combination you choose, or use the recommended aromatherapy blends.

Dealing with Change

Essential oils recommended for emotions connected with facing and handling change are black pepper, clary sage, cypress, frankincense, helichrysum, myrrh, St. John's wort, vitex, and ylang ylang. For instructions on using these essential oils, see page 212. Or use the following aromatherapy blend.

TRANSITION TONIC PERSONAL BLEND

⅛ ounce jojoba oil
3 drops frankincense oil
3 drops myrrh oil
1 drop clary sage oil
1 drop vitex oil

Add the essential oils to the jojoba oil and blend. Wear as a fragrance or inhale directly from the bottle as needed.

Compassion

Essential oils that encourage compassion are chamomile, helichrysum, and sandalwood. For instructions on using these essential oils, see page 212. Or use one or more of the aromatherapy blends that follow.

COMPASSION PERSONAL BLEND

⅛ ounce jojoba oil

4 drops chamomile oil

3 drops sandalwood oil

2 drops helichrysum oil

Add the essential oils to the jojoba oil and blend. Wear as a fragrance or inhale directly from the bottle as needed.

Concentration

Essential oils recommended for increasing concentration are basil, benzoin, black pepper, clary sage, cypress, elemi, eucalyptus, ginger, laurel, lemon, myrrh, patchouli, peppermint, rosemary, thyme, vetiver, and vitex. For instructions on using these essential oils, see page 212. Or use one or more of the aromatherapy blends that follow.

CONCENTRATION BATH BLEND

2 drops basil oil

2 drops laurel oil

1 drop eucalyptus oil

1 drop peppermint oil

Disperse the essential oils in a bathtub filled with warm water. Soak in the bath for twenty minutes. Repeat as needed.

CONCENTRATION DIFFUSER BLEND

20 drops lemon oil

10 drops cypress oil

8 drops clary sage oil

5 drops rosemary oil

Drop the essential oils into a small glass container with an airtight cover and combine. Add some of the blend to your diffuser or lamp as necessary.

Confidence

Essential oils recommended for boosting confidence are benzoin, bergamot, geranium, ginger, helichrysum, jasmine, laurel, lemon, marjoram, neroli, patchouli, peppermint, pine, rose, rosemary, tea tree, thyme, and ylang ylang. For instructions on using these essential oils, see page 212. Or use one or more of the aromatherapy blends that follow.

CONFIDENCE-BUILDING PERSONAL BLEND

⅛ ounce jojoba oil

3 drops neroli oil

2 drops jasmine absolute or enfleurage

2 drops rose oil

2 drops ylang ylang oil

1 drop benzoin resin

Add the essential oils to the jojoba oil and blend. Wear as a fragrance or inhale directly from the bottle as needed.

SELF-CONFIDENCE BATH
3 drops ylang ylang oil
2 drops bergamot oil
1 drop helichrysum oil

Disperse the essential oils in a bathtub filled with warm water. Soak in the bath for twenty minutes. Repeat as needed.

Courage

Essential oils recommended to heighten courage are black pepper, fennel, ginger, melissa, neroli, and thyme. For instructions on using these essential oils, see page 212. Or use the following aromatherapy blend.

COURAGE-BOOSTING BATH BLEND
3 drops thyme oil
2 drops fennel oil
1 drop black pepper oil
1 drop ginger oil

Disperse the essential oils in a bathtub filled with warm water. Soak in the bath for twenty minutes. Repeat as needed.

Creativity

Essential oils recommended for enhancing creativity are clary sage, coriander, fennel, geranium, helichrysum, jasmine, laurel, lavender, neroli, orange, patchouli, rose, rosewood, and ylang ylang. For instructions on using these essential oils, see page 212. Or use one or more of the aromatherapy blends that follow.

CREATIVITY PERFUME BLEND
⅛ ounce jojoba oil
4 drops rosewood oil
3 drops helichrysum oil
2 drops clary sage oil
1 drop neroli oil
1 drop rose oil

Add the essential oils to the jojoba oil and blend. Wear as a fragrance or inhale directly from the bottle as needed.

CREATIVITY DIFFUSER BLEND
15 drops orange oil
12 drops coriander oil
10 drops fennel oil
8 drops laurel oil
3 drops ylang ylang oil

Drop the essential oils into a small glass container with an airtight cover and combine. Add some of the blend to your diffuser or lamp as necessary.

Happiness/Joy

Essential oils recommended for promoting feelings of happiness and joy are basil, bergamot, coriander, jasmine, laurel, marjoram, neroli, orange, oregano, patchouli, peppermint, rose, and spruce. For instructions on using these essential oils, see page 212. Or use one or more of the aromatherapy blends that follow.

JOYOUS PERSONAL BLEND

⅛ ounce jojoba oil
3 drops bergamot oil
3 drops neroli oil
2 drops rose oil
1 drop laurel oil
1 drop orange oil

Add the essential oils to the jojoba oil and blend. Wear as a fragrance or inhale directly from the bottle as needed.

HAPPY BATH BLEND

3 drops bergamot oil
1 drop marjoram oil
1 drop oregano oil

Disperse the essential oils in a bathtub filled with warm water. Soak in the bath for twenty minutes. Repeat as needed.

JOYOUS DIFFUSER BLEND

20 drops bergamot oil
20 drops spruce oil
5 drops peppermint oil

Drop the essential oils into a small glass container with an airtight cover and combine. Add some of the blend to your diffuser or lamp as necessary.

Note: Bergamot and orange oils increase sensitivity to the sun. Omit them from your formula if you will expose your skin to sunlight.

Harmony/Balance

Essential oils recommended for deepening feelings of harmony and balance are bergamot, cedarwood, clary sage, coriander, elemi, eucalyptus, geranium, helichrysum, jasmine, lavender, lemon, melissa, orange, pine, rose, rosemary, rosewood, spruce, thyme, valerian, vetiver, and vitex. For instructions on using these essential oils, see page 212. Or use one or more of the aromatherapy blends that follow.

HARMONY PERSONAL BLEND

⅛ ounce jojoba oil
4 drops elemi oil
4 drops geranium oil
2 drops ylang ylang oil
1 drop vetiver oil

Add the essential oils to the jojoba oil and blend. Wear as a fragrance or inhale directly from the bottle as needed.

BALANCING BATH BLEND

3 drops lavender oil
2 drops geranium oil
1 drop cedarwood oil
1 drop coriander oil

Disperse the essential oils in a bathtub filled with warm water. Soak in the bath for twenty minutes. Repeat as needed.

EQUILIBRIUM DIFFUSER BLEND

20 drops lemon oil
15 drops elemi oil

15 drops rosewood oil

10 drops cedarwood oil

5 drops pine oil

Drop the essential oils into a small glass container with an airtight cover and combine. Add some of the blend to your diffuser or lamp as necessary.

Intuition

Essential oils recommended for enhancing intuition are clary sage, helichrysum, jasmine, rose, rosewood, and ylang ylang. For instructions on using these essential oils, see page 212. Or use the following aromatherapy blend.

INTUITION PERSONAL BLEND

⅛ ounce jojoba oil

4 drops helichrysum oil

4 drops rosewood oil

2 drops clary sage oil

1 drop rose oil

Add the essential oils to the jojoba oil and blend. Wear as a fragrance or inhale directly from the bottle, as needed.

Love

Essential oils recommended for deepening feelings of love are basil, benzoin, bergamot, coriander, ginger, jasmine, lavender, neroli, palmarosa, rose, rosemary, sandalwood, and ylang ylang. For instructions on using these essential oils, see page 212. Or use one or more of the aromatherapy blends that follow.

LOVE POTION PERSONAL BLEND

⅛ ounce jojoba oil

2 drops jasmine absolute or enfleurage

2 drops neroli oil

2 drops ylang ylang oil

1 drop benzoin resin

1 drop ginger oil

1 drop rose oil

Add the essential oils to the jojoba oil and blend. Wear as a fragrance or inhale directly from the bottle as needed.

LOVING BATH BLEND

3 drops ylang ylang oil

2 drops coriander oil

1 drop sandalwood oil

Disperse the essential oils in a bathtub filled with warm water. Soak in the bath for twenty minutes. Repeat as needed.

LOVE DIFFUSER BLEND

10 drops bergamot oil

10 drops ylang ylang oil

8 drops lavender oil

6 drops benzoin resin

6 drops palmarosa oil

4 drops ginger oil

Drop the essential oils into a small glass container with an airtight cover and combine. Add some of the blend to your diffuser or lamp as necessary.

Meditation

Essential oils recommended for heightening meditation include benzoin, black pepper, cedarwood, chamomile, clary sage, elemi, frankincense, helichrysum, jasmine, juniper, myrrh, rosewood, sandalwood, and vetiver. For instructions on using these essential oils, see page 212. Or use the following aromatherapy blend.

MEDITATION DIFFUSER BLEND
20 drops sandalwood oil
12 drops rosewood oil
10 drops elemi oil
5 drops frankincense oil
5 drops myrrh oil
5 drops vetiver oil
2 drops benzoin resin

Drop the essential oils into a small glass container with an airtight cover and combine. Add some of the blend to your diffuser or lamp as necessary.

Memory

Essential oils recommended for improving memory are basil, clary sage, coriander, fennel, ginger, laurel, peppermint, rosemary, spruce, and thyme. For instructions on using these essential oils, see page 212. Or use one or more of the aromatherapy blends that follow.

BRAIN TONIC BATH BLEND
3 drops rosemary oil
2 drops coriander oil
1 drop basil oil
1 drop thyme oil

Disperse the essential oils in a bathtub filled with warm water. Soak in the bath for twenty minutes. Repeat as needed.

MEMORY-JOGGER DIFFUSER BLEND
15 drops clary sage oil
10 drops coriander oil
10 drops spruce oil
8 drops ginger oil
3 drops peppermint oil

Drop the essential oils into a small glass container with an airtight cover and combine. Add some of the blend to your diffuser or lamp as necessary.

Peace/Serenity/Calmness

Essential oils recommended for deepening feelings of peace, serenity, and calmness are basil, benzoin, bergamot, cedarwood, chamomile, clary sage, coriander, cypress, elemi, fennel, frankincense, geranium, ginger, helichrysum, jasmine, lavender, lemon, marjoram, melissa, myrrh, neroli, patchouli, rose, rosewood, sandalwood, valerian, vitex, and ylang ylang. For instructions on using these essential oils, see page 212. Or use one or more of the aromatherapy blends that follow.

SERENITY PERSONAL BLEND

⅛ ounce jojoba oil

4 drops sandalwood oil

2 drops clary sage oil

2 drops melissa oil

2 drops rosewood oil

1 drop chamomile oil

1 drop neroli oil

Add the essential oils to the jojoba oil and blend. Wear as a fragrance or inhale directly from the bottle as needed.

COMPOSURE BATH BLEND

3 drops rosewood oil

2 drops clary sage oil

1 drop elemi oil

1 drop marjoram oil

Disperse the essential oils in a bathtub filled with warm water. Soak in the bath for twenty minutes. Repeat as needed.

CALMING DIFFUSER BLEND

18 drops lavender oil

15 drops rosewood oil

12 drops chamomile oil

12 drops geranium oil

10 drops clary sage oil

10 drops ylang ylang oil

Drop the essential oils into a small glass container with an airtight cover and combine. Add some of the blend to your diffuser or lamp as necessary.

Releasing the Past

Essential oils recommended to help you let go of the past are bergamot, black pepper, chamomile, cypress, fennel, frankincense, helichrysum, juniper, laurel, lavender, myrrh, rose, rosewood, and vitex. For instructions on using these essential oils, see page 212. Or use the following aromatherapy blend.

LETTING GO PERSONAL BLEND

⅛ ounce jojoba oil

3 drops frankincense oil

2 drops myrrh oil

2 drops rose oil

1 drop black pepper oil

1 drop helichrysum oil

Add the essential oils to the jojoba oil and blend. Wear as a fragrance or inhale directly from the bottle as needed.

Self-Esteem

Essential oils recommended for boosting self-esteem are benzoin, bergamot, cedarwood, cypress, ginger, helichrysum, jasmine, laurel, neroli, patchouli, peppermint, rose, rosemary, thyme, and ylang ylang. For instructions on using these essential oils, see page 212. Or use one or more of the aromatherapy blends that follow.

SELF-ESTEEM PERSONAL BLEND

⅛ ounce jojoba oil

6 drops ylang ylang oil

4 drops laurel oil

1 drop rose oil

Add the essential oils to the jojoba oil and blend. Wear as a fragrance or inhale directly from the bottle as needed.

ESTEEM-BOOSTING BATH

2 drops bergamot oil

1 drop cypress oil

1 drop patchouli oil

1 drop ylang ylang oil

Disperse the essential oils in a bathtub filled with warm water. Soak in the bath for twenty minutes. Repeat as needed.

Sexual Desire

Essential oils recommended for their aphrodisiac properties include basil, benzoin, black pepper, cedarwood, clary sage, coriander, fennel, ginger, jasmine, lavender, neroli, patchouli, peppermint, rose, rosewood, sandalwood, vetiver, and ylang ylang. For instructions on using these essential oils, see page 212. Or use one or more of the aromatherapy blends that follow.

ALL-PURPOSE APHRODISIAC PERSONAL BLEND

⅛ ounce jojoba oil

3 drops neroli oil

3 drops sandalwood oil

2 drops benzoin resin

2 drops jasmine absolute or enfleurage

1 drop rose oil

1 drop vetiver oil

Add the essential oils to the jojoba oil and blend. Wear as a fragrance or inhale directly from the bottle as needed.

SENSUALITY BATH

2 drops coriander oil

2 drops rosewood oil

2 drops ylang ylang oil

1 drop patchouli oil

Disperse the essential oils in a bathtub filled with warm water. Soak in the bath for twenty minutes. Repeat as needed.

SENSUAL DIFFUSER BLEND

10 drops clary sage oil

6 drops ylang ylang oil

4 drops coriander oil

4 drops ginger oil

2 drops vetiver oil

Drop the essential oils into a small glass container with an airtight cover and combine. Add some of the blend to your diffuser or lamp as necessary.

Spiritual Purity

Essential oils recommended for spiritual purification and cleansing are benzoin, cedarwood, elemi, eucalyptus, frankincense, ginger, jasmine, juniper, laurel, lemon, myrrh, neroli, orange, pine, rose, rosemary, sandalwood, and vetiver. For instructions on using these essential oils, see page 212. Or use the following aromatherapy blend.

PURIFYING BATH BLEND

2 drops juniper oil
2 drops myrrh oil
2 drops pine oil
1 drop elemi oil

Disperse the essential oils in a bathtub filled with warm water. Soak in the bath for twenty minutes. Repeat as needed.

Trust

Essential oils that nurture trust include cedarwood, jasmine, laurel, lemon, melissa, neroli, and rose. For instructions on using these essential oils, see page 212. Or use the following aromatherapy blend.

TRUSTING PERSONAL BLEND

⅛ ounce jojoba oil
3 drops laurel oil
2 drops lemon oil
2 drops melissa oil
1 drop rose oil

Add the essential oils to the jojoba oil and blend. Wear as a fragrance or inhale directly from the bottle as needed.

FATIGUE

Fatigue is the condition of not having enough energy to function to the point that you need to stop and rest or sleep. Fatigue indicates a weakened immune system; it compromises the body's ability to ward off illness or disease. Other symptoms may include dizziness, headaches, nausea, or nervousness. Mental weariness can also accompany physical fatigue.

Fatigue is a signal that your body needs to conserve its energy or strength. It can mean simply that you are expending more energy than your body produces. Fatigue can also be a symptom of an underlying health problem. Adrenal malfunction, allergies, anemia, candidiasis, depression, diabetes, hormonal imbalances, hypoglycemia, low blood pressure, poor absorption of nutrients, nutritional deficiencies, poor diet, sluggish lymph system, stress, and thyroid disorders can all produce fatigue, as can virtually any infectious illness. In some cases, fatigue can be the first sign of a developing physical or emotional problem. Often fatigue can contribute to emotional issues directed inwardly, such as anger, blame, depression, disgust, fear, guilt, hatred, helplessness, and hopelessness. When emotional tension and stress compound fatigue, emotional or nervous exhaustion may result.

HELPFUL TREATMENTS

If you are bothered by fatigue, you should see a health-care professional to check for low blood pressure and to rule out physical illness as the cause of your sluggishness. If illness is the cause of your fatigue, your doctor can recommend appropriate treatment. Begin a program to improve your immunity. (*See also* WEAKENED IMMUNE SYSTEM.)

If you can find no underlying illness or other cause for your fatigue, begin a regimen including regular exercise, a healthy diet focusing on fresh fruits and vegetables, nutritional supplementation, relaxation, and regular, restful sleep. This approach may be sufficient to restore your energy. Avoid such energy-depleting habits as smoking, drinking, overworking, taking drugs, and worrying. Learn ways to manage stress and balance your emotions. Reduce your responsibilities, if possible. If you do all of these things and your fatigue continues for more than several months, chronic fatigue syndrome may be a possibility. (*See also* CHRONIC FATIGUE SYNDROME.)

Aromatherapy can help you to increase your energy, improve your body's immune response, and reduce stress. Energizing and balancing essential oils such as basil, bergamot, cedarwood, chamomile, clary sage, coriander, elemi, frankincense, geranium, ginger, helichrysum, laurel, lavender, lemon, marjoram, orange, oregano, patchouli, peppermint, pine, rosemary, spruce, tea tree, thyme, and vetiver can regulate your energy level.

Take a Fatigue-Fighting Bath every morning. Apply Energizing Body Oil over your body once or twice daily and breathe in Energy Inhalant Oil during the day, as needed. You can also disperse Energy-Boosting Diffuser Blend in your home or office.

AROMATHERAPY BLENDS

You can prepare the aromatherapy blends below using pure essential oils. For a more detailed explanation of how to put together and use these blends, see Part Three: Ways to Use Aromatherapy. To review general guidelines for using essential oils, see page 142.

FATIGUE-FIGHTING BATH

2 drops orange oil
1 drop peppermint oil
1 drop rosemary oil
1 drop thyme oil

Disperse all the ingredients in a bathtub filled with warm water and soak in the tub for twenty to thirty minutes. Repeat as necessary.

ENERGIZING BODY OIL

2 ounces carrier oil
4 drops rosemary oil
3 drops geranium oil
3 drops lemon oil
2 drops coriander oil

Place the carrier oil in a clean container, add the essential oils, and gently turn the container over several times or roll it between your hands to blend. Massage the oil into your skin once a day, as needed.

ENERGY INHALANT OIL

8 drops spruce oil

6 drops elemi oil

4 drops patchouli oil

2 drops basil oil

1 drop laurel oil

Add the oils to a small glass bottle with an airtight cover and blend well. Inhale directly from the bottle any time you need a boost of energy.

ENERGY-BOOSTING DIFFUSER BLEND

15 drops spruce oil

12 drops pine oil

10 drops lemon oil

10 drops orange oil

2 drops elemi oil

Combine all the ingredients in a small glass bottle with an airtight cover. Add some of the mixture to your diffuser or lamp bowl as desired.

GAS, INTESTINAL

See INDIGESTION.

GUM DISEASE

When the gums or the tissues supporting the teeth become damaged or inflamed, gum disease (periodontal disease) can threaten oral health. Most cases of periodontal disease are related to poor oral hygiene. Plaque, a sticky bacterial substance, adheres to the teeth, especially along the gum line. When

minerals present in saliva combine with plaque, it hardens into tartar, which pushes the gums back; the bacteria in the tartar can then cause infection of the gum tissue. Periodontal disease may also arise from or be aggravated by faulty dental work, the presence of mercury amalgam fillings, mouth-breathing, the use of cigarettes or chewing tobacco, and grinding one's teeth. Systemic disorders such as anemia, collagen diseases, diabetes, impaired immunity, leukemia, and vitamin deficiencies can cause periodontal disease as well.

Gingivitis, or inflammation of the gums, is the most common form of periodontal disease. The gums swell, become sensitive, and bleed easily. The breath may smell offensive. If gingivitis is not treated, periodontitis may develop. In periodontitis, the tissue surrounding the teeth becomes inflamed, and the bones supporting the teeth gradually deteriorate. Finally, the gums recede and weaken; teeth become loose and may fall out. Periodontitis is the major cause of tooth loss in adults.

HELPFUL TREATMENTS

Good oral hygiene is the best way to prevent gum problems (see Oral Hygiene on page 233). If you already have gum problems, good oral hygiene may reverse some of the damage and prevent the problem from progressing further. You should also see your dentist for proper treatment.

Essential oils can complement your

dentist's treatment to minimize the pain and discomfort of periodontal disease. Lemon, myrrh, orange, rose, and tea tree oils aid gingivitis; cypress, myrrh, and tea tree are the best essential oils for the more advanced problems associated with periodontitis. Cypress, lemon, and tea tree oils help prevent bleeding gums; basil, fennel, and thyme oils can help fight gum infections; and basil, bergamot, lemon, myrrh, orange, and tea tree oils help heal mouth ulcers. All of these essential oils help to restore gum health and prevent additional problems.

Once or twice daily, after brushing your teeth, rub Gingivitis Gum Massage Oil into your gums to promote circulation and encourage gum health. Alternate this treatment with the use of Gum-Strengthening Mouthwash or Infection-Fighting Mouthwash.

AROMATHERAPY BLENDS

You can prepare the aromatherapy blends below using pure essential oils. For a more detailed explanation of how to put together and use these blends, see Part Three: Ways to Use Aromatherapy. To review general guidelines for using essential oils, see page 142.

GINGIVITIS GUM MASSAGE OIL

½ ounce carrier oil
4 drops tea tree oil
2 drops myrrh oil
1 drop lemon oil
1 drop orange oil

Place the carrier oil in a clean container, add the essential oils, and turn the container over a few times or gently roll it between your hands to blend. Once or twice daily, after brushing your teeth, massage a couple of drops into your gums.

GUM-STRENGTHENING MOUTHWASH

8 ounces distilled water
2 drops myrrh oil
2 drops tea tree oil
1 drop peppermint oil

Pour the water into a bottle and add the essential oils to the water. Turn upside down several times to blend. After brushing your teeth, rinse your mouth thoroughly with about ½ ounce of the mixture. Blend well before each use.

INFECTION-FIGHTING MOUTHWASH

8 ounces distilled water
2 drops basil oil
2 drops niaouli oil
2 drops thyme oil

Pour the water into a bottle, add the essential oils, and turn the bottle upside down several times to blend. After brushing your teeth, rinse your mouth thoroughly, using about ½ ounce of the mouthwash. Blend well before each use.

Oral Hygiene

Good oral hygiene combines proper home care with the professional care of your dentist and oral hygienist to keep your teeth and gums healthy. Proper brushing after eating removes plaque, a soft and sticky colorless film composed of bacteria and mucus. Plaque coats your teeth, attacks tooth enamel, and contributes to cavities. Take your time when brushing, and make sure you brush your tongue as well as your teeth. It is better to give your mouth one complete brushing each day than to brush several times quickly and miss certain areas again and again. Use a soft-bristle toothbrush, and replace it frequently (approximately every three months). Daily flossing also removes plaque and discourages the formation of tartar, the hardened deposits that form on the teeth when calcium from your saliva combines with plaque. If you have any doubts about proper brushing or flossing technique, ask your dentist or dental hygienist.

When combined with good home care, regular dental checkups and professional cleanings can prevent cavities and most dental problems. Most dentists recommend a cleaning and a checkup every six months. You should also consult your dentist between scheduled visits if you suspect you may be developing any tooth or gum problems.

Aromatherapy can be a valuable addition to your oral hygiene program. Lemon, myrrh, orange, peppermint, and tea tree oils fight the bacteria that cause plaque. Myrrh oil also helps preserve or restore gum health, while peppermint, orange, and lemon oils freshen breath. Many manufacturers fortify toothpastes, mouthwashes, dental flosses, and toothpicks with essential oils.

You can use the aromatherapy blends below to help you maintain good dental health. Therapeutic Breath-Freshening Mouthwash will freshen your breath as it contributes to gum health. Gum Therapy Oil will help maintain or improve the condition of your gums.

THERAPEUTIC BREATH-FRESHENING MOUTHWASH

8 ounces distilled water
2 drops myrrh oil
2 drops tea tree oil
1 drop peppermint oil

Mix all the ingredients together in a clean bottle. Swish about ½ ounce around in your mouth after brushing your teeth or after meals as needed. Shake well before using.

GUM THERAPY OIL
⅛ ounce carrier oil
10 drops tea tree oil
6 drops myrrh oil
3 drops lemon oil
1 drop peppermint oil

Place the carrier oil in a clean container, add the essential oils, and blend. Massage the mixture into your gums once a day, after brushing your teeth and rinsing your mouth with mouthwash.

HAIR AND SCALP PROBLEMS

A healthy head of hair begins with a healthy scalp. Normal hair is shiny, silky, and full of body. It is neither too dry nor too oily. Hair and scalp problems often result from imbalances in the body caused by nutritional deficiencies, poor diet, or stress. Sometimes heredity and environmental factors, such as the chemicals found in hair dyes and perm solutions or heat from electric styling appliances, play a role as well. The most common hair- and scalp-related problems include dry hair, oily hair, dandruff, and hair loss.

Most hair and scalp problems respond to a healthier diet and to the use of appropriate hair-care products. When nutritional deficiencies are corrected, hair and scalp conditions usually improve. No matter what problems you experience with your hair, you will benefit by eliminating all fatty and fried foods from your diet and by keeping your hair and scalp clean.

Aromatherapy hair-care treatments help improve the condition of your hair and scalp by stimulating circulation to your scalp and by adding luster and shine to your hair. They can also help by balancing your scalp's oil secretions. (*See also* HAIR CARE AND CREATING HAIR-CARE PRODUCTS in Part Three.)

Normal Hair

If your hair is normal, you already have a proper balance of oil secretions. You can maintain this balance and keep your hair looking healthy and shiny with chamomile, lavender, thyme, and ylang ylang oils. Use Normal Hair Conditioning Treatment as needed.

NORMAL HAIR CONDITIONING
TREATMENT
1 ounce jojoba oil or coconut oil
4 drops lavender oil
2 drops chamomile oil
1 drop ylang ylang oil

Add all the oils to the carrier oil. Turn the bottle upside down several times or roll it between your hands to blend. Once or twice a month massage the mixture into your scalp and hair. Wrap your hair in a towel for one hour. Then shampoo as usual.

Dry Hair

Dry hair appears dull and lifeless. The sebaceous, or oil, glands in the scalp secrete insufficient oil to lubricate the hair. Lack of nutritious oil in the diet can contribute to dry hair, as can a poor diet or nutritional deficiencies.

Many external factors can dry out your hair. The overuse of curling irons, electric curlers, hair dryers, hair dyes, hair-styling products, and perms all can dry out and even damage your hair. If you have dry hair, give your hair a rest from electric appliances, hair dyes, and perms.

Essential oils that help improve the condition of dry hair are cedarwood, chamomile, clary sage, lavender, and rosemary. Several times a week, apply Dry Hair Conditioning Treatment to your hair and scalp.

DRY HAIR CONDITIONING TREATMENT
2 ounces jojoba oil or coconut oil
3 drops cedarwood oil
3 drops clary sage oil
3 drops lavender oil

Place the oil in a clean container and add the essential oils. Turn the container upside down several times or roll it between your hands to blend. Once a week (or more, as needed), massage some of the treatment into your scalp and hair. Wrap your hair in a towel. Leave it on for thirty to forty-five minutes or overnight. Then shampoo your hair. After shampooing, you can massage a few drops of Dry Hair Conditioning Treatment into wet hair, particularly on dry or split ends.

Oily Hair
Oily hair can appear greasy and may cling to the scalp. Just as underactive sebaceous glands in the scalp lead to dry hair, oil glands that secrete too much oil cause oily hair. Other contributing factors may include a diet high in fats, refined carbohydrates, and sugar; the use of hair conditioners or hair-styling gels; hormonal imbalances; and infrequent washing of the hair.

Oily hair often responds to dietary changes. If you have oily hair, reduce your fat intake and eliminate all fried foods, refined carbohydrates, and sugar from your diet. Essential oils such as bergamot, cedarwood, clary sage, cypress, juniper, lavender, lemon, patchouli, pine, rosemary, tea tree, thyme, and ylang ylang can help reduce oiliness. Wash your hair every day. Afterward, massage Oily Hair Tonic into your scalp.

OILY HAIR TONIC
4 ounces pure grain alcohol or vodka
4 drops lemon oil
2 drops bergamot oil
2 drops cedarwood oil
2 drops pine oil
1 drop ylang ylang oil

Place the alcohol in a clean bottle. Add the essential oils. Turn the bottle upside down several times or roll it between your hands to blend. Apply to scalp once daily or more often to control oiliness. Blend well before each use. Do not inhale directly from the bottle. Never use isopropyl alcohol for aromatherapy purposes.

Dandruff

Dandruff can appear on both dry and oily scalps. It results from abnormal activity of the sebaceous, or oil-secreting, glands in the scalp. Fine white flakes of dead skin accumulate on the scalp and then fall off onto clothing.

People who have dandruff often have diets that are high in saturated fats and fried foods. Infrequent shampooing can contribute to the condition as well. Most commercial dandruff shampoos contain harsh chemicals and coal tar as active ingredients; they may control dandruff but rarely eliminate the underlying problem.

Essential oils that fight dandruff include cedarwood, clary sage, cypress, laurel, lemon, patchouli, pine, rosemary, and tea tree. Dandruff Scalp Treatment for Dry Hair helps to regulate the secretions of the sebaceous glands, thereby minimizing scalp problems.

DANDRUFF SCALP TREATMENT FOR DRY HAIR

2 ounces jojoba oil
6 drops tea tree oil
4 drops rosemary oil
3 drops cedarwood oil
3 drops pine oil

Place the jojoba oil in a clean container, add the essential oils, and blend. Massage some of the mixture into your clean scalp and leave it on for thirty minutes or overnight, then shampoo as usual. Repeat the treatment several times a week, as needed.

DANDRUFF-DIMINISHING TREATMENT FOR OILY HAIR

8 ounces pure grain alcohol or vodka
6 drops tea tree oil
4 drops cedarwood oil
3 drops pine oil
2 drops lemon oil
2 drops rosemary oil

Place the alcohol in a clean bottle. Add the essential oils. Turn the bottle upside down several times or roll it between your hands to blend. Apply to the scalp once daily or more often to control dandruff.

Blend well before each use. Do not inhale directly from the bottle. Do not use isopropyl alcohol with essential oils.

Hair Loss

Both men and women worry about hair loss. A daily loss of about 150 to 200 strands of hair is normal. If you lose more hair than that, you probably will not grow enough new hair to replace it, and the loss will become noticeable.

Hair loss can occur in patches or over the entire scalp or body. Most cases of hair loss, or *alopecia*, are probably related to aging, heredity, and hormones. In addition, sebum, or oil secretions, can build up on the scalp, plug the hair follicles, and interfere with new hair growth. Other causes of hair loss include chemotherapy or radiation treatments, cigarette smoking, diabetes, certain drugs, hypothyroidism, impaired circulation, poor diet, nutritional deficiencies, pregnancy, skin disorders such as psoriasis and seborrhea, and stress.

Hair loss is a problem that may not be reversible, but you can often prevent further loss of hair by reducing some of the contributing factors. Avoid stress as much as possible. Avoid using hair-styling products on your hair. These can clog hair follicles, thereby discouraging new hair growth.

Essential oils that slow down the loss of hair or stimulate the scalp to encourage growth of new hair include cedarwood, clary sage, rosemary, and ylang ylang. Massage Scalp-Stimulating Hair-Growth Formula into your scalp daily. Keep your hair and scalp clean by frequent shampooing. If you have oily hair, you may prefer to use Hair-Stimulating Tonic instead.

SCALP-STIMULATING HAIR-GROWTH FORMULA
1 ounce jojoba oil
3 drops clary sage oil
2 drops cedarwood oil
1 drop rosemary oil

Place the jojoba oil in a clean container and add the essential oils. Gently turn the container upside down several times or roll it between your hands to blend. Massage some of the mixture into your scalp daily.

Leave it on for thirty minutes or overnight, then shampoo as usual.

HAIR-STIMULATING TONIC
8 ounces pure grain alcohol or vodka
4 drops clary sage oil
3 drops cedarwood oil
3 drops ylang ylang oil

Place the alcohol in a clean bottle. Add the essential oils. Turn the bottle upside down several times or roll it between your hands to blend. Apply to clean scalp once daily or more often. Blend well before each use. Do not inhale directly from the bottle. Never use isopropyl alcohol for aromatherapy purposes.

HEADACHE
Headaches can take the form of a dull, throbbing pain or a sharp, stabbing pain, on one or both sides of the head. Sometimes the pain localizes in the temple area or behind the eyes. Blurred vision, pressure in the sinus cavities, and sensitivity to light can accompany headaches.

Most headaches result from tension. Tension produces muscle spasms in the head, neck, scalp, and shoulders that can interfere with circulation to the head. Feelings such as aggression, anxiety, anger, depression, fear, guilt, humiliation, rage, and rejection can cause or contribute to tension headaches, especially when these feelings are denied, ignored, or repressed. Headaches often increase irritability and can lead to insomnia.

Headaches may be related to any of a number of other health problems, including anemia, arthritis, brain disorders, candidiasis, constipation, digestive difficulties, eyestrain, fatigue, high blood pressure, head injury, low blood pressure, low blood sugar, nutritional imbalances, poor circulation, poor posture, premenstrual syndrome (PMS), sinusitis, spinal misalignment, stress, sun exposure, temporomandibular joint (TMJ) syndrome, or throat, nose, or eye disorders. They can also be triggered by certain foods and food additives, especially alcohol, caffeine, chocolate, dairy products, monosodium glutamate (MSG), refined and processed foods, sugar, and yeast, as well as by certain drugs or by exposure to cigarette smoke, certain smells, synthetic fragrances, chemicals, or environmental pollutants. Even being in a poorly ventilated room may cause a headache in some people.

Migraine is a type of headache that occurs when the arteries leading to the head bulge with excess blood, exerting pressure against the brain and the surrounding tissue. An abnormal flow of blood to the brain results, alternately constricting and dilating blood vessels. This first restricts the brain's blood supply and then floods the brain with blood. Pressure within the blood vessels can irritate nerve endings and contribute to the pain. The pain of a migraine may last for several hours or several days. While tension headaches are often relieved by a good night's sleep, this is not necessarily the case with migraines.

Migraines cause severe pain, sometimes beginning with a throbbing pain on one or both sides of the head. Some migraine sufferers experience visual auras—flashes of lights, hallucinatory-type effects, or holes in the field of vision—prior to the onset of a migraine. Nausea and vomiting, as well as stiffness and aches in the neck, often accompany migraines. Migraines can cause painful sensitivity to bright lights or sunlight.

Migraines are frequently related to food and environmental allergies. Foods that may trigger migraines include chicken, chocolate, corn, dairy products, fried foods, fruits, grains, nuts, potatoes, red meat, soy products, sugar, tomatoes, and yeast. Alcohol (especially red wines), caffeine, salt, monosodium glutamate (MSG), preservatives, and other food additives are common culprits as well. Changes in humidity, chemical sensitivities, poor circulation, constipation, a disturbance in one's sleep pattern, emotional upset, liver malfunction, nutritional imbalances, poor diet, sun exposure, and stress can bring on a migraine. In many women, migraines occur when hormones fluctuate during menopause or certain phases of the menstrual cycle. Self-inflicted stress, like that which comes from striving to be perfect, or feelings of anger, anxiety, depression, fear, frustration, or hatred can lead to migraines.

HELPFUL TREATMENTS

Headaches can be a symptom of an underlying illness; if you suffer from frequent or unusually severe headaches, consult with your health-care practitioner to rule out this possibility. In most cases, however, a headache—whether a tension headache or a migraine—indicates that your body needs to slow down and rest, or stop whatever you're doing at the moment. Painkillers may relieve the pain, but they do nothing to eliminate the cause of a headache; they may even mask symptoms that are your body's cry for changes in your behavior or lifestyle.

Low blood sugar can provoke headaches. Make sure that you eat regular, nutritious meals. You may wish to consult a nutritionist for advice about your diet and possible vitamin deficiencies. Focus on eating complex carbohydrates such as fresh vegetables and whole grains. Eliminate the most common dietary culprits: alcohol, artificial sweeteners, caffeine, dairy products (especially cheese), chicken, chocolate, fruits, processed meats, sugar, vinegar, and yeast products, as well as any other foods you suspect. After several weeks, if you find that you have fewer headaches, you can—gradually, and one at a time—reintroduce the banished foods back into your diet. If your headaches return, you can identify the responsible food or foods. If your headaches or migraines occur when you are hungry, or when you haven't eaten for a while, have your doctor check for hypoglycemia. You may need to eat small meals throughout the day to stabilize your blood sugar.

If you suspect that a misaligned spine is contributing to your headaches, visit a chiropractor for an evaluation and adjustment. Biofeedback, deep breathing techniques, meditation, relaxation, visualization, and yoga are other methods that are effective for many people, especially migraine sufferers. Avoid exposure to cigarette smoke, cleaning compounds, nail polish and polish remover, paints, and other chemicals, as well as anything with a synthetic fragrance or perfume.

Aromatherapy can help you avoid and reduce headaches by relaxing you physically and emotionally and by reducing stress. (*See also* STRESS.) It can also help with some of the underlying conditions that can lead to headaches, such as arthritis, candidiasis, constipation, digestive problems, fatigue, high or low blood pressure, premenstrual syndrome (PMS), poor circulation, sinusitis, and sluggish lymphatic system. (*See also* ARTHRITIS; CANDIDIASIS; CIRCULATION, POOR; CONSTIPATION; FATIGUE; HIGH BLOOD PRESSURE; INDIGESTION; LOW BLOOD PRESSURE; LYMPHATIC SYSTEM, SLUGGISH/SWOLLEN LYMPH GLANDS; PREMENSTRUAL SYNDROME [PMS]; SINUSITIS; *and* TEMPOROMANDIBULAR JOINT [TMJ] SYNDROME.)

Essential oils such as basil, chamomile, clary sage, coriander, eucalyptus, ginger, helichrysum, juniper, laurel, lavender, lemon, marjoram, melissa, oregano, peppermint, rose, rosemary, rosewood, St. John's wort, sandalwood, thyme, valerian, and vitex are helpful in preventing or easing headache or migraine pain. Apply Peppermint Pain Reliever to your forehead, neck, and shoulders whenever you feel a tension headache or a migraine coming on; it will help to reduce or eliminate the pain. At the first signs of headache or migraine, breathe in Inhalant for Headache for rapid relief. Bathe in Headache Relief Bath to relax your muscles and reduce muscular tension. Then apply an Icy Migraine Compress to your head to prevent a headache from progressing. You can repeat this regimen as necessary. To relieve muscular tension, rub Tension-Easing Massage Oil into your shoulders and neck. Apply a Warm Compress for Muscular Pain to your neck and shoulders. If at all possible, rest in bed until your symptoms subside.

AROMATHERAPY BLENDS

You can prepare the aromatherapy blends below using pure essential oils. For a more detailed explanation of how to put together and use these blends, see Part Three: Ways to Use Aromatherapy. To review general guidelines for using essential oils, see page 142.

PEPPERMINT PAIN RELIEVER

½ ounce carrier oil
6 drops peppermint oil

In a clean container, add the peppermint oil to the carrier oil and blend. At the first sign of a headache, apply the blend to the painful site, avoiding the eye area. Repeat the treatment as necessary.

INHALANT FOR HEADACHE—DAYTIME

10 drops peppermint oil
6 drops ginger oil
4 drops basil oil
2 drops eucalyptus oil

Add the oils to a small glass bottle with an airtight cover and blend. Inhale directly from the bottle as necessary to prevent or relieve the pain of headache or migraine.

INHALANT FOR HEADACHE—NIGHTTIME

10 drops lavender oil
8 drops chamomile oil
6 drops marjoram oil
1 drop valerian oil

Add the oils to a small glass bottle with an airtight cover and blend. Inhale directly from the bottle as necessary to prevent or ease the pain of headache or migraine.

HEADACHE RELIEF BATH

2 drops chamomile oil
2 drops lavender oil
2 drops marjoram oil
1 drop clary sage oil
1 drop coriander oil

Disperse the oils in a bathtub filled with warm water. Soak in the bath for twenty to thirty minutes. Repeat as necessary.

ICY MIGRAINE COMPRESS
1 quart ice-cold water
1 drop ginger oil
1 drop peppermint oil

Pour the water into a 2-quart glass bowl and add the essential oils. Soak a clean cloth in the water and apply it to your head, forehead, or neck at the first sign of a developing migraine. Avoid letting the compress come into contact with your eyes. You can apply an ice pack over the compress to keep it cool.

TENSION-EASING MASSAGE OIL
1 ounce carrier oil
3 drops marjoram oil
2 drops chamomile oil
2 drops lavender oil
1 drop helichrysum oil

Place the carrier oil in a clean container and add the essential oils. Gently turn the container upside down several times or roll it between your hands to blend all the ingredients together. Massage the mixture over your neck and shoulders to relieve muscular tension. Repeat as necessary.

WARM COMPRESS FOR MUSCULAR PAIN
1 quart hot water
1 drop ginger oil
1 drop peppermint oil
1 drop rosemary oil

Pour the water into a 2-quart glass bowl and disperse the oils in the water. Soak a clean cloth in the water and apply it to your neck and shoulders as needed.

HEARTBURN
See INDIGESTION.

HEMORRHOIDS
One-quarter of all adults suffer from hemorrhoids at some time in their lives. Hemorrhoids are dilated, stretched, or swollen veins that appear in or around the rectal opening. There may be blood clots within the veins, and sometimes hemorrhoids protrude out of the rectum. They may itch, tear, bleed, and cause extreme pain. In some cases, blood may be visible on the surface of the stools or on toilet paper.

Poor circulation and weakness of the blood vessels contribute to hemorrhoids. Straining during bowel movements can aggravate hemorrhoids or lead to their development. Other contributing factors include allergies, chronic constipation, lack of exercise, lifting heavy objects, obesity, poor nutrition, and standing or sitting for long periods of time. Pregnant women often get hemorrhoids as a result of the added pressure and weight on their pelvic veins.

HELPFUL TREATMENTS
A high-fiber diet reduces constipation and therefore reduces straining during elimination. Eating more fresh vegetables, whole grains, fruits, and legumes will promote

normal bowel movements. Make sure to drink plenty of pure water as well. Regular exercise also helps; begin an exercise program to improve your circulation. As much as possible, avoid standing or sitting in one position for prolonged periods of time.

Aromatherapy can help ease the discomfort of hemorrhoids by improving circulation, soothing the pain, and promoting the regeneration and healing of tissue. Essential oils that are effective in treating hemorrhoids include coriander, cypress, geranium, juniper, lavender, myrrh, niaouli, patchouli, tea tree, and vitex. Lavender, niaouli, or tea tree oil, applied topically, offers rapid relief in many instances.

A daily Hemorrhoid Sitz Bath can decrease discomfort, stimulate circulation, and promote healing. Apply Hemorrhoid Massage Oil throughout the day, as needed.

Aromatherapy Blends

You can prepare the aromatherapy blends below using pure essential oils. For a more detailed explanation of how to put together and use these blends, see Part Three: Ways to Use Aromatherapy. To review general guidelines for using essential oils, see page 142.

Hemorrhoid Sitz Bath

1 drop cypress oil
1 drop juniper oil
1 drop niaouli oil

Add the essential oils to a shallow tub filled with warm water. Sit hip-deep in the bath for twenty minutes.

Hemorrhoid Massage Oil

1 ounce jojoba oil
4 drops lavender oil
2 drops tea tree oil
1 drop coriander oil
1 drop myrrh oil

Place the jojoba oil in a clean container, add the essential oils, and gently turn the container upside down several times or roll it between your hands to blend. Apply the oil externally as needed.

HERPES VIRUS

The herpes viruses are a group of viruses that cause skin eruptions or blisters. Herpes simplex virus 1 (HSV1) causes cold sores. It is spread by direct contact with the fluids of a cold sore, fever blister, or skin eruption of someone who carries the virus. Herpes simplex virus 2 (HSV2) affects the genitals and typically is transmitted sexually. Other herpes viruses are responsible for chickenpox, shingles, and mononucleosis, among other illnesses. This section addresses oral and genital herpes, the problems caused by HSV1 and HSV2.

Once an individual contracts herpes, the virus remains in the body, usually lying dormant until some other factor—emotional upset, exposure to the sun, an infection, poor diet, spicy or oily foods, stress, or weakened immunity—triggers an outbreak. When this happens, small, painful, fluid-filled blisters form on and around the mouth or in the genital area within a few hours. Several days later, the blisters break, pus seeps out, and ulcers remain. It can take two to three weeks for them to heal completely. Certain foods, such as alcohol, caffeine, citrus fruits and juices, coffee, fried foods, nuts, popcorn, processed food, refined carbohydrates, spicy or hot foods, sugar, and those with high levels of arginine, can aggravate symptoms.

Helpful Treatments

Although there is no cure for herpes, you can take precautions to prevent outbreaks. The herpes virus thrives on low levels of the amino acid lysine and high levels of the amino acid arginine. If you have herpes, you should limit your consumption of foods that contain high levels of arginine. These include chicken, chocolate, corn (including popcorn), rice, carob, oats, dairy products, nuts, seeds, and whole-wheat products. When lysine levels exceed those of arginine, lysine suppresses the herpes virus. Foods high in lysine include eggs, fish, lima beans, potatoes, red meat, soy products, and yeast. Lysine is also available in supplement form. The B-complex vitamins, vitamins C and E, beta-carotene, and zinc supplements may also help control herpes. Boosting immunity will discourage the recurrence of herpes outbreaks.

Aromatherapy helps with herpes by improving immunity, relieving stress, and easing the pain and discomfort. Immediate treatment with essential oils such as bergamot, clary sage, cypress, eucalyptus, gera-nium, lavender, lemon, melissa, myrrh, niaouli, rose, St. John's wort, and tea tree will often reduce the severity as well as the length of an outbreak. If you take action immediately, you may even avert an attack. Melissa oil is renown for reducing the impact of herpes and discouraging future outbreaks. Make a dilute blend—1 drop of melissa in 100 drops of carrier oil and apply it frequently. At first signs of an oral herpes outbreak, apply a Cold Sore Compress frequently. Putting ice directly on the blister can sometimes halt its progress. Follow this with an application of Healing Oil for Herpes or Herpes Healing Tonic. Repeat these treatments regularly during the outbreak. For genital herpes, take a Herpes Sitz Bath two or three times a day as soon as symptoms first appear. Follow with a Cold Sore Compress and Healing Oil for Herpes. Repeat this regimen as often as necessary.

Aromatherapy Blends

You can prepare the aromatherapy blends below using pure essential oils. For a more detailed explanation of how to put together and use these blends, see Part Three: Ways to Use Aromatherapy. To review general guidelines for using essential oils, see page 142.

Cold Sore Compress

1 pint (16 ounces) cold or ice water
1 drop bergamot oil
1 drop lemon oil
1 drop tea tree oil

Pour the water into a 1-quart glass bowl, add the essential oils, and blend. Soak a clean cloth in the water to make a compress; apply the compress to the affected area. Repeat frequently.

HEALING OIL FOR HERPES
1 ounce jojoba oil
3 drops bergamot oil
3 drops niaouli oil
2 drops myrrh oil
2 drops tea tree oil

Mix all the ingredients together in a clean container. Apply the oil to the affected area after treatment with a Cold Sore Compress.

Note: Bergamot oil increases sensitivity to the sun, increasing the possibility of sunburn and uneven darkening of the skin. Omit it from the formula if your skin will be exposed to sunlight.

HERPES HEALING TONIC
1 ounce pure grain alcohol or vodka
4 drops tea tree oil
3 drops niaouli oil
2 drops eucalyptus oil
1 drop melissa oil

In a clean container, combine all the ingredients. Turn the bottle upside down several times to blend. Apply at the first signs of itching, which may signal an outbreak. Reapply frequently. Blend well before each use. Do not inhale directly from the bottle. Never use isopropyl alcohol for aromatherapy purposes.

HERPES SITZ BATH
2 drops niaouli oil
2 drops tea tree oil
1 drop eucalyptus oil
1 drop geranium oil

Disperse the oils in a shallow tub filled with warm water. Sit hip-deep in the water for twenty minutes. Repeat as necessary.

HIGH BLOOD PRESSURE

As blood courses through the arteries, it exerts pressure against the walls of the blood vessels. When the blood encounters more difficulty than normal flowing through the arteries, the pressure of the blood against the walls of the blood vessels rises. This condition is called high blood pressure, or hypertension. Hypertension commonly results when fatty deposits, or plaque, form inside the walls of blood vessels. They thicken the arterial walls and make them relatively rigid. While it is normal for blood pressure to rise in response to stress or physical exertion and then fall again when the stressful situation is over or activity ends, a person with hypertension will consistently show an elevated blood pressure (usually 140/90 or higher), even when at rest.

Alcohol, drugs, obesity or overweight, a lack of exercise, too much sodium in the diet, oral contraceptives, smoking, stress, and the regular consumption of stimulants such as coffee and tea can cause or contribute to high blood pressure. Heredity may also be a factor.

High blood pressure puts extra strain on the heart, forcing it to work harder to pump blood throughout the body. Over time, it can damage other internal organs, notably the kidneys and blood vessels. It can lead to heart attacks, kidney problems, and strokes.

HELPFUL TREATMENTS

In many cases, a low- or no-sodium, low-fat, caffeine-free, and alcohol-free diet can reduce blood pressure. Losing weight is usually helpful. (*See also* OBESITY AND OVERWEIGHT.) A diet that focuses on fresh fruits and vegetables and whole grains, which are high in nutrients and fiber, is recommended. Exercise and stress-reduction techniques can further reduce blood pressure. Many people with high blood pressure have difficulty relaxing. Because of the serious dangers associated with this condition, if your blood pressure is high and does not respond to dietary and lifestyle changes, you should consult a medical professional for treatment.

Aromatherapy massages and baths can help by calming and relaxing you. Certain essential oils—clary sage, laurel, lavender, lemon, marjoram, melissa, neroli, valerian, and ylang ylang—may actually lower blood pressure. Studies in England indicate that a massage with these oils can lower blood pressure for several days following the massage. Take a Blood Pressure–Reducing Bath every evening for its relaxing and calming benefits. Rub Hypertension Massage Oil over your body once or twice a day or have your massage therapist use it for massages. Disperse Diffuser Blend for Hypertension in your home or office or inhale it directly from the bottle during stressful situations.

AROMATHERAPY BLENDS

You can prepare the aromatherapy blends below using pure essential oils. For a more detailed explanation of how to put together and use these blends, see Part Three: Ways to Use Aromatherapy. To review general guidelines for using essential oils, see page 142.

BLOOD PRESSURE–REDUCING BATH

3 drops ylang ylang oil
2 drops clary sage oil
1 drop marjoram oil

Add the oils to a bathtub filled with warm water and soak in the bath for twenty minutes. Repeat daily or as necessary to reduce blood pressure.

HYPERTENSION MASSAGE OIL

1 ounce carrier oil
4 drops lavender oil
4 drops ylang ylang oil
1 drop melissa oil
1 drop neroli oil

Place the carrier oil in a clean container and add the essential oils. Gently turn the container upside down several times or roll it between your hands to blend. Massage the oil into your skin daily.

Diffuser Blend for Hypertension

15 drops clary sage oil
10 drops lavender oil
6 drops ylang ylang oil
4 drops marjoram oil

Drop the oils into a small glass bottle with an airtight cover and combine. Add some of the mixture to your diffuser or lamp bowl as necessary.

Cautions

Certain essential oils can elevate blood pressure. These include hyssop, peppermint, pine, rosemary, sage, and thyme oils. If you suffer from high blood pressure, you should avoid using these essential oils.

HYPERACTIVITY AND ATTENTION DEFICIT DISORDER

Hyperactivity usually affects children, although adults may be hyperactive as well. Some signs of hyperactivity include persistent impatience, impulsiveness, inability to sit still, a short attention span, aggressiveness, anger, clumsiness, emotional instability, failure to listen or follow directions, frequent frustration, headaches, lack of motor coordination, learning disabilities, lying, poor concentration, self-destructive behavior,

sleep disturbances, stomach pains, and temper tantrums.

The exact cause or causes of hyperactivity, known medically as attention deficit hyperactivity disorder, are unknown, but many cases appear to be related to one or more of the following: allergies to common foods such as corn, dairy products, eggs, soy, and wheat; reactions to food additives, especially sugar, salicylates, caffeine, artificial colors and flavorings, artificial sweeteners, nitrates, and preservatives, particularly BHA and BHT; exposure to environmental pollutants; food allergies and sensitivities, especially to foods with phosphates or with high phosphorus contents, such as meats, fats, and carbonated beverages; heavy metal poisoning from cadmium, copper, lead, manganese, or mercury, particularly the mercury found in "silver" dental amalgam fillings; hyperthyroidism; hypoglycemia; a poor diet, especially one that is deficient in protein; nutritional deficiencies, notably essential fatty acids; and vision or hearing loss. Heredity may play a role as well. A child may become hyperactive if his or her mother smoked or used alcohol or drugs during pregnancy, if there was prenatal trauma, or if the child was deprived of oxygen at birth.

Helpful Treatments

Diet can often successfully treat hyperactivity; dietary changes frequently bring about an immediate improvement. A person who is hyperactive should avoid all of the foods listed above that trigger hyperactivity. Other products to avoid include antacids; bacon; breath mints; candy; catsup; chewing gum; chocolate; cider vinegar; cough drops and throat lozenges; ham; hot dogs; ice cream; luncheon meats; margarine; milk; perfume; pills, including vitamins and nutritional supplements that are artificially colored or flavored; processed or "junk" foods; salt; soft drinks; soy sauce; and anything with artificial coloring, flavoring, or sweeteners. Read labels carefully. Some butter, cheeses, teas, and toothpastes, among other things, may contain these additives. Eliminating salicylates is a bit more difficult because these occur naturally in certain foods. Natural sources of salicylates that are best avoided include almonds, apples, apricots, berries, cherries, cucumbers, currants, oranges, peaches, plums, prunes, and tomatoes.

Essential fatty acids (EFAs) of linoleic and linolenic acids, taken internally, can help reduce hyperactivity in children. One British study reported that massaging evening primrose oil into the skin helped curb hyperactivity within five days. Other comparable sources of both EFAs are borage, flaxseed, and hemp oils. Skin can absorb EFAs readily, making massage soothing to emotions and body.

Aromatherapy can help calm and relax hyperactive individuals with such essential oils as benzoin, cedarwood, chamomile, clary sage, coriander, cypress, fennel, frankincense, laurel, lavender, marjoram, melissa, myrrh, neroli, oregano, rose, rosewood, St. John's wort, sandalwood, thyme, valerian, vetiver, and ylang ylang. For rapid relief, breathe in Instant Calm Inhalant. Disperse Diffuser Blend for Hyperactivity throughout the house or in the room or office of the person with this disorder. A daily bath in Relaxing Bath Blend can quickly calm down a person who is hyperactive, as will applying Calming Skin Oil with Essential Fatty Acids. Use Children's Bath Blend and Children's Skin Oil with Essential Fatty Acids for an infant or small child who is hyperactive.

AROMATHERAPY BLENDS

You can prepare the aromatherapy blends below using pure essential oils. For a more detailed explanation of how to put together and use these blends, see Part Three: Ways to Use Aromatherapy. To review general guidelines for using essential oils, see page 142.

INSTANT CALM INHALANT
10 drops chamomile oil
5 drops lavender oil
2 drops valerian oil

Add the essential oils to a small glass bottle with an airtight cover and blend. Inhale directly from the bottle as necessary to prevent or minimize hyperactivity.

DIFFUSER BLEND FOR HYPERACTIVITY
20 drops lavender oil
18 drops chamomile oil

10 drops rosewood oil

10 drops sandalwood oil

8 drops clary sage oil

6 drops thyme oil

6 drops ylang ylang oil

4 drops coriander oil

Blend all the oils together in a clean glass container. Use the mixture in your diffuser or lamp as necessary.

RELAXING BATH BLEND

3 drops lavender oil

2 drops marjoram oil

1 drop oregano oil

1 drop vetiver oil

Disperse the oils in a bathtub filled with warm water. Soak in the bath for ten to twenty minutes, or for as long as possible. Repeat as necessary.

CALMING SKIN OIL WITH ESSENTIAL FATTY ACIDS

1 ounce flaxseed oil

½ ounce borage oil

½ ounce hemp oil

4 drops chamomile oil

4 drops rosewood oil

2 drops laurel oil

1 drop melissa oil

1 drop rose oil

1 drop valerian oil

Place the carrier oils in a clean container and add the essential oils. Gently turn the container upside down several times or roll it between your hands to blend. Massage the oil into your skin once or more daily, as needed.

CHILDREN'S BATH BLEND

1 drop chamomile oil

1 drop lavender oil

Add the chamomile and lavender oils to a bathtub filled with warm water. Have the child soak in the bath for five to fifteen minutes (or for as long as you can persuade him or her to stay in the tub). Repeat as necessary.

CHILDREN'S SKIN OIL WITH ESSENTIAL FATTY ACIDS

1 ounce flaxseed oil

½ ounce borage oil

2 drops chamomile oil

2 drops lavender oil

1 drop valerian oil

In a clean container, add the essential oil to the carrier oils and blend. Massage the mixture into the child's skin once or more daily, as needed.

IMMUNE SYSTEM DISORDERS

See WEAKENED IMMUNE SYSTEM.

IMPOTENCE

Impotence is the inability of a man to achieve or maintain an erection or to complete the sexual act. Impotence may be an occasional, frequent, or permanent problem. Physical causes can include overall poor health; anatomical defects; diabetes; drug abuse; lower back problems; liver or kidney disorders; prostate problems; nervous system injury or disorders; and the use of alcohol, tobacco, and certain drugs, especially heart and blood pressure medications, antihistamines, and decongestants. However, most cases of impotence are related to psychological or emotional factors such as anxiety, depression, self-esteem, and relationship problems.

HELPFUL TREATMENTS

If you suffer from recurring impotence, you should visit your health-care provider to rule out any underlying medical problems or illness. If you suspect that stress is at the root of the problem, begin a stress management program. (*See also* STRESS.) If emotional or relationship problems are part of the problem, it may be helpful to seek individual or joint counseling. (*See also* EMOTIONAL ISSUES.)

Aromatherapy can help you overcome impotence by reducing stress and creating a sensual atmosphere for lovemaking. Certain essential oils have aphrodisiac properties and can stir sexual desire (see the recommendations for enhancing sexual desire on page 228). Benzoin, clary sage, coriander, fennel, ginger, jasmine, neroli, patchouli, rose, rosemary, rosewood, sandalwood, and ylang ylang all have reportedly helped many men overcome impotence.

Patchouli, rosewood, and vetiver help reduce anxiety about sexual performance. In addition, benzoin and vitex may help prevent premature ejaculation.

Bathe in Sexuality Bath—with your partner if possible. Afterward, massage each other with Sexuality Massage Oil. Disperse Sexuality Diffuser Blend throughout your bedroom or entire home.

AROMATHERAPY BLENDS

You can prepare the aromatherapy blends below using pure essential oils. For a more detailed explanation of how to put together and use these blends, see Part Three: Ways to Use Aromatherapy. To review general guidelines for using essential oils, see page 142.

SEXUALITY BATH

3 drops patchouli oil
2 drops clary sage oil
1 drop rosewood oil
1 drop ylang ylang oil

Add the essential oils to a bathtub filled with warm water. Soak in the bath, preferably with your partner, for fifteen to twenty minutes.

SEXUALITY MASSAGE OIL

2 ounces carrier oil
4 drops sandalwood oil
3 drops clary sage oil
3 drops ylang ylang oil
2 drops coriander oil
2 drops patchouli oil

2 drops rosewood oil
1 drop benzoin resin
1 drop ginger oil
1 drop vetiver oil

Place the carrier oil in a clean container and add the essential oils. Gently turn the container upside down several times or roll it between your hands to blend. Use the mixture to massage your partner's body. Then have your partner massage you.

Sexuality Diffuser Blend

20 drops sandalwood oil
12 drops clary sage oil
8 drops ylang ylang oil
6 drops rosewood oil
4 drops cedarwood oil
4 drops ginger oil
2 drops coriander oil

Combine all the ingredients in a small glass bottle with an airtight cover. Add some of the blend to your diffuser or lamp bowl as desired.

INCONTINENCE

Incontinence is the involuntary and uncontrollable release of urine. *Stress incontinence* occurs when coughing, laughing, or sneezing triggers a loss of urine. A strong urge to void your bladder along with an unexpected leakage indicates *urge incontinence*. *Mixed incontinence* combines stress incontinence and urge incontinence. A steady but weak stream or a frequent trickle of urine

along with the inability to empty the bladder signals *overflow incontinence*. Pain may accompany urination.

Aging and loss of muscle tone are common contributors to incontinence. Incontinence may also suggest a bladder infection, bladder stones, diabetes, kidney disorders, urinary tract infection or problems, or an infection of the reproductive system. Incontinence can be a symptom of allergies, emotional or psychological problems, nervous disorders, and possible structural damage to the urinary tract. During pregnancy, and even after delivery, women can experience incontinence. Frequently, it follows surgery.

In men, an enlarged prostate or other prostate problems can cause the bladder to retain urine until it overflows and leaks. Aging, alcohol consumption, central nervous system disorders, weakness of muscle structure supporting the bladder, medication, obesity, infection, or nerve damage can compound the problem. Incontinence is often a symptom of Alzheimer's disease or dementia.

Incontinence is common in menopausal and postmenopausal women. Aging reduces muscle tone; the uterus and pelvic wall may sag. This alters the angle of the urethra, which transports urine from the body. Due to decreased sensitivity in the area, a woman may no longer receive sensations that warn of a full bladder.

Diuretics, which are often prescribed for high blood pressure and are a chief ingredient in diet pills and other medications, decrease the water weight of the body by increasing the amount of urine excreted. This can stress and overwork the bladder. Other drugs can interfere with the normal discharge of urine by first causing it to be retained, then suddenly and urgently released, with little or no warning. Other pills, such as antidepressants, pain relievers, sedatives, and tranquilizers, reduce the sensation of the need to urinate and can result in incontinence.

Many people ignore signals that they need to urinate. Over time, holding on to urine even when you feel the signal, or delaying urination until it is more convenient, can weaken bladder muscles. Eventually, the muscles can no longer hold back. Also, inadequate intake of water to flush out the urinary tract can irritate the bladder and kidneys, thus contributing to recurrent bouts of cystitis, which further weaken the bladder.

Food and beverages are big factors in the frequency of urination. Expect a fuller bladder from foods with high water content, such as melons, citrus fruits, grapes, peaches, pineapples, plums, and other juicy fruits, as well as cucumbers and tomatoes. Coffee, tea, alcoholic beverages (particularly beer and wine), colas and other carbonated beverages, juices or other drinks with high sugar content, hot soups and beverages, sugary or spicy foods, sports beverages, and diet drinks with artificial colorings, flavorings, and sweeteners can irritate the bladder and stimulate frequent urination.

HELPFUL TREATMENTS

Most cases of incontinence can benefit from simple treatments. Become aware of what is causing your incontinence and make changes in your diet and lifestyle. When you first feel the urge to urinate, do so. Don't wait. Visit the toilet at regular intervals. Wear clothing that is quick and easy to manipulate to avoid delays when you need to use the bathroom. Plan your consumption of beverages to coincide with times when you are near a toilet. When you are unable to visit the toilet, reduce your intake of beverages. Always urinate before going out, especially if you are traveling in a car.

Remember to drink ample water over the course of the day, however. While drinking water increases the flow of urine, your body requires it to flush out toxins and wastes. When you are thirsty, make water your first choice. Water helps to purify your body, particularly the kidneys and bladder. Your system handles water better than other beverages. If you don't drink enough water, wastes will linger in your bladder and kidneys, which can lead to cystitis or irritation that can increase incontinence.

Exercises can help restore muscle tone and may be more effective than medication in minimizing or solving incontinence for both men and women. Squeeze the muscles around your bladder as if trying to prevent the passage of gas. Hold for three seconds, then relax for three seconds. Repeat this sequence up to 100 times every day. For women, this exercise also improves vaginal muscle tone and boosts circulation, which may help with some symptoms of menopause, such as vaginal dryness, thinning, and loss of muscle tone. You can do this exercise unobserved almost anytime—while doing the dishes, driving, standing in line, walking, or working. No one need know. If you are squeezing the correct muscles, this exercise will stop the flow of urine. You can do this to make sure you are exercising the correct muscles, but don't actually do the exercise while you are urinating. Practicing with an empty bladder is more effective.

Herbal urinary tonics such as buchu, cleavers, and dandelion may offer relief. Even though they also act as diuretics, they can strengthen the urinary system while eliminating wastes. The herbal forms of St. John's wort and valerian may help minimize incontinence. Other folk remedies include eating fresh cherries or drinking cherry juice concentrate with water but without sugar. Unsweetened cranberry juice concentrate mixed with water helps prevent bladder infections and maintain bladder health. Vitamin C keeps the urinary tract free of infections.

If you are taking any type of medication, ask your pharmacist or physician if the side effects can include increased urination or if the pill contains a diuretic. Any drug can aggravate an existing condition. For many people, a change of medication helps. Surgical procedures can provide relief.

Aromatherapy offers physical and emotional support for incontinence. Abdominal exercises help maintain or regain muscle tone. Essential oils that can tone the urinary tract include bergamot, cedarwood, cypress, elemi, eucalyptus, fennel, frankincense, juniper, and sandalwood oils. Apply Urinary Tonic Blend over your abdomen, back, and bladder and kidney areas twice daily, especially before doing incontinence exercises. Essential oils of St. John's wort and valerian may decrease episodes of incontinence. When related to menopause or hormone imbalances, patchouli, rose, and vitex may offer relief. Aromatherapy can relieve stress associated with incontinence. Essential oils that support the functions of the urinary tract and nurture confidence and esteem include benzoin, bergamot, cedarwood, cypress, juniper, rose, and tea tree oils. Choose Incontinence Control Blend for Men or for Women and use it regularly to discourage incontinence. Sitz baths encourage circulation and improve lymph flow to the groin and abdominal area as do massage with essential oils. Sit in an Incontinence Sitz Bath as often as possible.

AROMATHERAPY BLENDS

You can prepare the aromatherapy blends below using pure essential oils. For a more detailed explanation of how to put together and use these blends, see Part Three: Ways to Use Aromatherapy. To review general guidelines for using essential oils, see page 142.

URINARY TONIC BLEND

1 ounce carrier oil
3 drops bergamot oil
2 drops elemi oil
2 drops sandalwood oil

Place the carrier oil in a clean container and add the essential oils. Gently turn the container upside down several times or roll it between your hands to blend the ingredients together. Rub the mixture over the bladder and kidney areas twice daily or as needed.

INCONTINENCE CONTROL BLEND FOR MEN

1 ounce carrier oil
4 drops St. John's wort oil
3 drops sandalwood oil
2 drops cedarwood oil
1 drop valerian oil

Place the carrier oil in a clean container and add the essential oils. Gently turn the container upside down several times or roll it between your hands to blend the ingredients together. Rub the mixture over the bladder and kidneys twice daily or as needed.

INCONTINENCE CONTROL BLEND FOR WOMEN

1 ounce carrier oil
3 drops St. John's wort oil
2 drops bergamot oil
2 drops vitex oil
1 drop rose oil
1 drop valerian oil

Place the carrier oil in a clean container and add the essential oils. Gently turn the container upside down several times or roll it between your hands to blend the ingredients together. Rub the mixture over the bladder and kidneys twice daily or as needed.

INCONTINENCE SITZ BATH

2 drops bergamot oil
1 drop St. John's wort
1 drop sandalwood oil

Add the oils to a shallow tub filled with water. Sit hip-deep in the water for five to fifteen minutes.

INDIGESTION

Indigestion can take the form of bloating, constipation, diarrhea, gas, heartburn, nausea, or queasiness. Poor digestion may be a result of the aging process, anxiety, eating too quickly, emotional upset or stress, improper food combinations, food allergies, lack of digestive enzymes, low fiber intake, nutritional deficiencies, poor diet, failure to chew food thoroughly, overeating, overweight, pregnancy, eating spicy or hot foods, or stress. When the body's ability to digest food decreases, tiny particles of partially digested food can enter the bloodstream through the intestinal mucosa. This can cause autoimmune disorders, food allergies, joint problems, and abdominal aches and pains.

Gas, or flatulence, usually results from digestive enzyme deficiencies, poor diet, or poor eating habits such as eating too quickly, overeating, or swallowing foods without chewing them thoroughly. In addition, certain foods—notably legumes and carbonated beverages—and certain combinations of foods commonly cause gas.

Gastritis is an inflammation of the stomach or stomach lining that typically causes a burning sensation in the stomach, nausea, or vomiting. It is usually related to the consumption of a specific irritant such as alcohol, caffeine, tobacco, or certain drugs.

Heartburn is a tight, burning feeling in the middle of chest or the upper abdominal area that extends upward through the esophagus and causes unpleasant belching, bloating, or gas. Heartburn can be a result of anxiety, bacterial infection, eating too rapidly, gastritis, an imbalance of stomach acids, improper food combinations, nervousness, poor diet, stress, or ulcers. Heartburn can also result if the lining of the stomach becomes unable to produce the mucus that normally protects it from attack by stomach acid.

Nausea is a queasy, uneasy feeling and may result in vomiting. It often occurs after eating spoiled foods or foods that disagree with you. Anxiety, morning sickness, motion sickness, nervousness, and stress can also cause nausea.

HELPFUL TREATMENTS

Use a food diary to keep track of what you eat and how you feel afterward. This can help identify foods, or combinations of foods, that cause digestive distress. Always chew your food thoroughly. Certain food combinations can cause digestive difficulties. Avoid eating proteins with carbohydrates, fruits, sugars, or starches. Eat sweet fruits, such as bananas, dates, raisins, and dried fruits, either by themselves or in combination with the sub-acid fruits—grapes, papayas, mangoes, and fruits with cores or pits, such as apples, peaches, and pears. Eat acid fruits, including pineapples, citrus fruits, tomatoes, and most berries, either by themselves or in combination with sub-acid fruits; never combine them with sweet fruits. Always eat melons by themselves. You may wish to check with a nutritionist to determine whether you have any nutritional deficiencies and ask for suggestions to improve your diet.

Digestive enzymes, available in health-food stores, may be helpful. Eating a diet that centers on fresh, raw foods will provide more natural enzymes. If feelings of anxiety, nervousness, or stress are interfering with your digestion, find ways to reduce them. Many culinary herbs, such as basil, bay leaves (laurel), black pepper, cardamom, cilantro, coriander, cumin, fennel, ginger, marjoram, oregano, parsley, rosemary, sage, tarragon, and thyme, promote better digestion. You can often enhance both your dining pleasure and your digestion by seasoning your favorite dishes with these herbs.

Essential oils can help by aiding the digestive process, relieving gas, easing heartburn, and soothing nausea. Essential oils that improve digestion include basil, benzoin, bergamot, black pepper, chamomile, clary sage, coriander, fennel, frankincense, ginger, helichrysum, juniper, laurel, lavender, lemon, marjoram, melissa, myrrh, neroli, oregano, palmarosa, peppermint, rose, rosemary, thyme, valerian, and ylang ylang. Oils that relieve gas include basil, benzoin, black pepper, chamomile, clary sage, coriander, fennel, ginger, laurel, marjoram, myrrh, peppermint, rosemary, and thyme. For heartburn, use black pepper, chamomile, coriander, fennel, ginger, lemon, marjoram, and peppermint oils. Sandalwood and thyme oils are specifics for gastritis; basil, black pepper, coriander, fennel, ginger, melissa, peppermint, rose, rosewood, and sandalwood oils soothe nausea.

For any digestive difficulty, use All-Purpose Digest-Aid Oil to massage your abdomen twice a day.

AROMATHERAPY BLENDS

You can prepare the aromatherapy blend below using pure essential oils. For a more detailed explanation of how to put together and use this blend, see Part Three: Ways to Use Aromatherapy. To review general guidelines for using essential oils, see page 142.

ALL-PURPOSE DIGEST-AID OIL

2 ounces carrier oil
3 drops basil oil
2 drops laurel oil
2 drops rosemary oil
2 drops thyme oil
1 drop coriander oil
1 drop ginger oil
1 drop peppermint oil

Place the carrier oil in a clean container and add the essential oils. Gently turn the container upside down several times or roll it between your hands to blend the ingredients together. Rub the mixture over your entire abdominal area twice daily or as needed.

INSECT BITES

Most encounters with insects are nothing more than a nuisance. However, the bites and stings of many insects can cause pain, itching, redness, swelling, and soreness within a localized area. Allergic reactions can involve the entire body and may cause headache and fever. Certain insect bites can lead to infection.

HELPFUL TREATMENTS

Always cleanse insect bites thoroughly to prevent infection and apply Insect Repellent and Bite Oil immediately. Repeat as necessary. For stings, remove the stinger by gently scraping rather than by pulling it out. Immediately apply Insect Repellent and Bite Oil and place a cold compress or ice over the area to reduce itching and swelling. This formula is all-purpose and both repels insects and relieves the itching and swelling of insect bites. Apply the oil several times daily until the discomfort subsides. Aloe vera gel also can soothe bites. To prevent scarring, resist the urge to scratch insect bites.

Using an insect repellent deters insect bites and stings, thereby averting allergic reactions. Aromatherapy is a safe, natural way to ward off the attack of insects. Many essential oils, such as basil, bergamot, cedarwood, chamomile, cypress, eucalyptus, fennel, laurel, lavender, melissa, niaouli, patchouli, peppermint, pine, St. John's wort, sandalwood, spruce, tea tree, thyme, vetiver, and ylang ylang are useful in treating insect bites. They all possess repellent properties. Apply Insect Repellent and Bite Oil before you go outside to prevent insect bites.

AROMATHERAPY BLENDS

You can prepare the aromatherapy blend below using pure essential oils. For a more detailed explanation of how to put together and use this blend, see Part Three: Ways to Use Aromatherapy. To review general guidelines for using essential oils, see page 142.

INSECT REPELLENT AND BITE OIL

2 ounces carrier oil
3 drops eucalyptus oil
3 drops spruce oil
2 drops niaouli oil
2 drops patchouli oil
2 drops pine oil
2 drops vetiver oil

In a clean container, add the essential oils to the carrier oil and blend. Apply the oil to insect bites to help them heal. To repel insects, apply the oil to your skin before going outdoors.

INSOMNIA

Insomnia is the chronic inability to sleep, taking the form of difficulty falling asleep or remaining asleep throughout the night. Common causes of insomnia include emotional upset, excitement, stress, and worry. Dietary or eating habits can contribute, especially eating late at night, eating sweets or spicy or stimulating foods, eating a poor or high-sugar diet, eating poor combinations of foods, and overeating.

Taking prescription sleeping pills, even occasionally, interferes with normal sleep patterns and breathing. They can become habit-forming and lead to insomnia. Other possible causes of insomnia include asthma, indigestion, hypoglycemia, muscular aches and pains, the consumption of caffeine or certain drugs, exercising too close to bedtime, and nutritional deficiencies, especially a copper or iron deficiency.

HELPFUL TREATMENTS

If you suffer from insomnia, consider visiting your health-care professional to rule out or obtain treatment for any underlying health problems. Avoid caffeine. If you feel you must consume foods and beverages that contain caffeine, do so before noon. Avoid sugar and spicy or stimulating foods. Exercise early in the day since exercising before bedtime can invigorate you and prevent you from falling asleep.

Meditating or reading before bedtime often helps many people fall asleep. Bathing in Dead Sea salts or mineral bath salts before bedtime relaxes muscles and promotes calmness. Enhance your relaxation by playing soft music and drinking a cup of sleep-inducing herbal tea thirty minutes before bedtime. Catnip, chamomile, hops, skullcap, spearmint, and valerian root teas are good choices.

Aromatherapy can calm your nerves and help you sleep more soundly. Many essential oils such as basil, chamomile, coriander, lavender, marjoram, melissa, neroli, orange, oregano, rose, St. John's wort, sandalwood, spruce, thyme, valerian, vetiver, and ylang ylang reduce stress and promote relaxation, making it easier to fall asleep.

Before bedtime, enjoy a leisurely bath in Bedtime Bath Blend. Put Good Night Diffuser Blend in your diffuser. Following your bath, massage your skin with Nighttime Massage Oil. Apply Sweet Slumber Personal Blend before bedtime. Spray your pillow and sheets with Sweet Dreams Pillow Spray.

AROMATHERAPY BLENDS

You can prepare the aromatherapy blends below using pure essential oils. For a more detailed explanation of how to put together and use these blends, see Part Three: Ways to Use Aromatherapy. To review general guidelines for using essential oils, see page 142.

BEDTIME BATH BLEND

½ to 1 cup Dead Sea salts (optional)
4 drops chamomile oil
2 drops marjoram oil
2 drops ylang ylang oil

Add the ingredients to a bathtub filled with warm water and disperse well. Soak in the bath for twenty minutes.

GOOD NIGHT DIFFUSER BLEND

20 drops lavender oil
8 drops German chamomile oil
8 drops marjoram oil
6 drops ylang ylang oil

Add the oils to a clean glass bottle and gently turn the container upside down several times or roll it between your hands to combine. Add some of the blend to your diffuser or lamp bowl as necessary.

NIGHTTIME MASSAGE OIL

2 ounces carrier oil
5 drops lavender oil
4 drops ylang ylang oil
2 drops vetiver oil
1 drop melissa oil
1 drop valerian oil

Place the carrier oil in a clean container, add the essential oils, and blend. Massage the oil into your skin before bedtime as needed.

SWEET SLUMBER PERSONAL BLEND
⅛ ounce jojoba oil
6 drops sandalwood oil
2 drops neroli oil
2 drops ylang ylang oil
1 drop coriander oil
1 drop vetiver oil

Blend the oils together well in a clean container. Apply a few drops to your pulse points before bedtime.

SWEET DREAMS PILLOW SPRAY
4 ounces distilled water
3 drops lavender oil
2 drops chamomile oil
2 drops rose oil
1 drop neroli oil

Pour the water into a spray bottle, add the essential oils, and turn the bottle upside down several times to blend. Spray the mixture on your pillow and sheets or in your room before bedtime. Blend well before each use.

JOCK ITCH

Jock itch (known to doctors as *tinea cruris*) is the common name for a ringworm infection that appears on the groin, particularly in men. The fungal organism that causes it belongs to the same family as the fungus that causes athlete's foot. Like other fungi, it thrives in moist, dark, warm places. Inflamed bumps appear on the upper inner thigh. As these bumps dry out, they turn into a scaly rash that causes painful and embarrassing itching. Friction between the legs further irritates the skin. Wearing tight pants or undershorts, particularly ones made from synthetic fabrics, can contribute to jock itch. Contact with an infected towel, article of clothing, or athletic supporter, especially when these items are shared, can spread the infection.

HELPFUL TREATMENTS
If you are suffering from jock itch, keep the groin area clean and dry. Wash all clothing that comes into contact with the affected area after each wearing. Never share clothing or athletic supporters.

Essential oils such as cypress, laurel, lavender, myrrh, niaouli, oregano, patchouli, spruce, tea tree, and thyme fight fungi and can help control jock itch. Take a Jock Itch Bath at the first signs of jock itch; repeat once or twice daily until the symptoms subside. Apply Jock Itch Oil to the affected area twice daily. Coconut oil may discourage the growth of fungi.

AROMATHERAPY BLENDS
You can prepare the aromatherapy blends below using pure essential oils. For a more

detailed explanation of how to put together and use these blends, see Part Three: Ways to Use Aromatherapy. To review general guidelines for using essential oils, see page 142.

JOCK ITCH BATH

3 drops spruce oil
2 drops niaouli oil
2 drops patchouli oil
1 drop myrrh oil

Add the essential oils to a bathtub filled with warm water. Soak in the bath for fifteen to twenty minutes. Repeat daily, as needed.

JOCK ITCH OIL

1 ounce coconut oil
3 drops tea tree oil
3 drops thyme oil
1 drop laurel oil
1 drop myrrh oil

Place the carrier oil in a clean container and add the essential oils. Gently turn the container upside down several times or roll it between your hands to blend. Apply the mixture to the affected area several times daily, as needed.

LOW BLOOD PRESSURE

Low blood pressure, or hypotension, is a condition in which the blood does not pump through the blood vessels with as much force as normal. Less common than high blood pressure, it poses little threat to health, unless severe. However, it can be inconvenient. When the brain does not receive a steady, sufficient supply of blood, you may feel dizzy or faint, especially upon rising. People with low blood pressure often chill or tire easily. Low blood pressure can indicate inadequate function of the adrenal glands.

HELPFUL TREATMENTS

If you have low blood pressure, always move from a lying position to a sitting position, and from sitting to standing, slowly, to prevent dizziness. Pace yourself. Dress warmly to prevent chills, particularly from air conditioning. Regular exercise, massage, and skin brushing will also help by improving circulation.

Aromatherapy can help by raising blood pressure, stimulating circulation, preventing or minimizing dizziness, and helping to overcome fatigue. Peppermint, pine, rosemary, and thyme oils can elevate low blood pressure and stimulate circulation. Basil, black pepper, coriander, and peppermint oils also reduce the possibility of fainting. Coriander and ginger oils can reduce dizziness. Spruce oil tones the adrenal glands, which maintain blood pressure.

Before bathing, dry-brush your skin to stimulate circulation. (*See* SKIN BRUSHING in Part Three.) Follow this with a Low Blood Pressure Bath daily. Afterward, massage Low Blood Pressure and Dizziness Massage Oil into your skin.

AROMATHERAPY BLENDS

You can prepare the aromatherapy blends below using pure essential oils. For a more detailed explanation of how to put together and use these blends, see Part Three: Ways to Use Aromatherapy. To review general guidelines for using essential oils, see page 142.

LOW BLOOD PRESSURE BATH

3 drops rosemary oil
2 drops thyme oil
1 drop peppermint oil

Add the essential oils to a bathtub filled with warm water. Soak in the bath for fifteen to twenty minutes. Repeat daily.

LOW BLOOD PRESSURE AND DIZZINESS MASSAGE OIL

1 ounce carrier oil
4 drops pine oil
3 drops spruce oil
2 drops coriander oil
1 drop thyme oil

Place the carrier oil in a clean container and add the essential oils. Gently turn the container upside down several times or roll it between your hands to blend. Massage the oil over your skin daily. Apply over the kidneys to tone the adrenal glands.

CAUTIONS

Certain essential oils can depress blood pressure. These include clary sage, laurel, lavender, lemon, marjoram, melissa, neroli, valerian, and ylang ylang. If your blood pressure is already low, you should avoid using these oils.

LYMPHATIC SYSTEM, SLUGGISH/SWOLLEN LYMPH GLANDS

The lymphatic system is a major component of the immune system. The health of your lymphatic system determines your body's ability to fight invaders and maintain health. Sluggish lymphatic health is often an overlooked factor in illness and disease. As the waste treatment facility for the body, it collects wastes and toxins throughout the body for dispersal and disposal. The lymphatic system also maintains the body's fluid balance by absorbing excess fluids and returning them to the bloodstream for distribution throughout the body. It supports the circulatory system; its activities and condition affect the abilities of the blood to perform its many duties. The lymphatic system also produces lymphocytes, white blood cells that scavenge lymph fluids to eliminate foreign matter and microorganisms responsible for disease and infection.

The primary components of the lymphatic system include the bone marrow and the thymus. The thymus lies beneath the breastbone, or sternum. It produces T cells, a key type of lymphocytes that defends against invading microbes. It also produces hormones and works with the endocrine system.

The secondary components of the lymphatic system are the spleen; the lymph nodes, located throughout the body but especially in the armpits, breast, groin, knees, and neck; the appendix; Peyer's patch, in the small intestines; the tonsils; and mucous membranes throughout the body.

The lymphatic system relies entirely upon bodily movements and contraction of the muscles to "push" fluid through veins and valves. Modern sedentary lifestyles don't offer ample opportunities to stimulate lymphatic circulation. Without exercise or massage, lymphatic circulation slows. Wastes linger and lodge in cells throughout the body. Stress further depletes immunity, and muscle tension can inhibit proper flow of both blood and lymphatic fluids throughout muscle and body. An insufficient intake of water slows the processes of the lymphatic system, interfering with the body's prompt response to foreign invasion and with the proper elimination of wastes.

Sluggish lymphatic circulation may manifest as allergies, cellulite, chronic fatigue syndrome, emotional disturbances, fat, fatigue, general malaise, headaches, illness, overweight, pain, recurring infections, slow healing of wounds, and weakened immunity. Swollen lymph glands usually occur in the neck or throat, the tonsils, the armpits, or the groin. Lymph glands swell as part of the immune response. As lymphocytes rush to the scene to fight infection, they cause swelling, tenderness, and pain. Other areas that may become enlarged or inflamed include the abdomen, breasts, elbows, knees, and even the ankles.

HELPFUL TREATMENTS

Movement and exercise are essential. Massage, even light touching or tapping on the areas of lymphatic tissue, can stimulate circulation and encourage the removal of wastes. (*See* MASSAGE in Part Three.) Tapping gently on the upper breastbone stimulates the thymus to improve immunity and lymph activity. Skin brushing stimulates the lymph system to eliminate wastes more effectively. (*See* SKIN BRUSHING in Part Three.)

Drinking lots of pure water—64 ounces a day—helps to flush the toxins and wastes from your system. Herbal lymphatic-system tonics include cleavers, echinacea, and Oregon grape root, which may be taken as teas, tinctures, or capsules. Eating a diet consisting of whole healthy foods will improve overall health. Focus on fresh fruits and vegetables, eating them raw whenever possible.

Aromatherapy can help by encouraging the circulation of both lymph and blood. It detoxifies cells, thereby releasing the buildup of toxins and wastes that burden the whole body. It improves immunity. Essential oils that can improve lymph functions include basil, coriander, cypress, eucalyptus, frankincense, geranium, juniper, laurel, lemon, marjoram, oregano, rosemary, and thyme. One of the best essential oils for lymphatic massage is laurel oil. Essential oils complement massage or skin brushing and produce a synergistic effect. Daily aroma-therapy baths relax your body and mind. They also reduce stress while stimulating circulation and releasing wastes.

AROMATHERAPY BLENDS

You can prepare the aromatherapy blends below using pure essential oils. For a more detailed explanation of how to put together and use these blends, see Part Three: Ways to Use Aromatherapy. To review general guidelines for using essential oils, see page 142.

LYMPH MASSAGE OIL

1 ounce carrier oil
6 drops laurel oil
2 drops cypress oil
2 drops lemon oil

Place the carrier oil in a clean container and add the essential oils. Turn the container upside down several times or roll it between your hands to blend. Gently massage the oil over your lymph glands to stimulate lymphatic circulation or to soothe swollen glands.

LYMPH-STIMULATING BATH

3 drops lemon oil
2 drops laurel oil
1 drop coriander oil

Disperse the essential oils well in a bathtub filled with warm water. Enjoy a leisurely soak for twenty to thirty minutes daily or as needed.

MENOPAUSE-RELATED PROBLEMS

Menopause marks the "change of life" for women, with the gradual cessation of their menstrual cycles. Some women start this change in their middle to late thirties, but the majority of women usually begin during their forties or fifties. Although this transition should be gradual and smooth, many women experience much difficulty. Symptoms such as depression, heavy periods or prolonged bleeding, hot flashes, insomnia, irregular cycles, and night sweats can continue for several years. Mood swings, personality changes, and even a loss of libido can accompany menopause. Other common complaints include bloating, circulatory problems, constipation, discomfort of the bladder, incontinence, and varicose veins. Skin loses elasticity, and moisture levels drop, contributing to dryness and wrinkles. Vaginal thinning and dryness may make intercourse painful. Memory loss, inability to concentrate, disorientation, and forgetfulness may occur. Changes in libido are common. As a result of hormonal imbalances and changes from menopause, osteoporosis—or the demineralization of bones and reduction of bone mass and density—may develop. Other causes of osteoporosis include aging, high levels of steroids, lack of exercise, poor diet, and malnutrition.

Many women claim that hot flashes are the most troublesome symptom of menopause. Hot flashes happen when blood vessels erratically dilate and constrict. Blood flow increases, body temperature rises, and the heart pumps faster. Sweating usually accompanies hot flashes.

Along with the physical symptoms of menopause, many women experience a fear of growing old, feeling less feminine, or losing their looks. Indeed, skin loses elasticity, and dehydration results. While it is natural to have these concerns, maintaining a bright, optimistic attitude can ease your apprehensions. To a large degree, menopause is what you make it; your expectations of what you will encounter will influence your experience. You can improve with age and enter this new phase of your life with joy and enthusiasm. Besides, there are benefits: You no longer have to worry about unplanned pregnancy; if you've had PMS or painful periods, or have had to interrupt your normal activities because of menstrual difficulties, you now can enjoy a new freedom. Many women welcome these changes.

HELPFUL TREATMENTS

A healthy diet, an active lifestyle, and time out for relaxation and stress reduction can make the transition smoother. Women in Japan complain little of menopausal symptoms. Scientists speculate that diet is the key: Foods common in the Japanese diets such as miso, soybeans, and tofu all contain plant hormones that can balance the body's hormones. Dates, flaxseeds, and pomegranates are other sources of phytoestrogens.

Borage, evening primrose oil, and other oils high in essential fatty acids—flaxseed and hemp—provide additional relief for some women. Gamma-oryzanol, a derivative of rice bran, can relieve symptoms.

Many women take calcium supplements or consume extra or even excessive amounts of milk and dairy products, although some experts speculate that the bones do not absorb this calcium. Some studies cite an increase in osteoporosis as a result of large consumption of dairy products. Perform this test on your calcium supplements to determine if your body is absorbing them: Put a tablet in a cup of vinegar, stirring every few minutes. If it doesn't dissolve within thirty minutes, it won't dissolve in your body.

Not every woman can benefit from hormone replacement therapy (HRT). Almost half of the women who take HRT stop treatment after six months. According to physicians, the prevention of osteoporosis is one of HRT's big benefits, yet some findings suggest that hormone usage must continue for more than seven years to show results. If HRT ends, bone density can decline rapidly, and other symptoms can return as well, sometimes more severe than they were before the HRT. Taking HRT can increase the risk of breast, uterine, and ovarian cancers, as well as lupus. In addition, changes in liver metabolism can occur because the body cannot assimilate and eliminate the synthetic or engineered forms of estrogen most often used in HRT. Other side effects include blood clots, fluid retention, and high blood pressure. Recently, researchers and women have been paying more attention to progesterone, as well as the importance of achieving a balance between estrogen and progesterone levels.

Aromatherapy can help to make the passage smoother by diminishing many of the discomforts you may experience. Used as a precautionary measure, aromatherapy may prevent many symptoms and make your transition smoother. Chamomile, cypress, jasmine, melissa, neroli, orange, patchouli, rose, St. John's wort, valerian, vitex, and ylang ylang oils calm both the body and mind. Clary sage, coriander, fennel, geranium, lavender, pine, rose, spruce, vetiver, and vitex oils restore hormonal balance.

Though ancient physicians such as Hippocrates recommended vitex, or chaste tree, for menopausal problems more than two thousand years ago, only relatively recently have distillers begun producing the essential oil. If vitex were a drug, the medical field would proclaim it a miracle cure. In its way, it is.

Simply smelling vitex several times throughout the day can minimize or eliminate most of the problems associated with the change of life. Vitex works by balancing hormonal secretion in the pituitary gland, where it prompts your body to release the amounts of progesterone and estrogen that it needs. This eliminates the guesswork of HRT, the success of which depends on finding the right medication at the right dosage that will relieve symptoms without creating serious health conditions or severe side effects that are worse than the symptoms. Rose is a feminine and nurturing oil that restores confidence, comforts the emotions, and regulates the menstrual cycle. Essential oils that can avert or minimize hot flashes are clary sage, cypress, patchouli, peppermint, rose, and vitex. Add a drop to a cool hand bath and soak your hands for ten to fifteen minutes.

Breathe in Hormone Helper Inhalant directly from the bottle several times daily, particularly when you feel a hot flash coming on or when you need an emotional boost. If you prefer, you can inhale vitex oil directly from the bottle. Pamper yourself with Menopause-Balancing Bath as you relax and restore balance to your life. Keep cool with Cool Flash Spray or Cool-Down Compress Blend. You may substitute chamomile, fennel, peppermint, or rose hydrosol. Massage Menopause-Balancing Body Oil into your skin every day to fight fluid retention, restore balance, and ease your transition. Borage and evening primrose oils as carrier oils may relieve some of the symptoms of menopause. Dab on Femininity Personal Fragrance throughout the day and celebrate your femininity.

AROMATHERAPY BLENDS

You can prepare the aromatherapy blends below using pure essential oils. For a more detailed explanation of how to put together and use these blends, see Part Three: Ways to

Use Aromatherapy. To review general guidelines for using essential oils, see page 142.

HORMONE HELPER INHALANT
6 drops clary sage oil
6 drops vitex oil
2 drops rose oil

Add the essential oils to a small glass bottle with an airtight cover and blend. Inhale directly from the bottle as necessary to relieve the symptoms of menopause.

MENOPAUSE-BALANCING BATH
2 drops chamomile oil
2 drops clary sage oil
1 drop fennel oil
1 drop geranium oil

Disperse the essential oils in a bathtub filled with warm water. Soak in the bath for twenty to thirty minutes.

COOL FLASH SPRAY
8 ounces distilled water
2 drops clary sage oil
1 drop patchouli oil
1 drop peppermint oil

Pour the water into a spray bottle, add the essential oils, and turn the bottle over several times to blend. Spritz yourself whenever you feel a hot flash coming. Refrigerate the spray for an even more cooling effect. Blend well before each use.

COOL-DOWN COMPRESS BLEND
6 drops chamomile oil
6 drops clary sage oil
4 drops lavender oil
4 drops orange oil
2 drops geranium oil
2 drops patchouli oil

Add the essential oils to a small glass bottle and blend. Add 1 to 2 drops of the essential oil blend to 1 quart of cool water. Soak a clean cloth in the water and apply it to your face, forehead, back of your neck, chest, or other areas of your body to prevent or cool down hot flashes. If you wish, you can apply an ice pack over the compress to keep it cool. Do not let the compress come in contact with your eyes.

MENOPAUSE-BALANCING BODY OIL
1½ ounces sesame oil
½ ounce borage oil
4 drops clary sage oil
3 drops geranium oil
3 drops vitex oil
2 drops orange oil
1 drop coriander oil
1 drop fennel oil
1 drop patchouli oil

Place the carrier oil in a clean container and add the essential oils. Gently turn the container upside down several times or roll it between your hands to blend. Apply the mixture over your entire body, especially on bloated areas.

FEMININITY PERSONAL FRAGRANCE
⅛ ounce jojoba oil
3 drops clary sage oil
2 drops geranium oil
2 drops German chamomile oil
2 drops vitex oil
1 drop coriander oil
1 drop jasmine absolute or enfleurage
1 drop rose oil

In a clean container, add the essential oils to the jojoba oil and combine well. Wear on pulse points as a fragrance or inhale it directly from the bottle frequently throughout the day.

MENSTRUAL PROBLEMS

For most young women, menstruation begins sometime between the ages of eleven and fifteen. Every twenty-one to thirty-five days during her reproductive years, a healthy woman's ovaries will release an egg. If the egg is not fertilized, the woman will shed the lining of her uterus about two weeks later. This shedding is known as menstruation. A woman's monthly menstrual flow normally lasts three to seven days; the entire menstrual cycle continues until menopause, which usually occurs during her forties or fifties.

Although menstruation itself should not necessarily be painful, about two-thirds of menstruating women experience some sort of difficulty or pain each month with their menstrual cycle. Numerous women complain of premenstrual syndrome, or

PMS. (*See also* PREMENSTRUAL SYNDROME.) Below are causes of and suggestions for the most common menstrual complaints: Menstrual Cramps, Heavy Menstrual Flow, and Scant or Irregular Menstrual Periods.

Menstrual Cramps

Painful periods, or *dysmenorrhea,* commonly involve abdominal and back pain; sometimes diarrhea, headaches, nausea, nervousness, and vomiting accompany cramping. Medical researchers are not certain about the cause of cramping, but many believe that high levels of prostaglandins, which are hormones secreted by the uterine lining prior to menstruation, may be involved. These hormones can trigger contractions or spasms of the smooth muscle of the uterus. Alternately, low levels of progesterone may cause dysmenorrhea. Other physiologic factors, such as emotional or psychological stress, abnormal positioning of the uterus, or obstructions that block the menstrual discharge, can cause complications. In addition, when the uterus swells and constricts in spasms, it restricts blood flow into the pelvic region and diminishes the supply of oxygen to those tissues. This can contribute to cramping.

Look at your lifestyle, especially diet, to discover and address the causes of cramping. Pay attention to diet, especially to adequate levels of dietary fiber and fluids, which promote regularity, since constipation often intensifies the pain of menstrual cramps. Avoid sugar, fats—especially cooked fats—and any other foods that cause gas or make the lower abdomen uncomfortable.

Foods high in plant hormones, or phytohormones, such as soybeans and miso, help regulate the body's own hormones. Others foods containing phytohormones include apples, brown rice, carrots, green beans, flaxseeds, fennel, legumes, peas, potatoes, rye, sesame seeds, tarragon, whole wheat, and yams. Eliminate alcohol, caffeine, and cigarettes, particularly the week preceding menstruation. Fast food and junk food can bloat and constipate you. Animal products and byproducts are frequently laden with residues of growth hormones, antibiotics, and other medications considered vital for keeping livestock and poultry healthy; these can interfere with your own hormones. Many prescription drugs, including antibiotics and birth control pills, alter levels of essential fatty acids (EFAs) and prompt hormonal shifts and imbalances. Unrefined vegetable oils such as flaxseed and hemp have essential fatty acids and offer relief while restoring balance within your body.

A regular exercise program is also beneficial. However, during the time you are experiencing cramps, take it easy and forego strenuous exercise. Instead, do yoga or light stretching or take a walk. Wear loose clothing that doesn't hinder circulation. Attitude affects your periods, especially if you dislike having your period or feel cursed for being a woman. If your periods are extremely painful, consult your physician about the possibility of an underlying health problem.

Licorice and dong quai are the leading herbs for restoring hormonal and glandular harmony. Rose petal and red hibiscus teas soothe cramps and help restore hormonal balance.

Aromatherapy can help minimize menstrual pain by easing cramps, regulating menstrual cycles, and soothing the emotions. It can also help relieve other symptoms of PMS. (*See also* PREMENSTRUAL SYNDROME.) Basil, chamomile, clary sage, cypress, fennel, geranium, ginger, helichrysum, juniper, marjoram, melissa, neroli, peppermint, rose, vitex, and ylang ylang oils help relieve pain, reduce swelling, and soothe the muscle spasms of cramps.

Vitex restores hormonal balance within your body and therefore can help regulate your menstrual cycles and minimize or eliminate painful cramps. Throughout the month, breathe in vitex oil one or more times daily. Several days before you anticipate your period, begin bathing daily in Cramp Relief Bath. Repeat as often as necessary to reduce cramps. Apply Menstrual Cramp Massage Oil or Rose Cramp Relief Oil to your abdomen and back starting several days prior to your period, before pain and cramping begin, if possible. You also can smooth Rose Cramp Relief Oil over your body or use as an inhalant to soothe emotions. Cramp-Soothing Compress, placed on your abdomen or lower back, can ease cramping.

You can prepare the aromatherapy blends below using pure essential oils. For a more detailed explanation of how to put together and use these blends, see Part Three: Ways to Use Aromatherapy. To review general guidelines for using essential oils, see page 142.

CRAMP RELIEF BATH
2 drops marjoram oil
2 drops ylang ylang oil
1 drop fennel oil
1 drop rose oil

Disperse the oils in a bathtub filled with warm water. Soak in the bath for twenty to thirty minutes. Repeat as necessary.

MENSTRUAL CRAMP MASSAGE OIL
2 ounces carrier oil
4 drops chamomile oil
4 drops marjoram oil
4 drops ylang ylang oil
3 drops cypress oil
1 drop helichrysum oil

Place the carrier oil in a clean container, add the essential oils, and blend by gently turning the container upside down several times or rolling it between your hands. Massage the oil over your abdomen and back as necessary.

ROSE CRAMP RELIEF OIL
½ ounce carrier oil
6 drops rose oil

Place the carrier oil in a clean container. Add the rose oil and blend. Beginning several days before the anticipated onset of your period, massage the oil over your abdomen and back. Repeat as necessary.

CRAMP-SOOTHING COMPRESS
1 quart cool water
1 drop chamomile oil
1 drop geranium oil
1 drop helichrysum oil
1 drop juniper oil

Pour the water into a 2-quart glass bowl and add the essential oils. Soak a clean cloth in the water and apply it to your abdomen. Repeat as necessary.

Heavy Menstrual Flow

Some women experience heavy menstrual flow or unusually long menstrual periods (also known as *hypermenorrhea* or *menorrhagia*) along with clotting each month during their menstrual cycles. If this continues for a prolonged time, doctors consider it dysfunctional uterine bleeding. Hormonal imbalances and thyroid disorders are two health problems that can cause heavy menstrual flow. It may also be a sign of endometriosis, fibroid tumors, pelvic infection, or other female reproductive problems. Over time, heavy periods can lead to iron deficiency anemia and other nutritional deficiencies.

If you have unusually heavy periods, consult your health-care professional to rule out the possibility of an underlying health problem and to check for nutritional deficiencies, especially anemia.

Consider the dietary suggestions mentioned under Menstrual Cramps. Regular exercise may be helpful, but avoid strenuous exercise while you are having your period.

Aromatherapy can help regulate menstrual cycles and reduce menstrual flow. Vitex oil helps regulate the balance of estrogen and progesterone. Essential oils that minimize heavy flow are cypress, frankincense, geranium, rose, and vitex. Bathe in Flow-Minimizing Bath twice a day, as necessary. Massage Flow-Minimizing Oil over your abdomen frequently. Apply a Cool Cypress Compress over your abdominal area as needed to reduce heavy flow. If your flow is heavy, you should avoid using basil, clary sage, coriander, jasmine, juniper, myrrh, and thyme oils during your period. These essential oils encourage menstrual flow.

You can prepare the aromatherapy blends below using pure essential oils. For a more detailed explanation of how to put together and use these blends, see Part Three: Ways to Use Aromatherapy. To review general guidelines for using essential oils, see page 142.

FLOW-MINIMIZING BATH
2 drops cypress oil
1 drop frankincense oil
1 drop geranium oil
1 drop rose oil

Add the oils to a bathtub filled with warm water. Soak in the bath for twenty to thirty minutes daily, or as needed.

FLOW-MINIMIZING OIL
2 ounces carrier oil
6 drops cypress oil
4 drops geranium oil
3 drops frankincense oil
1 drop vitex oil

Place the carrier oil in a clean container, add the essential oils, and blend. Massage the oil frequently over your abdomen and back, beginning, if possible, before the onset of your period.

COOL CYPRESS COMPRESS
1 quart cold water
4 drops cypress oil

Add the cypress oil to a 2-quart glass bowl containing 1 quart of cold water and mix well. Soak a clean cloth in the water and apply it to the abdominal area. Repeat as needed.

Scant or Irregular Menstrual Periods
Amenorrhea, or lack of menstruation not due to pregnancy or menopause or during lactation and breast-feeding, frequently results from emotional stress, particularly during major life changes. Other causes or contributory factors include anorexia nervosa, depression, emotional stress, extreme

physical exertion, fatigue, hypoglycemia, illness, low protein intake, nutritional deficiencies, poor diet, shock, sports training, travel and jet lag, sudden or extreme weight loss, and a very low ratio of body fat to muscle. An abnormal development of the ovaries or uterus can cause amenorrhea.

Consider the dietary recommendations discussed under Menstrual Cramps. Initiate a daily exercise program. Have your body-fat proportion checked to discover if it is below normal. Often vegetarian or vegan women whose body fat drops below 18 percent may cease to menstruate. Examine your lifestyle for sources of stress and reduce it wherever possible. You may want to consider having a thorough physical examination to rule out illness as a factor.

Aromatherapy can help encourage menstrual flow and regulate menstrual cycles. If your period is scant or late, and not due to pregnancy, the emmenagogue oils—basil, cedarwood, chamomile, clary sage, coriander, fennel, jasmine, juniper, laurel, marjoram, myrrh, oregano, peppermint, and thyme oils—can help start or increase your flow. Aromatherapy also helps to reduce stress that is contributing to irregularity. (*See also* STRESS.) Bathe daily in a Period-Promoting Bath. Massage Flow-Inducing Oil over your abdomen and back.

To help normalize your menstrual cycles, use hormone- or cycle-regulating oils: chamomile, clary sage, coriander, fennel, geranium, jasmine, juniper, pine, rose, spruce, vetiver, and vitex oils. Massage Cycle-Regulating Oil into your skin, particularly on your abdomen and back, daily. Once or twice a week, take a Cycle-Regulating Bath. Wear Harmonious Hormone Personal Perfume daily.

You can prepare the aromatherapy blends below using pure essential oils. For a more detailed explanation of how to put together and use these blends, see Part Three: Ways to Use Aromatherapy. To review general guidelines for using essential oils, see page 142.

PERIOD-PROMOTING BATH

2 drops clary sage oil
1 drop cedarwood oil
1 drop coriander oil
1 drop myrrh oil

Disperse the oils in a bathtub filled with warm water. Soak in the bath for twenty to thirty minutes.

FLOW-INDUCING OIL

2 ounces carrier oil
6 drops clary sage oil
4 drops juniper oil
2 drops coriander oil
2 drops laurel oil

In a clean container, add the essential oils to the carrier oil and blend. Massage the oil over your abdomen and lower back several times daily.

CYCLE-REGULATING OIL

2 ounces carrier oil

6 drops chamomile oil

6 drops clary sage oil

4 drops spruce oil

3 drops vitex oil

2 drops fennel oil

2 drops rose oil

2 drops vetiver oil

Place the carrier oil in a clean container and add the essential oils. Gently turn the container upside down several times or roll it between your hands to blend. Massage the oil into your skin daily.

CYCLE-REGULATING BATH

2 drops clary sage oil

2 drops geranium oil

1 drop coriander oil

1 drop fennel oil

Add the essential oils to a bathtub filled with warm water. Soak in the bath for fifteen to twenty minutes.

HARMONIOUS HORMONE
PERSONAL PERFUME

⅛ ounce jojoba oil

4 drops clary sage oil

3 drops geranium oil

2 drops rose oil

2 drops vetiver oil

2 drops vitex oil

In a small bottle, add the essential oils to the jojoba oil and blend. Apply the mixture as a fragrance every day.

MIGRAINE

See HEADACHE.

MORNING SICKNESS

An estimated half of all pregnant women experience morning sickness in the beginning of pregnancy. Although women with morning sickness often feel nauseous or may vomit upon rising in the morning, the condition unfortunately can occur intermittently throughout the day.

Bouts of morning sickness can continue for two weeks to three months or longer. Changes in hormone levels and metabolism, along with the liver's inability to process increased amounts of hormones, account for most cases of morning sickness. Emotional factors can intensify episodes of nausea or vomiting.

HELPFUL TREATMENTS

Eat dry toast or crackers first thing in the morning to prevent nausea and vomiting. During the day, eat smaller meals at more frequent intervals to keep some food in your stomach at all times. Drinking ginger tea can discourage the queasiness of morning sickness.

Aromatherapy can help alleviate the discomfort of morning sickness. Inhale ginger or rose oil directly from the bottle or use Morning Sickness Inhalant Blend. Melissa and sandalwood oils ease queasiness and nausea, reduce vomiting, and can soothe the digestive tract as well as the nerves.

AROMATHERAPY BLENDS

You can prepare the aromatherapy blend below using pure essential oils. For a more detailed explanation of how to put together and use this blend, see Part Three: Ways to Use Aromatherapy. To review general guidelines for using essential oils, see page 142.

MORNING SICKNESS
INHALANT BLEND
4 drops ginger oil
1 drop melissa oil
1 drop rose oil

Add the essential oils to a small glass bottle with an airtight cover and blend. Inhale directly from the bottle as necessary to fight nausea and prevent vomiting.

CAUTIONS

Essential oils are highly concentrated and can have powerful effects. Some essential oils stimulate menstrual flow and/or uterine contractions and are therefore not recommended for use during pregnancy. These include basil, cedarwood, chamomile, clary sage, coriander, fennel, jasmine, juniper, laurel, marjoram, myrrh, oregano, peppermint, spruce, and thyme. You should consult with your health-care practitioner before using any essential oils during pregnancy.

MOTION SICKNESS

Motion sickness can cause tremendous discomfort for some travelers. They may exhibit such symptoms as headaches, nausea, queasiness, and vomiting while driving, flying, sailing, or riding as a passenger. Other complaints include cold sweats, dizziness, fear, loss of appetite, sleepiness, and even lack of coordination in extreme cases. Sometimes symptoms persist for several hours after travel ends.

When certain postures or movements rotate a mechanism in the inner ear in different directions simultaneously, motion sickness occurs. This mechanism, called the vestibular apparatus, helps maintain equilibrium. These rotations disrupt normal balance and also send messages to the brain that conflict with the nerve impulses sent by the other sensory organs.

HELPFUL TREATMENTS

If you tend to suffer from motion sickness, stay as still as possible and in a position that minimizes movement while traveling. Avoid reading or observing passing scenery. Some people find that focusing their eyes on a point on the horizon is helpful; fresh air may also offer relief. Motion sickness is easier to prevent than to cure. Drink ginger tea or take ginger capsules before embarking on a trip. Most mainstream over-the-counter and prescription motion-sickness remedies can cause side effects, especially drowsiness. Scientific studies have shown that ginger is equally effective, or even more so.

Use aromatherapy to minimize discomfort and prevent nausea. Chamomile, ginger, melissa, oregano, and peppermint are the best essential oils for treating motion sickness. Ginger, oregano, and peppermint oils help prevent nausea and vomiting, while chamomile and melissa oils calm the nerves, quell queasiness, and soothe the stomach. Inhaling any of these oils directly from the bottle may avert an attack of motion sickness. Other oils that minimize nausea include basil, black pepper, coriander, fennel, and rose. Breathe in Motion Sickness Inhalant Blend, beginning at least one hour before travel. Continue inhaling it every fifteen to thirty minutes throughout your trip.

AROMATHERAPY BLENDS

You can prepare the aromatherapy blends below using pure essential oils. For a more detailed explanation of how to put together and use these blends, see Part Three: Ways to Use Aromatherapy. To review general guidelines for using essential oils, see page 142.

MOTION SICKNESS INHALANT BLEND
10 drops ginger oil
10 drops peppermint oil

Add the oils to a small glass bottle with an airtight cover and blend. Inhale directly from the bottle, beginning an hour before travel. Repeat frequently.

MUSCULAR ACHES, PAINS, AND INJURIES

Muscular aches and pains may result from a strenuous workout, overexertion of muscles, illness, poor posture, or simply using your muscles without warming them up. Muscular aches and pains function as warning signals sent by your body to prevent serious injury by keeping you from using or overusing stressed muscles. If this signal is ignored, injury often occurs. Types of muscle injuries include a tear in the muscle tissue, fluid retention in or around the muscle, muscle spasms, or overstretching of the connective tissue surrounding the muscle.

Aches and pains can be localized in particular muscle groups, such as the neck or shoulders, as a result of injury, overuse, strain, trauma, or even emotional tension. They can cause burning, hot or cold sensations, numbness, tingling, and weakness in the muscles. Chronic muscular aches and pains may be a sign of a type of soft tissue rheumatism that affects the muscles, ligaments, tendons, or joints. Symptoms may include muscle aches, fatigue, pain, and stiffness, as well as the development of painful points on certain muscles. In addition to muscular problems, this condition—like any kind of chronic pain—can lead to anxiety, depression, headaches, and sleep disturbances.

HELPFUL TREATMENTS

To help prevent aches, pains, and injuries, warm up your muscles before engaging in strenuous physical activity, whether work, exercise, or sports. Be aware of your posture during exercise. Try not to exceed your body's capabilities. Set reasonable fitness goals and work up to them gradually.

Massage Preventive Sports Rub into your muscles before working out to reduce or eliminate injuries, sore muscles, and strain. After exercise or physical work, take an After-Sports Bath. Then apply either Deep Heat Tingling Rub or Post-Workout Rub to your muscles to ease or prevent soreness, as needed.

Immediately treat any suspected injury to the muscles by applying ice or a cold compress. Use a cold Muscle-Strain Compress for bruises, inflammation, sprains, swelling, and tennis elbow. After an injury that results in bruising, apply Bruise Blend several times a day to promote healing. Seek medical attention immediately for any serious injury.

For chronic muscular pain, use warm or hot compresses. Apply a hot Chronic Pain Compress to minimize the discomfort of chronic muscle aches or old injuries. Acupressure, acupuncture, hypnosis, massage, and relaxation techniques offer relief for many people with chronic muscular pain. If you have a tendency to injure the same spots again and again, physical therapy may help you to retrain your muscles.

Aromatherapy can comfort both acute and chronic muscular aches and pains. Many essential oils, including basil, bergamot, black pepper, chamomile, clary sage, coriander, cypress, eucalyptus, helichrysum, juniper, lavender, marjoram, rosemary, thyme, and vetiver can be used to relieve pain, reduce swelling, and ease muscle spasms. If you suffer from chronic muscular aches and pains, take a Chronic Pain Relief Bath daily or several times a week. In the morning, apply Daytime Muscle Ache Oil for an invigorating treatment. In the evening, rub on Nighttime Muscle Relief Oil for a relaxing effect. As carrier oils, flaxseed and hemp can relieve muscle aches and joint pains, while almond, borage, calophyllum inophyllum, evening primrose, flaxseed, and hemp oils can reduce inflammation.

AROMATHERAPY BLENDS

You can prepare the aromatherapy blends below using pure essential oils. For a more detailed explanation of how to put together and use these blends, see Part Three: Ways to Use Aromatherapy. To review general guidelines for using essential oils, see page 142.

PREVENTIVE SPORTS RUB

1 ounce carrier oil
3 drops basil oil
3 drops rosemary oil
2 drops peppermint oil
1 drop ginger oil

Place the carrier oil in a clean container and add the essential oils. Gently turn the container upside down several times or roll it between your hands to blend. Massage the mixture into your muscles before physical activity.

AFTER-SPORTS BATH
1 cup Dead Sea salts (optional)
¼ cup seaweed or algae powder (optional)
3 drops lavender oil
2 drops chamomile oil
2 drops marjoram oil
1 drop helichrysum oil

Disperse the essential oils, and the Dead Sea salts and seaweed or algae powder, if desired, in a bathtub filled with warm water. After physical exertion, soak in the bath for twenty minutes.

DEEP HEAT TINGLING RUB
½ ounce flaxseed oil
½ ounce hemp oil
3 drops peppermint oil
2 drops ginger oil
1 drop black pepper oil

In a clean container, mix the carrier oils. Add the essential oils and blend. Use this rub to massage sore muscles following physical activity.

POST-WORKOUT RUB
1 ounce hemp oil
10 drops calophyllum inophyllum oil
3 drops chamomile oil
3 drops marjoram oil
2 drops thyme oil
1 drop vetiver oil

Place the carrier oils in a clean container, add the essential oils, and blend. After physical exertion, massage the mixture into your muscles and joints to prevent stiffness and pain.

MUSCLE-STRAIN COMPRESS
1 quart cold water
2 drops chamomile oil
1 drop marjoram oil

Pour the water into a 2-quart glass bowl, add the essential oils, and blend. Saturate a clean cloth in the water and apply it to the affected area as needed. If you wish, you can apply an ice pack over the compress to keep it from getting warm.

BRUISE BLEND
½ ounce flaxseed oil
½ ounce hemp oil
6 drops calophyllum inophyllum oil
3 drops geranium oil
2 drops helichrysum oil
2 drops juniper oil
1 drop ginger oil

In a clean container, combine the carrier oils. Add the essential oils and blend well by gently turning the container upside down several times or rolling it between your hands. After an injury, massage the blend over the bruised area several times daily.

CHRONIC PAIN COMPRESS

1 quart hot water
2 drops helichrysum oil
1 drop chamomile oil

Pour the water into a 2-quart bowl and disperse the oils in the water. Saturate a clean cloth in the water and apply it to the affected areas as needed.

CHRONIC PAIN RELIEF BATH

2 drops clary sage oil
2 drops juniper oil
1 drop coriander oil
1 drop vetiver oil

Add the essential oils to a bathtub filled with warm water. Soak in the bath for twenty to thirty minutes.

DAYTIME MUSCLE ACHE OIL

2 ounces almond oil
1 ounce flaxseed oil
10 drops rosemary oil
8 drops eucalyptus oil
6 drops cypress oil
4 drops peppermint oil
3 drops thyme oil

Place the carrier oils in a clean container and add the essential oils. Gently turn the container upside down several times or roll it between your hands to blend. Massage the oil into sore muscles as needed.

NIGHTTIME MUSCLE RELIEF OIL

2 ounces almond oil
1 ounce hemp oil
10 drops chamomile oil
10 drops marjoram oil
4 drops clary sage oil
4 drops coriander oil
4 drops ylang ylang oil

In a clean container, combine the carrier oils. Add the essential oils and blend well. At bedtime, apply the oil to sore muscles as needed.

OBESITY AND OVERWEIGHT

A weight gain of a few pounds over normal makes you overweight. If your body weight exceeds the optimum weight for your age, bone structure, height, and sex by 20 to 30 percent or more, overweight becomes obesity. Weight gain occurs when the intake of calories exceeds the output. Calories that aren't used immediately settle as fat in the 30 to 40 billion fat cells of the average body. Storing fat is an ancient survival mechanism that kept hunter-gatherers alive during lean times; modern people rarely require it.

Excess weight burdens the entire body and can result in pain in the ankles, back, hips, knees, and shoulders. It crowds the internal organs. Obesity compromises immunity and can lead to the development of circulatory disorders, diabetes, gallbladder problems, heart problems, high blood pressure, kidney disease, and stroke. Additionally, excess weight generates enormous emotional and psychological issues, as the obsession to be thin pervades our culture.

Up to half of all adults in America are on diets at any one time. Though they spend over $30 billion annually on dieting, they don't keep the weight off. In less than one year, about 95 percent of dieters regain the weight they lose; many put on additional pounds. Yet people hesitate to admit that dieting doesn't work.

Adults are not the only ones with weight problems. One-fourth of American teens are overweight enough to be candidates for health problems later in life: Even if they slim down and stay slim, they remain at increased risk for heart attack, stroke, colon cancer, gout, and other illnesses. More and more children become obese due to poor eating habits learned at home and to bad food choices. Society's obsession with thinness doesn't help, either. Emotionally, some teens feel too helpless and hopeless to ever achieve the ideal of slim and trim.

Poor nutrition and poor eating habits are the biggest culprits in overweight and obesity. Billboards, magazine ads, and television commercials aggressively promote processed and junk foods that are laden with calories and chemicals and have little or no nutrition. The body has difficulty digesting, assimilating, and eliminating these substances. Instead, it stores them in the body as fat and wastes. Empty calories bloat our bodies but leave us hungry for nourishment. For all their bulk and body weight, Americans are severely malnourished. Each year as weights rise, health steadily declines.

Many people eat out of habit even when they aren't hungry. More and more Americans eat on the run, frequenting fast-food takeout places. They wash down wads of half-chewed foods with soda or, worse, with alcoholic beverages, which add calories and slow the burning of fats stored in body. Fad dieting or continuous dieting often contributes to overweight; the imbalance of foods permitted on the diet, plus feelings of deprivation coupled with the constant feeling of hunger, leads people to abandon the diet. In addition, reducing calories often slows metabolism, making weight loss more difficult as the body burns fewer calories in an attempt to conserve energy.

An inadequate intake of water can contribute to overweight. The body is more than 70 percent water and requires about 64 ounces of pure water every day to function properly. Without sufficient water, the metabolism slows, allowing excess weight to accumulate. Thin people almost always drink lots of water.

Diseases and disorders such as diabetes, hypoglycemia, and endocrine disorders can contribute to weight problems. Anxiety, boredom, depression, obsessive and/or compulsive behavior, and other emotional issues are often factors in overweight. Many people who experienced physical or sexual abuse or trauma in childhood become obese. Psychologically, they may seek to build boundaries around their bodies or to insulate themselves from other people. Many people also find comfort in food as a substitute for love.

HELPFUL TREATMENTS

Lifestyle changes are necessary for weight loss and management. Controlling and maintaining a healthy weight depend not on dieting but on daily choices of healthy and nutritious foods throughout your life. Eating more vegetables—especially raw ones—can provide a feeling of fullness with very few calories and little fat. Avoid fried and greasy foods. Learning and following positive eating habits help establish permanent lifestyle patterns to control weight. (See Positive Eating Habits on page 279.)

Aromatherapy can help with some underlying problems by, for instance, subduing stress and regulating appetite. (*See also* APPETITE DISTURBANCES *and* STRESS.) Some essential oils can help to keep your skin toned during weight loss. Nurturing your body and mind with essential oils during weight loss can provide support and strength while helping you to maintain your resolve and determination.

Essential oils such as basil, bergamot, cedar, coriander, cypress, fennel, geranium, ginger, juniper, laurel, lemon, myrrh, orange, palmarosa, patchouli, rosemary, spruce, thyme, and vetiver can help restore balance to your body by supporting the digestion and assimilation of food, stimulating sluggish metabolism, improving blood and lymphatic circulation, and encouraging elimination of wastes. (*See also* CIRCULATION, POOR; *and* LYMPHATIC SYSTEM, SLUGGISH/ SWOLLEN LYMPH GLANDS.)

Aromatherapy can provide emotional support during weight loss. Essential oils that provide strength and boost willpower include cedarwood, cypress, fennel, lemon, marjoram, myrrh, neroli, and rosemary. (*See also* EMOTIONAL ISSUES.) Soaking in an aromatic bath such as Weight-Loss Nurturing Bath can ease stress, relax your mind, and stimulate circulation and elimination of wastes as you nurture yourself. Follow this with an application of Skin-Toning Oil to keep your skin supple and pliant during weight loss. Throughout the day, inhale Weight-Loss Inhalant to boost your metabolism, regulate your appetite, and reaffirm your commitment to yourself and your body.

AROMATHERAPY BLENDS

You can prepare the aromatherapy blends below using pure essential oils. For a more detailed explanation of how to put together and use these blends, see Part Three: Ways to Use Aromatherapy. To review general guidelines for using essential oils, see page 142.

Positive Eating Habits

The key to achieving and maintaining a healthy weight is not dieting, but daily adherence to healthy eating and lifestyle habits. The following are guidelines that can help:

• Seek slow weight loss. Rapid loss rarely lasts, nor is it healthy.

• Don't count calories, but do make your calories count. Choose foods that provide the most nutrition for the calories.

• Drink lots of water—at least 64 ounces every day. Choose water first if you are thirsty. Drink one or two glasses of water thirty minutes before meals.

• Before you begin eating, take a minute to relax and reflect on your food and your health.

• Don't skip meals.

• Eat only when you are hungry. Eat slowly and enjoy each bite. Chew thoroughly. Put only the amount of food you want to eat on your plate. After that, stop and leave the table.

• Eat the largest meal for breakfast or lunch, not dinner.

• Avoid eating anything late at night.

• Wear tight-fitting clothing or a belt to let you know when your stomach has expanded enough and to remind you to stop eating.

• Stay away from the kitchen and the refrigerator until mealtime. Break the habit of associating visiting the kitchen with needing to eat something. Put reminders on the refrigerator.

• Don't shop on an empty stomach. Purchase only nutritious foods. You can't eat junk food or forbidden foods if you don't buy them.

• Find supportive friends who won't sabotage your efforts. Most of all, support yourself.

• Don't chew gum. It triggers the flow of digestive juices that signal hunger.

• Adjust your attitude about your body, your diet, and your health. The thoughts you put in your mind are as important as the foods you put in your mouth.

• Learn to love your body as it is now.

• Increase your activity level to avoid boredom and daydreaming about food. Find constructive ways to fill up your life.

WEIGHT-LOSS NURTURING BATH

3 drops cypress oil
2 drops coriander oil
2 drops fennel oil
1 drop laurel oil

Disperse the oils in a bathtub filled with warm water. Soak in the bath for twenty to thirty minutes. Repeat daily.

SKIN-TONING OIL

2 ounces carrier oil

6 drops geranium oil

4 drops orange oil

4 drops patchouli oil

2 drops laurel oil

Place the carrier oil in a clean container and add the essential oils. Gently turn the container upside down several times or roll it between your hands to blend. Apply the mixture over your entire body.

WEIGHT-LOSS INHALANT

6 drops fennel oil

3 drops ginger oil

2 drops rosemary oil

1 drop black pepper oil

Add the essential oils to a small glass bottle with an airtight cover and blend. Inhale directly from the bottle as necessary.

PREMENSTRUAL SYNDROME (PMS)

Many women experience emotional, mental, and physical discomfort and distress each month, usually starting one to two weeks before menstruation begins. They suffer from premenstrual syndrome, or PMS, with its 150 or more possible symptoms.

The most common physical symptoms of PMS include backaches, blemishes, bloating and fluid retention, cramps, faintness, fatigue or lethargy, headaches, swollen or tender breasts, insomnia, nausea, poor concentration, and a swollen abdomen. (*See also* ACNE; BACKACHE AND BACK PROBLEMS; FATIGUE; HEADACHE; INSOMNIA; *and* MENSTRUAL PROBLEMS.) Mentally and emotionally, PMS may produce aggression, anger, anxiety, depression, irritability, mood swings, nervousness, personality changes, increased sensitivity, suicidal thoughts, and violent actions. (*See also* ANXIETY; DEPRESSION; *and* EMOTIONAL ISSUES.)

The precise cause or causes of PMS are not well understood, but the syndrome may be related to hormonal imbalance, especially high levels of estrogen and low levels of progesterone, as well as rapid fluctuations in hormone levels. Hypoglycemia, nutritional deficiencies, poor absorption of nutrients, thyroid imbalances, food allergies, and candidiasis all can contribute to the discomforts of PMS as well.

HELPFUL TREATMENTS

Diet can help control many aspects of PMS. Foods high in phytoestrogens such as soybeans and miso help regulate hormones. Others foods containing phytoestrogens include apples, brown rice, carrots, green beans, flaxseeds, fennel, legumes, peas, potatoes, rye, sesame seeds, tarragon, whole wheat, and yams.

Some women have had success using nutritional supplements—vitamin A, the B vitamins (especially vitamin B_6 and folic acid), calcium, magnesium, essential fatty acids, and borage or evening primrose oil—to control PMS. Following a healthy diet that is low in sodium and sugar and contains no alcohol, animal products or byproducts, caffeine, chocolate, or processed foods can reduce the severity of symptoms. If you suffer from PMS, concentrate on eating a diet of primarily fresh vegetables and fruits and whole grains. Drink eight to ten glasses of pure, clean water daily throughout the month.

Aromatherapy helps to minimize the discomforts of PMS in several ways. It can reduce bloating and puffiness, ease emotional upset, and relieve many of the physical and emotional symptoms associated with PMS. Chamomile, coriander, cypress, fennel, geranium, juniper, laurel, marjoram, orange, patchouli, and thyme oils help reduce bloating and fluid retention. Essential oils that decrease general symptoms of PMS include benzoin, chamomile, clary sage, coriander, fennel, geranium, juniper, marjoram, neroli, rose, vetiver, vitex, and ylang ylang. Emotionally soothing and comforting essential oils include benzoin, chamomile, jasmine, melissa, neroli, rose, and ylang ylang.

Vitex oil balances the levels of estrogen and progesterone secreted by the pituitary gland, thereby relieving or minimizing many of the symptoms of PMS. Studies show that women who take one drop daily find amazing and rapid relief from PMS. Most women experience remarkable reduction in symptoms of PMS simply by inhaling vitex oil, or Hormone Help Inhalant, directly from the bottle several times a day throughout the month. Bathe in PMS Bath Blend daily for one to two weeks before your period begins. Apply PMS Body Oil to your skin every day. Use PMS Personal Blend as a fragrance throughout the month or as desired. If you suffer from fluid retention or bloating, bathe in Fluid-Retention Bath at the first sign of puffiness and once or twice daily thereafter, as needed. Apply Fluid-Retention Massage Formula over your abdomen several times daily. Borage and evening primrose oil, internally or externally, can reduce symptoms of PMS. Placing a high priority on pampering yourself when you feel down from the effects of PMS will give you an emotional boost, as well as encourage you to take better care of yourself.

AROMATHERAPY BLENDS

You can prepare the aromatherapy blends below using pure essential oils. For a more detailed explanation of how to put together and use these blends, see Part Three: Ways to Use Aromatherapy. To review general guidelines for using essential oils, see page 142.

HORMONE HELP INHALANT

6 drops vitex oil
3 drops geranium oil
1 drop rose oil

Add the essential oils to a small glass bottle with an airtight cover and blend. Inhale directly from the bottle as necessary to relieve the symptoms of PMS.

PMS Bath Blend
2 drops chamomile oil
2 drops geranium oil
2 drops marjoram oil
1 drop cypress oil

Disperse the essential oils in a bathtub filled with warm water. Soak in the bath for twenty to thirty minutes. Repeat as necessary.

PMS Body Oil
4 ounces carrier oil
6 drops chamomile oil
6 drops clary sage oil
4 drops coriander oil
4 drops fennel oil
4 drops vitex oil
3 drops ylang ylang oil

Place the carrier oil in a clean container, add the essential oils, and blend. Massage the oil over your body daily, as needed.

PMS Personal Blend
⅛ ounce jojoba oil
3 drops clary sage oil
2 drops geranium oil
2 drops neroli oil
2 drops vitex oil
1 drop benzoin resin
1 drop rose oil

In a clean container, add the essential oils to the jojoba oil and combine. Wear the blend as a fragrance.

Fluid-Retention Bath
3 drops cypress oil
2 drops chamomile oil
2 drops patchouli oil

Disperse the oils in a bathtub filled with warm water. Soak in the bath for fifteen to twenty minutes. Repeat as needed.

Fluid-Retention Massage Formula
2 ounces carrier oil
6 drops chamomile oil
3 drops coriander oil
3 drops patchouli oil
2 drops cypress oil

Place the carrier oil in a clean container, add the essential oils, and blend well. Massage the oil over swollen or bloated areas as necessary.

PROSTATE PROBLEMS
The prostate gland is part of the male reproductive system. Situated beneath the bladder and encircling the urethra, it controls the release of urine. The prostate gland also secretes seminal fluid.

An estimated one-third to one-half of all men over the age of fifty have an enlarged prostate gland or other prostate problems. An enlarged prostate, or benign prostatic hypertrophy, is an overgrowth of the prostate. The precise cause is not known. Changes in hormone levels that accompany aging are possibly a factor. Alcohol and stress may accelerate the development of the problem. If the prostate becomes sufficiently enlarged, it begins to press against the urethra and can interfere with urination, making it impossible to empty the bladder completely. As a result, the frequency of urination and feelings of urgency increase, particularly during the night; however, urination may require much effort, and the flow of urine may become weaker. The retention of urine in the bladder also increases the possibility of bladder infections and incontinence. If allowed to continue for prolonged periods of time, this can damage the kidneys.

Prostatitis is the inflammation or infection of the prostate gland. Like an enlarged prostate, a prostate that is inflamed as the result of infection can block the flow of urine from the bladder, and the infection may migrate, via the urethra and the bladder, into the kidneys. Chronic inflammation of the prostate can weaken the bladder, making it more susceptible to infection.

Some cases of prostatitis are caused by bacterial infection; an infection elsewhere in the body can spread to the urinary tract. In other cases, the cause is unknown. Some researchers suspect that men who have had vasectomies are more likely to develop prostate infections. Other possible complicating factors include hormonal imbalances, lack of exercise, zinc deficiency, failure to eliminate toxins properly, poor circulation, poor diet, and the consumption of alcohol, antihistamines, caffeine, high-acid foods, and

too little dietary fiber. Symptoms can include difficulty urinating, a diminishing volume or flow of urine, a frequent need or desire to urinate, incontinence, the need to get up during the night to urinate, and pain or a burning sensation while urinating. Fatigue, fever, lethargy, and pain in the legs, lower abdomen, or lower back can also be symptoms of prostatitis.

Prostatitis is often associated with cystitis. Diminished sex drive, impotence, and premature ejaculation may accompany prostatitis. If untreated, the condition can lead to obstruction of the bladder and severe health consequences.

HELPFUL TREATMENTS

If you are suffering from the symptoms of an enlarged prostate or prostate infection, consult your health-care provider. Because symptoms of prostate enlargement are similar to those of prostate cancer, a professional evaluation may provide early detection. Dietary changes can bring about relief of many prostate problems and possibly prevent them from developing into more serious conditions. Eat a diet consisting of fresh vegetables, whole grains, nuts, seeds, legumes, brown rice, and sources of polyunsaturated fatty acids, such as unrefined olive, pumpkin seed, sesame, and sunflower oils.

Supplementing your diet with essential fatty acids, ginseng, pumpkin seeds, brewer's yeast, vitamin B_6, and/or zinc may also help. Avoid all alcohol, caffeine, fried or greasy foods, and refined carbohydrates. Also avoid contact with pesticides. Increase your intake of water to two or three quarts per day, and be sure to get regular exercise.

Aromatherapy can reduce anxiety and stress, increase urination, and fight infection in the urinary tract. Essential oils that can help with prostate problems are benzoin, bergamot, black pepper, cedarwood, chamomile, cypress, elemi, eucalyptus, fennel, frankincense, geranium, jasmine, juniper, lemon, myrrh, niaouli, orange, patchouli, pine, rose, sandalwood, spruce, tea tree, and thyme. A Prostate Sitz Bath can diminish some of the discomfort. Alternating hot and cold sitz baths improves circulation to the prostate. After a sitz bath, apply Prostate Massage Oil to your abdomen, lower back, and groin area.

AROMATHERAPY BLENDS

You can prepare the aromatherapy blends below using pure essential oils. For a more detailed explanation of how to put together and use these blends, see Part Three: Ways to Use Aromatherapy. To review general guidelines for using essential oils, see page 142.

PROSTATE SITZ BATH
1 drop cypress oil
1 drop sandalwood oil
1 drop spruce oil

Add the oils to a shallow tub filled with water. Sit hip-deep in the water for five to fifteen minutes. Alternate between using hot and cold water. Use this treatment daily or as needed.

PROSTATE MASSAGE OIL
1 ounce carrier oil
4 drops cedarwood oil
2 drops lemon oil
1 drop juniper oil
1 drop pine oil

Place the carrier oil in a clean container and add the essential oils. Gently turn the container upside down several times or roll it between your hands to blend. Massage the mixture over your abdomen, lower back, and groin area. Repeat once or twice daily, as necessary.

PSORIASIS

Psoriasis appears as bright-red, inflamed skin with raised dry, silvery scales. The new skin cells of psoriasis sufferers grow about five times faster than the old cells are shed. Crusty patches of skin result, usually appearing on the elbows, knees, lower back, buttocks, nails, scalp, or chest. In severe cases, psoriasis can cover the entire body.

Heredity plays a major role in the development of psoriasis, while emotional factors and stress often determine the frequency and severity of outbreaks. Bacterial infections, drugs, illnesses, liver dysfunction, skin injuries, sunburn, surgery, and certain viruses can also trigger or aggravate outbreaks of psoriasis.

HELPFUL TREATMENTS

Sunshine often reduces the symptoms of psoriasis, as does a vacation away from sources of stress. Some sufferers notice an improvement within three months after supplementing their diets with borage oil, flaxseed oil, soy lecithin, or wheat germ oil. Many people bathe in Dead Sea salts to keep their psoriasis under control. Adding essential oils to the Dead Sea salts increases their effectiveness. Massaging carrier oils such as borage, evening primrose, flaxseed, hazelnut, hemp, jojoba, or sesame oils can provide relief. Apple cider vinegar, especially when added to an aromatherapy bath, can calm the skin.

Aromatherapy can often control psoriasis by diminishing stress, reducing inflammation, and soothing and softening the skin. The essential oils of benzoin, bergamot, cedarwood, chamomile, clary sage, helichrysum, juniper, lavender, melissa, myrrh, neroli, orange, oregano, patchouli, pine, rose, rosemary, rosewood, St. John's wort, sandalwood, spruce, tea tree, thyme, and ylang ylang reduce itching, inflammation, and irritation as they soothe the skin.

For rough areas, use Psoriasis Skin Scrub several times weekly to smooth and soften skin and to remove dead skin. Bathe in Soothing Psoriasis Bath daily or several times a week until symptoms improve, then once a week to maintain results. Apply Psoriasis Skin Oil to the affected areas several times daily.

AROMATHERAPY BLENDS

You can prepare the aromatherapy blends below using pure essential oils. For a more detailed explanation of how to put together and use these blends, see Part Three: Ways to Use Aromatherapy. To review general guidelines for using essential oils, see page 142.

PSORIASIS SKIN SCRUB

2 tablespoons blue cornmeal, flaxseed meal,
or hazelnut meal
1 tablespoon honey
1 drop bergamot oil
1 drop helichrysum oil
1 drop spruce oil

In a small bowl, blend all the ingredients together into a paste, adding a few drops of water if necessary for the proper consistency. Massage the paste over the affected areas for several minutes. Rinse thoroughly and apply Psoriasis Skin Oil. Use this treatment several times weekly or even daily to ease symptoms of psoriasis. If large areas of the body are affected, you may double or triple the formula to yield larger amounts of scrub.

SOOTHING PSORIASIS BATH

2 cups Dead Sea salts
2 drops chamomile oil
2 drops helichrysum oil
1 drop bergamot oil
1 drop spruce oil

Disperse all the ingredients in a bathtub filled with warm water. Soak in the water for thirty minutes. Repeat several times a week until symptoms improve, then once a week to maintain results.

PSORIASIS SKIN OIL
1 ounce jojoba oil
½ ounce flaxseed oil
½ ounce hemp oil
10 drops borage oil
4 drops bergamot oil
3 drops chamomile oil
2 drops helichrysum oil
2 drops neroli oil

Mix the carrier oils together in a clean container. Add the essential oils and gently turn the container upside down several times or roll it between your hands to blend. Apply the mixture to the affected areas as needed.

Note: Bergamot oil increases sensitivity to the sun. Omit it from the formula if your skin will be exposed to sunlight.

SCALP PROBLEMS
See HAIR AND SCALP PROBLEMS.

SCIATICA
The sciatic nerve is the largest nerve in the body, running from the sacrum, through the hip, down the back of the thigh, through the knee, and into the foot. Degenerated or ruptured disks can compress the root of the sciatic nerve along the lum-bar (lower-back) spine. The discomfort of sciatica may manifest as aching, burning, stabbing, throbbing, or tingling pain that travels along the sciatic nerve. Lifting heavy objects improperly is a common cause, as is misalignment of the spine, especially in the lumbar region. Poor posture can lead to sciatica. Other sources are abnormal stress on joints or strain on muscles; constipation; injury to the back, foot, knee, or hip; pregnancy or childbirth; pressure of an internal organ on the spine; spasms in the buttock muscle; and emotional stress and tension. Bony deposits on spinal vertebrae can pinch the sciatic nerve roots.

HELPFUL TREATMENTS
Determine the source of your pain and how you can correct the conditions that contribute to sciatica. Recognize pain as a signal from your brain that you are using your body incorrectly. Relaxing your muscles and your mind and reducing stress, whether physical or emotional, can begin to relieve your discomfort.

Nutrition helps. Foods that contain thiamine, or vitamin B_1, and magnesium relax muscles. These include dark-green leafy vegetables, yellow vegetables, whole grains, and raw seeds and nuts. Avoid caffeine, chocolate, and refined sugar.

Chiropractic manipulation can sometimes correct the problem. Improving your posture, particularly while lifting and moving objects, can prevent further discomfort. (See Proper Posture on page 183.) Physical therapy can help to improve your posture and to reeducate your muscles to move more efficiently. Traction can open up collapsed spaces between the disks.

Treatments that can be used to relieve pain include acupressure; application of heating pads; clay packs; compresses; hydrotherapy, or water therapy, such as baths, sitz baths, or whirlpool baths; contrast hydrotherapy (taking hot baths followed by cold baths); and massage.

Aromatherapy can help by controlling pain, minimizing stress, reducing inflammation, and relaxing muscles. It can also stimulate circulation, thereby improving the delivery of nutrients to the area and the removal of wastes away from it. Basil, black pepper, cedarwood, chamomile, coriander, cypress, eucalyptus, geranium, helichrysum, juniper, laurel, lavender, lemon, marjoram, oregano, peppermint, pine, rosemary, St. John's wort, spruce, valerian, vetiver, and ylang ylang are essential oils that can relieve the discomfort of sciatica.

Relax your muscles and your mind by sitting in Sciatica Soak once a day. Apply a Warming Sciatica Compress and then a Cooling Sciatica Compress to stimulate circulation, relax muscles, and reduce inflammation. Apply Sciatica-Soothing Massage Oil to affected areas as needed to prevent or control pain.

AROMATHERAPY BLENDS
You can prepare the aromatherapy blends below using pure essential oils. For a more detailed explanation of how to put together and use these blends, see Part Three: Ways to Use Aromatherapy. To review general guidelines for using essential oils, see page 142.

SCIATICA SOAK
½ to 1 cup Dead Sea salts
3 drops marjoram oil
2 drops eucalyptus oil
2 drops thyme oil

Disperse the essential oils, and the Dead Sea salts, if desired, in a bathtub filled with warm water. Soak for twenty minutes once daily to relax back muscles.

WARMING SCIATICA COMPRESS
1 quart hot water
1 drop coriander oil
1 drop juniper oil

Pour the water into a 2-quart glass bowl, add the essential oils, and blend. Saturate a clean cloth in the water and apply it to the affected area as needed.

COOLING SCIATICA COMPRESS
1 quart cold water
1 drop eucalyptus oil
1 drop peppermint oil

Pour the water into a 2-quart glass bowl, add the essential oils, and blend. Saturate a clean cloth in the water and apply it to the affected area as needed.

SCIATICA-SOOTHING MASSAGE OIL

2 ounces carrier oil

3 drops geranium oil

3 drops laurel oil

3 drops spruce oil

2 drops helichrysum oil

2 drops St. John's wort oil

In a clean container, add the essential oils to the carrier oil and blend. Massage into sore muscles, especially around the spine, as needed.

SEBORRHEA

Seborrhea, or seborrheic dermatitis, affects areas of skin with abundant oil glands, such as the chest, ears, eyebrows, face, nose, and scalp. When these glands secrete abnormal amounts of oil (or sebum) and the skin cells grow at a faster than normal rate, the ducts through which the sebum normally flows to the surface of the skin can become blocked. The glands then produce even more oil. Red eruptions with thick crusting and scaliness appear on the skin. The oily, pinkish-yellow scales resemble dandruff and may itch and flake.

A diet high in fats and sugar, food allergies, heredity, hormonal imbalances, infection, nutritional deficiencies, stress, and a yeast organism called *Pityrosporon orbiculare*, which is normally present in hair follicles, may contribute to the development of seborrhea. In infants, seborrhea on the scalp is called "cradle cap."

HELPFUL TREATMENTS

Use an elimination diet or consult a nutritionist to determine if you have food allergies or nutritional deficiencies. Eating a healthy diet that focuses on fresh vegetables and fruits and whole grains often helps to control seborrhea. Avoid chocolate, dairy products, fried or greasy foods, nuts, refined foods, sugar, and white flour. Supplements of vitamin A, the B vitamins (especially vitamin B_6 and biotin), flaxseed oil, and zinc may offer relief for some people with seborrhea.

Jojoba oil has a chemical composition very similar to human sebum. It can help regulate sebum secretion and restore the correct balance of oil to the skin and scalp. Therefore, it makes an ideal treatment when used alone or as a carrier oil in aromatherapy blends that treat seborrhea. Other therapeutic oils for skin application include borage, flaxseed, and hemp.

Essential oils that help with seborrhea include cedarwood, clary sage, geranium, juniper, niaouli, oregano, patchouli, pine, rosemary, spruce, and tea tree. For seborrhea on the scalp, massage Seborrhea Scalp Soother into your scalp daily. For seborrhea on the face or other parts of the body, apply Seborrhea Skin Oil daily, as necessary.

AROMATHERAPY BLENDS

You can prepare the aromatherapy blends below using pure essential oils. For a more detailed explanation of how to put together and use these blends, see Part Three: Ways to

Use Aromatherapy. To review general guidelines for using essential oils, see page 142.

Seborrhea Scalp Soother
1 ounce jojoba oil
2 drops cedarwood oil
2 drops pine oil
2 drops rosemary oil
2 drops tea tree oil

Place the jojoba oil in a clean container and add the essential oils. Gently turn the container upside down several times or roll it between your hands to blend. Massage the mixture into your clean scalp and leave it on for fifteen to thirty minutes or overnight. Shampoo as usual. After shampooing, if your hair or scalp feels dry, you may massage a few drops into wet hair and scalp.

Seborrhea Skin Oil
1 ounce jojoba oil
3 drops clary sage oil
2 drops geranium oil
1 drop patchouli oil
1 drop spruce oil

In a clean container, add the essential oils to the jojoba oil and blend. Massage the oil over the affected areas one or more times daily, as needed.

SINUSITIS
Sinusitis is an inflammation or infection of the sinus cavities, which are open spaces in the skull that are located above the eyes, behind the bridge of the nose, beneath the cheekbones, and in the upper nose. Sinusitis often accompanies or follows a cold or an upper respiratory infection. Because the sinus cavities are connected to the nose and nasal passages, infections can easily spread into the sinuses. The sinus cavities become inflamed and filled with mucus; this blocks normal drainage and may impair breathing. Pressure builds within the sinuses, creating a dull or throbbing ache behind the forehead, around the eyes, or in the cheeks. Other symptoms of sinusitis may include headache, fever, earache, loss of the sense of smell, bad breath, and even toothache.

Allergies may trigger sinusitis. Hay fever and food allergies, especially an allergy to milk and dairy products, often cause allergic sinusitis. An injury to your nasal passages or chronic insult from exposure to cigarette smoke, drugs, environmental pollutants, fragrances, and other irritants can cause or contribute to sinusitis, as can the presence of tiny growths in the nasal passages called "polyps." Exposure to dampness and the consumption of certain foods, such as wheat, dairy products, sugar, and refined carbohydrates, may make a person more susceptible to sinusitis.

Helpful Treatments
If you are prone to sinusitis, investigate the cause or causes of your condition. Experiment with an elimination diet to discover if food allergies are a factor. Dairy and wheat products are two of the most common

troublemakers; start by eliminating them from your diet. Avoid contact with noxious chemicals, environmental pollutants, and synthetic fragrances.

During an acute attack of sinusitis, eliminate dairy products, sugar, and wheat from your diet. Drink adequate amounts of water. If your sinusitis does not improve within several days, you should consult your health-care practitioner to rule out the possibility of recurring infection.

Aromatherapy can help to clear sinusitis by combating infection, opening up nasal passages, reducing congestion, and relieving pain and discomfort. Basil, benzoin, cedarwood, eucalyptus, ginger, helichrysum, lavender, marjoram, niaouli, oregano, peppermint, pine, rosemary, sandalwood, tea tree, and thyme oils soothe sinus inflammation and ease discomfort. For instant relief, breathe Sinus Inhalant directly from the bottle whenever necessary. Prepare a Sinus Steam Inhalation several times daily. A Sinus Foot Bath will also help to open sinuses and restore normal breathing.

AROMATHERAPY BLENDS

You can prepare the aromatherapy blends below using pure essential oils. For a more detailed explanation of how to put together and use these blends, see Part Three: Ways to Use Aromatherapy. To review general guidelines for using essential oils, see page 142.

SINUS INHALANT

10 drops eucalyptus oil

5 drops cedarwood oil

5 drops oregano oil

3 drops niaouli oil

Drop the oils into a small glass bottle with an airtight cover. Blend by gently turning the container upside down several times or rolling it between your hands. Breathe directly from the bottle as needed.

SINUS STEAM INHALATION

1 quart steaming water

1 drop eucalyptus oil

1 drop ginger oil

1 drop tea tree oil

1 drop thyme oil

Pour the water into a 2-quart glass bowl and disperse the essential oils in the water. Hold your head over the bowl and drape a towel over both your head and the bowl to capture the steam. Breathe in the vapors for five to ten minutes. Repeat as necessary.

SINUS FOOT BATH

1 drop ginger oil

1 drop pine oil

1 drop rosemary oil

Add the oils to a shallow tub or foot bath filled with warm water. Soak your feet in the water for fifteen to thirty minutes. Repeat as needed.

SKIN PROBLEMS
AND SKIN CARE

Healthy skin is clear and radiant, with a smooth and soft texture. The muscles that support the skin are firm, supple, and resilient; the skin surface looks moist and is neither too oily nor too dry. Its coloring is even, and the pores are only slightly visible.

If your skin doesn't look or feel like this, you may have a skin problem. Maintaining healthy and attractive skin is a challenge with the stresses of modern life, pollution, and poor nutrition. Fortunately, aromatherapy and a good skin-care routine can improve the condition of your skin and make the most of your natural assets.

Your skin serves as more than an attractive covering for your body. Skin is the largest organ of the body. As a vital part of your immune system, your skin offers the first line of defense from outside invaders. It protects you from environmental assaults, such as cold, heat, pollution, sun, and wind, and prevents most foreign chemicals and water from entering your body. It regulates your body temperature and insulates your internal organs. Through perspiration, it releases heat when you become too warm. Your skin is also an organ of elimination. Excess wastes that your kidneys, lungs, and intestines cannot process may be expelled through the skin.

Skin health relies on good blood and lymph circulation and an adequate supply of water. These factors become increasingly important with age. Poor circulation prevents the normal cellular exchange of nutrients and wastes. If circulation to the skin is sluggish, the cells fail to receive sufficient nourishment, and wastes build up. The production of new skin cells slows down, and premature aging may begin. Blemishes or acne can occur. Broken capillaries or varicose veins may appear. Boosting circulation to your skin cells can restore a healthy, radiant glow to your complexion while warding off signs of premature aging.

Water is critical for healthy skin. Your body consists of about 70 percent water, and your skin cells need a constant supply of fresh water to function properly and to continue looking moist and youthful. Dehydrated skin cells show up as lines, wrinkles, and dry, dull skin.

Skin is commonly classified as normal, dry, or oily. To determine your skin type, perform the following test in the morning before cleansing your face: Blot your forehead, your nose, your chin, and your cheeks, each with a separate single layer of facial tissue. Then examine the tissues. Oily spots on the tissue reveal an oily area. No oil on a tissue indicates a dry area. Normal skin may leave a minimal amount of oil on the tissues.

Although these are the most common skin types, normal, dry, and oily skins are not the only classifications of skin type. Mature skin is skin that has begun to show signs of aging, such as lines and wrinkles. Combination skin has both dry and oily areas. Usually, the area known as the

T-zone—the forehead, nose, and chin—is oily, while the cheeks and throat are dry. Combination skin may require a two-part approach to skin care in which you treat each area with products designed for that skin type.

Sensitive skin can be either dry or oily. It is usually very fragile and delicate and requires special treatment. Many cosmetics are too harsh for sensitive skin and will often irritate it, causing blemishes, broken capillaries, chapping or cracking, irritation, or rashes. If you have sensitive skin, you should be extremely careful about skin care and the products you use.

As you get older, your skin changes. As skin matures, it becomes thinner and more fragile, more susceptible to broken capillaries, bruising, and other injuries. Discolorations or variations in pigment may appear. However, much of what people accept as normal or inevitable signs of aging is actually premature aging. Lines and wrinkles and dry or sagging skin are the first signs of premature aging. All skin will develop lines and wrinkles eventually, but if you follow a natural skin-care routine and live a healthy lifestyle, you skin should look relatively line-free until you are in your late thirties or early forties, or even longer.

Lines and wrinkles may also result from years of repeating the same facial expressions, such as smiling, frowning, pouting, pursing your lips, raising your eyebrows, and squinting. These repeated expressions eventually etch their marks into your skin.

Gravity also has an effect. Many factors can accelerate the development of lines and wrinkles: the consumption of alcohol; exposure to cigarette smoke, both firsthand and secondhand, and other environmental pollutants; chronic constipation; dehydration; illness; certain drugs; harsh cosmetics; hormone imbalances; bad dental work; lack of good skin care; poor diet; nutritional deficiencies; improper posture; a sedentary lifestyle; sluggish blood or lymph circulation; stress; and overexposure to the sun. Heredity and coloring also are factors. Fair skin and dry complexions usually age sooner than dark skin and oily complexions.

A good skin-care regimen can help any type of skin at any age. (See Taking Care of Your Skin on page 298.) Whether you are treating problem skin or want to maintain healthy, normal skin, you should drink eight to twelve glasses of pure, clean water every day, and eat plenty of fresh fruits and vegetables to get the nutrients your skin needs. Avoid unprotected exposure to the sun. Sesame oil is a natural sunscreen, and coconut and olive oils also provide some protection. Wear protective clothing, hats, and sunglasses. Choose skin-care products that are suited to your skin type.

Use the formulas in this section to make your own simple aromatherapy skin-care products easily and inexpensively. They will not be as elaborate or refined as commercial products, but they will be pure and will contain no preservatives, artificial colorings, fragrances, or any other unnecessary ingredients. You will know the quality and the levels of the essential oils they contain because you made them yourself. Best of all, they will work. It may seem like a little more trouble at first; some of the products have to be made just before each application. However, when you notice the improvement in the condition of your skin, you will probably decide that the rewards are well worth any extra effort.

Normal Skin

Normal skin is the ideal skin type, neither too dry nor too oily. It is moist and clear, with a smooth texture and even color. Normal skin appears soft and is firm to the touch. Pores may be perceptible but are not large.

Essential oils that are helpful for normal skin include cedarwood, clary sage, elemi, frankincense, geranium, jasmine, lavender, neroli, palmarosa, patchouli, rose, rosemary, rosewood, sandalwood, and vetiver. To maintain healthy normal skin, use the aromatherapy blends below in your skin-care regimen. Or see SKIN CARE AND CREATING SKIN-CARE PRODUCTS in Part Three. For a quick review of general guidelines for using essential oils, see page 142.

HONEY AND CLAY CLEANSER FOR NORMAL SKIN

1 teaspoon French green clay powder
1 teaspoon honey
1 drop lavender oil
1 drop rosemary oil

Blend all the ingredients into a paste in your palm. Massage into your skin until it feels clean. Rinse with warm water.

NORMAL SKIN TONER

8 ounces distilled water
1 drop lavender oil
1 drop palmarosa oil
1 drop rosewood oil

Pour the distilled water into a clean bottle and add the essential oils. Turn the bottle upside down several times to blend. Apply the toner to your skin with a cotton ball after cleansing. Blend well before each use.

FACIAL OIL FOR NORMAL OR SENSITIVE SKIN

1 ounce jojoba oil
2 drops neroli oil
2 drops rose oil
1 drop sandalwood oil

Place the jojoba oil in a clean container and add the essential oils. Gently turn the container upside down several times or roll it between your hands to blend. Apply several drops to your face twice daily, after cleansing and toning.

FACIAL MASK FOR NORMAL OR OILY SKIN

1 teaspoon French green clay powder
1 teaspoon honey (approximately)
1 drop palmarosa oil
1 drop rosewood oil

In the palm of your hand, combine the essential oils with the green clay and honey and blend well. Apply the mixture to clean facial skin and relax for fifteen minutes. Rinse well. Use this mask once a week.

Dry, Mature, and Prematurely Aging Skin

Dry skin lacks oil and moisture and may appear scaly or flaky. It is usually thin, even transparent, with few or no visible pores. Dry skin usually feels tight after washing. It may lack suppleness and resiliency. Dry skin is relatively problem-free during youth, but it may show signs of aging sooner than normal or oily skin. Essential oils that benefit dry skin include benzoin, bergamot, cedarwood, clary sage, elemi, fennel, frankincense, geranium, jasmine, lavender, myrrh, neroli, palmarosa, patchouli, rose, rosemary, rosewood, sandalwood, and vetiver. If your skin is dry, use the aromatherapy blends in this section as part of your regular skin-care regimen. Or see SKIN CARE AND CREATING SKIN-CARE PRODUCTS in Part Three for other ways to use essential oils in your skin-care routine.

Mature or prematurely aging skin is often thin and transparent, and is usually dry or dehydrated. The coloring may be uneven. The skin may also have lost some of its muscle tone and may sag. Lines, wrinkles, dryness, and loss of elasticity characterize mature skin or prematurely aging skin.

If you feel that your skin is aging prematurely, examine your lifestyle for possible contributing factors. The most common ones are sun exposure, poor diet, insufficient water intake, improper skin care, repeated facial expressions, and nutritional deficiencies. Many lines and wrinkles are preventable. You can even minimize existing ones by changing your habits and your lifestyle. Watch yourself in the mirror. Do your lines correspond to certain facial expressions you make regularly? You can gain control over those expressions and the lines they cause by becoming aware of them. If you can stop making them, you can often reduce the depth of the lines and certainly prevent them from becoming deeper. You may also wish to consult a nutritionist about improving your diet and discovering any nutritional deficiencies you may have.

Mature or prematurely aging skin can benefit from clary sage, elemi, fennel, frankincense, geranium, helichrysum, jasmine, lemon, myrrh, neroli, palmarosa, peppermint, rose, rosemary, rosewood, sandalwood, vetiver, and ylang ylang oils. Fennel, frankincense, myrrh, palmarosa, patchouli, rose, rosemary, rosewood, sandalwood, and ylang ylang are noted for warding off wrinkles and minimizing premature aging. Use the aromatherapy blends in this section to make skin-care products that are appropriate for your skin type, and apply Rejuvenating Facial Oil to your skin twice a day to encourage the formation of new skin cells. Or see SKIN CARE AND CREATING SKIN-CARE PRODUCTS in Part Three for other ways to incorporate the benefits of essential oils into your skin-care routine and create custom cosmetics. For a quick review of general guidelines for using essential oils, see page 142.

JOJOBA OIL CLEANSER FOR DRY SKIN
1 ounce jojoba oil
2 drops myrrh oil
1 drop benzoin resin
1 drop fennel oil
1 drop frankincense oil
1 drop patchouli oil

Place the jojoba oil in a clean container and add the essential oils. Gently turn the container upside down several times or roll it between your hands to blend. Massage the cleanser into your skin. Gently wipe it off with a warm, wet washcloth.

DRY SKIN TONER
8 ounces distilled water
1 drop frankincense oil
1 drop rosewood oil
1 drop vetiver oil

Pour the water into a clean bottle, add the essential oils, and turn the bottle upside down several times to combine. Apply the toner to your skin with a cotton ball after cleansing. Blend well before each use.

FACIAL OIL FOR DRY OR MATURE SKIN
1 ounce jojoba oil
3 drops palmarosa oil
2 drops frankincense oil
2 drops myrrh oil
1 drop rose oil

In a clean container, add the essential oils to the jojoba oil and combine. Apply several drops of oil to your face, twice daily, after cleansing and toning, and at other times as needed.

FACIAL MASK FOR DRY OR MATURE SKIN
2 teaspoons honey
1 drop frankincense oil
1 drop sandalwood oil

In the palm of your hand, add the sandalwood and frankincense oil to the honey and blend well. Apply the mask to clean skin. Relax for fifteen minutes, then rinse thoroughly. Use this mask once a week.

REJUVENATING FACIAL OIL
1½ ounces jojoba oil
10 drops borage oil
3 drops neroli oil
3 drops rosewood oil
3 drops ylang ylang oil
2 drops clary sage oil
2 drops sandalwood oil
1 drop myrrh oil

Mix the carrier oils together. Add the essential oils and blend. Massage several drops of oil into your skin every morning and evening after cleansing and toning.

Oily Skin

Oily skin usually has a shiny appearance because its overactive oil glands produce excess oil. The pores are often enlarged and clog easily, so the skin must be kept extremely clean to avoid blemishes. Although oily skin is acne-prone during the teen and early adult years, its natural oils help it to maintain youthfulness longer than dry skin.

Essential oils that can improve the condition of oily skin include bergamot, cedarwood, clary sage, cypress, elemi, eucalyptus, frankincense, geranium, jasmine, juniper, lemon, neroli, niaouli, orange, palmarosa, patchouli, peppermint, rosemary, rosewood, sandalwood, tea tree, thyme, vetiver, and ylang ylang. To help regulate oily skin and keep it clear, use the aromatherapy blends in this section in your skin-care regimen (*see also* page 293 for Facial Mask for Normal or Oily Skin). Or see SKIN CARE AND CREATING SKIN-CARE PRODUCTS in Part Three.

CLAY CLEANSER FOR OILY SKIN

1 teaspoon French green clay powder
1 teaspoon water
1 drop ylang ylang oil

Hold the green clay powder in the palm of your hand. Add the water and essential oil. Blend well to make a paste. Massage the cleanser into your skin until it feels clean. Rinse with warm water.

OILY SKIN TONER

8 ounces distilled water
1 drop clary sage oil
1 drop geranium oil

Pour the water into a clean bottle, add the essential oils, and turn the bottle upside down several times to blend. Apply the toner to your skin with a cotton ball after cleansing. Blend well before each use.

FACIAL OIL FOR OILY SKIN

1 ounce jojoba oil
3 drops cypress oil
2 drops lemon oil
1 drop clary sage oil
1 drop geranium oil
1 drop niaouli oil

Place the jojoba oil in a clean container and add the essential oils. Gently turn the container upside down several times or roll it between your hands to blend. Apply one or two drops of oil to your face twice daily after cleansing and toning.

OILY SKIN TONIC

4 ounces pure grain alcohol or vodka
4 drops elemi oil
2 drops palmarosa oil
1 drop patchouli oil

Place the alcohol in a clean bottle. Add the essential oils. Turn the bottle upside down several times or roll it between your hands to blend. Apply to face once daily or more often to control oiliness. Blend well before each use. Do not inhale directly from the bottle. Never use isopropyl alcohol for aromatherapy purposes.

Chapped or Cracked Skin

Skin that is chapped or cracked is extremely dry and dehydrated. It may lack both oil and moisture. Skin conditions such as dermatitis; exposure to cold, sun, wind, or harsh chemicals or cosmetics; and dietary factors such as an insufficient intake of oil, essential fatty acids, water, or certain nutrients (especially vitamin A) all can cause chapped or cracked skin.

If your skin has chapped or cracked areas, make sure you are getting enough water. Every day eat about one tablespoon of unrefined vegetable oil. Choose flaxseed, hazelnut, hemp, sesame, or sunflower oil. Add the oil to your salads or vegetable dishes. Consult a nutritionist if you suspect a nutritional deficiency. Protect yourself from the weather, the sun, harsh chemicals, and detergents.

Essential oils that can soothe and help heal chapped and cracked skin are benzoin, bergamot, frankincense, myrrh, patchouli, and vetiver. Apply Chapped Skin Oil to the affected areas at least twice daily.

CHAPPED SKIN OIL

1 ounce jojoba oil
3 drops benzoin resin
2 drops frankincense oil
2 drops myrrh oil
1 drop vetiver oil

In a clean container, add the essential oils to the jojoba oil and blend. Apply the oil to chapped areas as necessary.

All Skin Types

Some skin-care products can be beneficial regardless of whether your skin is normal, dry, or oily. The following aromatherapy blends are recommended for all skin types.

ALL-PURPOSE SKIN SCRUB

1 teaspoon almond meal or blue cornmeal
1 teaspoon honey (approximately)
1 drop lavender oil
1 drop ylang ylang oil

Blend all the ingredients together into a paste in your palm. After cleansing and before toning, massage the scrub into your skin for one minute, then rinse thoroughly. Use one to three times a week, depending on your skin type. (See Taking Care of Your Skin on page 298.)

FLORAL FACIAL MIST

8 ounces distilled water
3 drops lavender oil
2 drops rosewood oil
1 drop chamomile oil
1 drop clary sage oil
1 drop geranium oil

Taking Care of Your Skin

Your face is usually the first part of you that the rest of the world sees. It makes a lasting impression on other people and often determines their perception of you. You want your face to look its very best, and attractive skin makes a major contribution toward looking good.

Taking good care of your skin is your best assurance for maintaining healthy, youthful skin. Skin care is simple when you know what to do and when you establish a regular routine. The immediate and long-range benefits of a consistent daily skin-care program—a healthy, radiant complexion that looks good now and for years to come—are well worth the commitment.

Simple skin care involves seven basic steps. You need to do some procedures, such as cleansing, toning, and moisturizing, twice a day.

Others—scrubbing, steaming, and applying masks—you can do about once a week. Misting can be done as often as you like. A skin-care routine may seem like extra work initially, especially if you haven't been caring for your skin. But once you become adjusted to your new program, it will feel as normal as brushing your teeth or taking a shower.

The seven basic steps of a good skin-care regimen are:

1. Cleansing. Cleansing removes dirt and impurities from the surface of the skin. Cleansing is increasingly important for maintaining good skin today, as the level of environmental pollutants rises. Cleanse your skin once in the morning to remove wastes your skin generates during sleep, and again at night to remove bacteria, oils, makeup, dirt, and any other residues that collect on your face during the day. Use a cleanser formulated for your skin type. Dry skin cleansers moisturize as they clean skin; oily skin cleansers remove excess oil as they cleanse.

2. Scrubbing. A facial scrub gently exfoliates (sloughs off) dead skin cells that can contribute to blackheads, blemishes, dryness, and wrinkles. It also boosts circulation to your face and gives your complexion a healthy glow. Scrubs can be made from almond, corn, flaxseed, hazelnut, or jojoba meals, or from any kind of grain that gently removes dead skin cells.

Avoid abrasive scrubs that can scratch or irritate your skin. One to three times a week, gently massage the scrub into your skin after cleansing. Scrubs are appropriate for all skin types except sensitive skin or skin with broken capillaries. If you have either of those conditions, you should avoid using scrubs.

3. Toning. A toner removes residues left on your skin by your cleanser, mask, scrub, or tap water. A toner leaves your face moist, allowing for better absorption of your moisturizer or facial oil. After cleansing, scrubbing, or removing a mask, moisten a cotton ball with toner and glide it over your face and neck. Repeat this procedure until no traces of dirt remain. Men can splash their faces with toner or after-shave after cleansing or shaving. Gentle toners are made with floral or herbal waters. Avoid toners or astringents that contain alcohol, which can dry and ir-ritate your skin.

4. Moisturizing. Moisturizers or fa-cial oils create a protective barrier be-tween your skin and the atmosphere, bacteria, makeup, and smog. They plump up your surface skin cells, pre-vent moisture loss, and give your skin a smooth, soft appearance. Every skin, even oily skin, needs a moisturizer or facial oil to protect it. Select one for-mulated for your skin type. Apply a small amount of moisturizer or several drops of facial oil to your face after cleansing and toning. If your skin is dry, you may wish to apply moisturizer or facial oil at other times, too, espe-cially after misting (see below).

5. Misting. A facial mist replenishes the moisture that your skin constantly loses to the atmosphere, especially with air conditioning and heating and in dry climates. Facial mists usually contain herbal or floral waters. Avoid products that contain synthetic ingredients and alcohol. Spray your face as often as you like.

6. Steaming. Facial steaming once a week will deep-cleanse your pores, moisturize your skin, and improve cir-culation to your face. To steam your face, add 1 to 3 drops of an essential oil or blend of essential oils appropriate for your skin type to a glass bowl contain-ing 1 quart of steaming water. Capture the steam by draping a towel over your head to create a "tent" and hold your face over the bowl for five to ten minutes. Follow with a scrub or facial mask.

7. Masks. A facial mask can nourish your skin, replenish moisture, normal-ize oil secretions, and invigorate your complexion. Once a week, apply a mask for your skin type and relax for ten to fifteen minutes. Both the mask and the relaxation will improve the condition of your skin. Rinse off with warm water. Apply toner and facial oil.

Pour the distilled water into a spray bottle, add the essential oils, and turn the bottle upside down several times to blend. Spray your skin with the mist frequently during the day. Blend well before each use.

All-Purpose Aftershave

8 ounces distilled water
2 drops cedarwood oil
2 drops cypress oil
1 drop elemi oil
1 drop sandalwood oil

Add the essential oils to the water and blend. Splash the mixture on your skin after shaving. Blend well before each use.

Cautions

Any undiluted essential oil can potentially irritate the skin. Some oils, even diluted, can irritate sensitive skin. These include basil, bitter fennel, black pepper, cajeput, camphor, cardamom, cedarwood, cinnamon, citronella, clove, elemi, eucalyptus, fir, ginger, laurel, lemon, lemongrass, lemon verbena, melissa, parsley, pennyroyal, peppermint, pimento, pine, niaouli, oregano, rosemary, sassafras, savory, tea tree, thuja, thyme, and wintergreen. Perform a test on a patch of skin before using any essential oil. If your skin is sensitive, you may wish to use the above essential oils at lower levels than generally recommended, or simply avoid using them.

SORE THROAT

A sore throat usually starts as a scratchy, aching, or swollen feeling inside the throat. The throat may become red and inflamed; the lymph nodes in the neck may feel tender. Swallowing or talking may be difficult or painful. Fatigue, fever, headache, and/or nausea may accompany a sore throat, especially when it signals the beginning of a cold or the flu.

Viral or bacterial infections produce most sore throats. Other possible causes include allergies, asthma, and local irritation from exposure to cigarette smoke, environmental pollutants, or other irritants. Nutritional deficiencies, fatigue, and a weakened immune system may make a person more susceptible to illnesses that can cause a sore throat.

Helpful Treatments

Most sore throats respond well to bed rest, nutritional supplements, and an increased consumption of liquids, especially water and warm herbal teas. Taking supplements of vitamin A, vitamin C, bioflavonoids, and zinc can speed your recovery. The herbs echinacea, garlic, and goldenseal also help. Avoid eating foods containing sugar when you have a sore throat, because sugar encourages the growth of bacteria.

Benzoin, bergamot, clary sage, eucalyptus, geranium, ginger, laurel, lavender, lemon, marjoram, myrrh, niaouli, oregano, pine, rose, sandalwood, tea tree, and thyme are essential oils that can soothe your sore throat and accelerate healing. One drop of laurel or lavender oil, put in the back of your throat when it first feels sore, can often alleviate or minimize pain and scratchiness. Repeat frequently until all symptoms subside. In addition, several times a day, massage Sore Throat Massage Oil or Geranium Throat Rub over your throat and neck area to soothe the pain and to prevent the spread of infection. Gargle frequently with Sore Throat Gargle. Apply a warm Throat-Soothing Compress several times during the day.

AROMATHERAPY BLENDS

You can prepare the aromatherapy blends below using pure essential oils. For a more detailed explanation of how to put together and use these blends, see Part Three: Ways to Use Aromatherapy. To review general guidelines for using essential oils, see page 142.

SORE THROAT MASSAGE OIL

1 ounce jojoba oil
3 drops geranium oil
2 drops eucalyptus oil
2 drops lavender oil
1 drop thyme oil

Place the jojoba oil in a clean container and add the essential oils. Turn the container upside down several times or roll it between your hands to blend. Gently massage the oil over your neck and throat to soothe a sore throat or swollen glands.

GERANIUM THROAT RUB

½ ounce jojoba oil
5 drops geranium oil

Blend the geranium oil into the jojoba oil. Massage the mixture over the throat area. Repeat as necessary.

SORE THROAT GARGLE

Add 1 drop of ginger, lavender, lemon, or tea tree oil to a glass of warm water and mix thoroughly. Gargle. Repeat every two hours or as needed.

THROAT-SOOTHING COMPRESS

1 quart hot water
2 drops niaouli oil
1 drop geranium oil
1 drop pine oil

Pour the water into a 2-quart glass bowl and disperse the essential oils in the water. Saturate a clean cloth in the water. Apply the compress to your throat and neck as needed.

STRESS

Stress is the general term for a disturbance of your physical or emotional balance. Virtually any type of change can cause stress. Changes in climate, deadlines, exposure to environmental pollutants or toxins, family conflicts, financial or job pressures, and physical or emotional trauma all cause stress. Stress is linked with most diseases as either a causative or contributing factor. Some common conditions that are closely associated with stress are asthma, autoimmune diseases, cancer, cardiovascular disease, depression, diabetes, digestive disorders, headaches, high blood pressure, menstrual difficulties, premenstrual syndrome, ulcers, and weakened immunity.

When you encounter stress, your body releases hormones to stimulate physiological changes—the "fight-or-flight" response—that prepare you to deal with a threat. Digestion ceases, your heart rate increases, and your blood pressure rises. Breathing becomes more rapid; palms may sweat. Your body releases fats and sugars into the bloodstream, making cholesterol and blood sugar levels rise. The muscles become more rigid; blood prepares to clot.

In the modern world, only rarely do people need to fight or flee in response to the things triggering stress reactions, yet these bodily reactions still occur. They can continue for hours after the fight-or-flight phase ends. This extreme physical reaction takes a toll on your body, nerves, and emotions. When stress is constant or prolonged, your body has little chance to recover. Stress overloads your organs and immune system, weakening your body's immune response. Constant or repeated stress eventually may exhaust one or more organs.

The inability to relax, the attempt to maintain too many commitments, overwork, and poor nutrition, especially a high-sugar diet that contains too many refined foods and sweets, will aggravate stress. The consumption of alcohol, tobacco, caffeine, and other drugs also can make the situation worse. Whether stress results from a major disaster or a minor annoyance, its impact is the same: Stress lowers immunity, elevates blood pressure, and raises cholesterol levels; it depletes your body's supply of vitamins and minerals, including vitamin A, the B vitamins, vitamin C, vitamin D, vitamin E, calcium, iron, magnesium, molybdenum, potassium, sulfur, and zinc. Stress also exhausts your physical, mental, and emotional energies. Stress-induced problems such as backache, diarrhea, diverticulosis, fatigue, hair loss, headaches, heartburn, high blood pressure, impotence, indigestion, insomnia, muscular aches, and ulcers can interfere with your life. Emotional signs of stress may include anger, anxiety, depression, emotional exhaustion, fear, hostility, impatience, irritability, lethargy, and mental fatigue.

HELPFUL TREATMENTS

Since stress is a fact of life, the best antistress strategies involve learning to avoid, manage, minimize, or eliminate stress-provoking situations. Stress management includes anything that relaxes you and takes your mind off the sources of your stress. Biofeedback, deep-breathing techniques, exercise, meditation, relaxation and visualization techniques, writing in a journal, and yoga can help control or counteract stress. When you are experiencing stress, stop for a moment and consider what is happening and why. Relax. Take time out for yourself. Avoid taking on too many responsibilities or new commitments. Diet is important, too. Eat plenty of fresh vegetables, complex carbohydrates, and whole grains, as well as fruits, seeds, nuts, and protein. Avoid alcohol, caffeine, cigarettes, drugs, refined or processed foods, and sugar. If you suspect that nutritional deficiencies are contributing to your stress, seek advice from a nutritionist.

Stress reduction is one of aromatherapy's specialties. Aromatherapy treatments can calm and relax you, offering you an opportunity to slow down and determine what is causing your stress so that you can decide on a plan of action. Essential oils such as bergamot, chamomile, jasmine, lavender, marjoram, rose, valerian, and ylang ylang will relax you. Basil, benzoin, cedarwood, geranium, juniper, orange, peppermint, pine, rosemary, and spruce oils will recharge, revitalize, and stimulate you. Geranium, pine, rosemary, and spruce oils strengthen the adrenal glands, which will feel the effects of stress. Spruce counteracts many of the adverse effects of the fight-or-flight reaction to stress. Other essential oils with general stress-reducing properties include clary sage, coriander, cypress, elemi, fennel, frankincense, helichrysum, marjoram, neroli, palmarosa, patchouli, rosewood, sandalwood, tea tree, and vetiver.

Aromatherapy can boost immunity, which becomes compromised by stress. In addition, it provides relief for some of the stress-related conditions mentioned above. Taking time out for yourself is a key factor in combating stress, and aromatherapy offers you wonderful ways to do just that. Aromatherapy baths, diffuser blends, fragrances, inhalants, massage oils, and treatments for skin, hair, and body all let you pamper yourself and improve the condition of your body as you reduce stress. Breathe in Stress-Away Inhalant frequently to minimize or avert stress throughout the day. Take a Stress-Reducing Bath whenever you feel stressed. Apply Stress-Soothing Massage Oil to your skin daily. Arrange to receive massages with it, if possible. Use Stress-Buster Diffuser Blend in your home or office to keep stress under control.

AROMATHERAPY BLENDS

You can prepare the aromatherapy blends below using pure essential oils. For a more detailed explanation of how to put together and use these blends, see Part Three: Ways to Use Aromatherapy. To review general guidelines for using essential oils, see page 142.

STRESS-AWAY INHALANT

6 drops spruce oil
5 drops clary sage oil
3 drops rosewood oil

Add the oils to a small glass bottle with an airtight cover and blend. Inhale directly from the bottle as necessary to prevent or minimize stress.

STRESS-REDUCING BATH

2 drops lavender oil
1 drop cypress oil
1 drop geranium oil
1 drop pine oil
1 drop vetiver oil

Disperse the essential oils in a bathtub filled with warm water. Enjoy a leisurely soak for twenty to thirty minutes.

STRESS-SOOTHING MASSAGE OIL

2 ounces carrier oil
4 drops chamomile oil
4 drops spruce oil
3 drops marjoram oil
2 drops elemi oil
2 drops ylang ylang oil

Place the carrier oil in a clean container, add the essential oils, and gently turn the container upside down several times or roll it between your hands to blend. Massage the oil into your skin daily.

STRESS-BUSTER DIFFUSER BLEND

10 drops clary sage oil
10 drops geranium oil
10 drops spruce oil
8 drops bergamot oil
8 drops elemi oil
6 drops rosewood oil
3 drops coriander oil

Combine all the oils in a small glass bottle with an airtight cover. Add some of the mixture to your diffuser or lamp bowl as necessary.

STRETCH MARKS

Stretch marks are thin, narrow, wavy reddish-pink, purple, or silvery sunken streaks or lines that form when the skin stretches to accommodate an increase in body size. As the skin stretches, the collagen and elastic fibers in the deep layers of the skin weaken and lose their normal crisscross structure, becoming thinner and straighter. Initially, stretch marks appear as parallel grooves that are slightly raised. They give the surface skin a loosely wrinkled appearance. Over time, they may flatten out and fade to a white or silvery-white color.

Stretch marks—medically known as *striae atrophicae, striae gravidarum, striae distensae, lineae atrophicae,* or *linear atrophy*—are usually associated with pregnancy. However, they may also result from obesity; bodybuilding or weight training; rapid growth, especially during puberty and adolescence; an endocrine disorder known as Cushing's syndrome; the topical application of steroid creams; or prolonged treatment with corticosteroid drugs.

Most commonly, stretch marks occur during pregnancy on the abdomen, breasts, buttocks, hips, lower back, thighs, and waist, although they may appear on any area of skin that experiences rapid growth or expansion.

HELPFUL TREATMENTS

Preventing stretch marks is easier than eliminating them. If you expect a weight gain or an increase in size, such as with pregnancy or a bodybuilding program, or weight loss during dieting, plan ahead by keeping your skin well lubricated. Essential oils that help prevent stretch marks are cypress, lavender, neroli, and vetiver. Patchouli helps skin to retain or regain its firmness during fluctuations in weight. In addition, cocoa butter, flaxseed oil, hazelnut oil, rose hip seed oil, vitamin E oil, and wheat germ oil are useful in preventing stretch marks. If stretch marks do develop, benzoin, bergamot, frankincense, helichrysum, lemon, neroli, palmarosa, patchouli, and rosewood oils may minimize their appearance over time. Cocoa butter helps minimize stretch marks as do flaxseed and wheat germ oils.

Massage Stretch Mark Prevention Oil into your skin daily to prevent or to minimize the appearance of stretch marks. If you already have stretch marks, long-term daily treatment with Stretch Mark Reducing Oil may help them fade. Only surgery can remove them.

AROMATHERAPY BLENDS

You can prepare the aromatherapy blend below using pure essential oils. For a more detailed explanation of how to put together and use these blends, see Part Three: Ways to Use Aromatherapy. To review general guidelines for using essential oils, see page 142.

STRETCH MARK PREVENTION OIL

1 ounce cocoa butter, melted
½ ounce flaxseed oil
¼ ounce rose hip seed oil
¼ ounce wheat germ oil
8 drops lavender oil
4 drops neroli oil
2 drops vetiver oil

Blend the melted cocoa butter with the carrier oils. Transfer the mixture to a clean jar. As it begins to cool and solidify, add the essential oils. Allow the mixture to cool to a comfortable temperature before using it. Massage the oil into your skin once or twice daily.

STRETCH MARK REDUCING OIL

1 ounce cocoa butter, melted
½ ounce flaxseed oil
½ ounce hemp oil
6 drops patchouli oil
4 drops rosewood oil
2 drops palmarosa oil
2 drops vetiver oil

Blend the melted cocoa butter with the carrier oils. Transfer the mixture to a clean jar. As it begins to cool and solidify, add the essential oils. Allow the mixture to cool to a comfortable temperature before using it. Massage the oil into your skin once or twice daily.

SUNBURN

Sunburn is the skin's response to overexposure to the ultraviolet (UV) rays of the sun. The skin becomes pink or red and may feel tight and dry. It may become sore and swell with inflammation. In severe cases, the skin may blister and peel. Although sunburned skin often turns into a suntan, any time the skin burns or tans, it is suffering damage. Sunburns, even one severe occurrence, can predispose a person to developing skin cancer later in life.

Sunburn and sun exposure have a weakening and suppressing action on the immune system. The skin is the immune system's first barrier against outside threats; sunburned skin compromises your body's ability to defend itself. Some scientists say that one hour of exposure can weaken immunity for up to two weeks and that the damage is cumulative.

Helpful Treatments

When it comes to sunburn, prevention and precaution are more important than treatment. Minimize exposure to the sun, especially during the midday hours between 10:00 A.M. and 3:00 P.M., when the sun's rays are strongest.

Sunscreens can provide a false sense of security about protection from the sun, and they cannot guard against the immune-weakening effect the sun has on your body. Additionally, some dermatologists believe that harsh chemicals contained in sunscreens with high sun protection factor

(SPF) ratings actually encourage the formation of cancer cells on skin. These doctors discourage the use of sunscreens for people with moderate- to dark-colored skin. Instead, they recommend protective clothing and the gradual increase in exposure of the skin to the sun.

Skin specialists suggest that certain vegetable oils may provide some protection against the sun. Sesame oil can reduce the burning ability of the sun by about 30 percent, while coconut and olive oils block about 20 percent of the burning rays. Aloe vera can also inhibit about 20 percent of the sun's rays. Though this is lower than the protection achieved with commercial sunscreens, the risks and potential side effects are far fewer. Research indicates that helichrysum oil effectively screens out some of the sun's damaging rays. Adding it to a base of sesame, olive, and coconut oils can boost its protective capabilities. Niaouli oil also may prevent burning.

Apply Natural Sunscreen Oil before exposure to the sun. Reapply frequently if you are swimming or perspiring. By using common sense, wearing protective clothing, and limiting the length of exposure, you can protect your skin and immune system with safer alternatives to commercial sunscreens.

If you do choose to use a commercial sunscreen, apply it to all exposed skin thirty minutes before going outdoors. It requires this time to penetrate your skin. Waiting until you are in the sun before applying sunscreen leaves your skin unprotected for a time. When swimming or exercising, reapply sunscreen frequently. Cover as much of your body as possible with protective clothing. Wear a hat and sunglasses that filter out UV rays. After spending time in the sun, thoroughly remove commercial sunscreen by showering or bathing. Apply after-sun products to reduce the drying effects the sun has on your skin.

If you do develop sunburn, aromatherapy can help relieve some of the discomfort and may minimize the damage to your skin. Chamomile, eucalyptus, helichrysum, lavender, niaouli, patchouli, peppermint, and St. John's wort oils are especially helpful for soothing sunburn pain and cooling burned skin. Aloe vera gel, apple cider vinegar, buttermilk, oatmeal, and yogurt are home remedies that relieve the sting of sunburn, soothe skin, and prevent dryness. Bathe in a Sunburn-Soothing Bath as soon as possible to help draw out the heat from your sunburn. To relieve sunburn pain and the dry, tight feeling and to discourage peeling of the skin, apply Lavender Sunburn Oil or Sunburn Relief Skin Oil to the affected areas several times daily.

AROMATHERAPY BLENDS

You can prepare the aromatherapy blends below using pure essential oils. For a more detailed explanation of how to put together and use these blends, see Part Three: Ways to Use Aromatherapy. To review general guidelines for using essential oils, see page 142.

NATURAL SUNSCREEN OIL

1 ounce sesame oil

½ ounce coconut oil, melted

½ ounce olive oil

10 drops helichrysum oil

5 drops lavender oil

3 drops chamomile oil

In a clean container, add the essential oils to the carrier oils. Gently turn the container upside down several times or roll it between your hands to blend. Apply to the skin before exposure to the sun. Repeat application as needed.

SUNBURN-SOOTHING BATH

½ cup apple cider vinegar (optional)

4 drops lavender oil

2 drops chamomile oil

1 drop eucalyptus oil

1 drop peppermint oil

Disperse the vinegar and the essential oils in a bathtub filled with cool water. If you wish, you can add ice cubes to keep the water cool. Soak for fifteen to twenty minutes. Repeat every few hours until the pain subsides.

LAVENDER SUNBURN OIL

2 ounces carrier oil

15 drops lavender oil

Place the carrier oil in a clean container and add the lavender oil. Blend well. Apply the oil frequently to sunburned skin.

SUNBURN RELIEF SKIN OIL

2 ounces sesame oil

6 drops lavender oil

5 drops helichrysum oil

4 drops chamomile oil

2 drops patchouli oil

In a clean container, add the essential oils to the carrier oil. Gently turn the container upside down several times or roll it between your hands to blend. Apply often to the affected areas.

SWOLLEN GLANDS

See LYMPHATIC SYSTEM, SLUGGISH/SWOLLEN LYMPH GLANDS.

TEETHING

See TOOTHACHE.

TEMPOROMANDIBULAR JOINT (TMJ) SYNDROME

Temporomandibular joint (TMJ) syndrome is a disorder of the joint between the lower jawbone, or mandible, and the bone of the side of the skull. More than 10 million Americans experience difficulty and pain as this joint clicks, grinds, or pops while they chew or open and close their mouths, although most cases are never treated. Complications and symptoms can include blurred vision; dizziness; headaches; pain in the ears, jaw, neck, and shoulders; pressure behind the eyes; ringing in the ears; sinus problems; and toothache.

When the cartilage that cushions this joint becomes displaced or worn, the bones begin to rub against each other instead of gliding smoothly. Malocclusion, or bad bite, and stress are common causes. Tooth grinding, especially during sleep, or clenching the jaw can contribute, as can arthritis, bad dental work, muscle tension, or silver amalgam (mercury) fillings. Even the repeated insertion of hypodermic needles for dental anesthesia can be a factor. Bad posture, chewing gum, cradling the telephone between the jaw and shoulder, favoring one side of the mouth for chewing, thumb-sucking, and whiplash or other injury to the head, face, jaw, or neck are other contributing causes. People with hypoglycemia often experience TMJ syndrome because, when their blood sugar levels drop, they tend to clench and grind their teeth.

To determine if you have TMJ syndrome, perform the following test: Place the tips of your little fingers in your ears to block outside sounds. Slowly open, then close your mouth. If you hear or feel clicking, popping, or grinding, your jaw may be misaligned.

HELPFUL TREATMENTS

Conventional treatment for TMJ syndrome ranges from jaw exercises and drug therapy to dental procedures and, in severe cases, surgery. If you suspect TMJ syndrome, get your bite checked, since malocclusion can contribute to other problems—earache, headache, and sinus congestion, as well as the formation of wrinkles around the mouth and sagging facial skin.

Relaxation techniques can release stress and muscular tension. Breathing soothes you and your muscles. Yoga position for the face can help as can regular meditation. Evaluate what is causing your stress and tension and find ways to reduce or control them.

Massage helps. Using your fingertips, gently tap the muscles around the jaw joint to release tension, relax the muscles, and stimulate circulation to the area. Acupressure also helps. Use your thumb to apply light pressure while you open and close your mouth. Whenever you think about it, leave your mouth slightly open. This relaxes all the muscles. Putting your tongue between your teeth prevents you from grinding your teeth or clenching your jaw.

Aromatherapy can help on several levels. It can relax your body and mind. It can reduce stress. It can minimize inflammation and swelling in the joint. It helps regulate breathing while improving circulation. Essential oils that provide relief include benzoin, chamomile, coriander, cypress, eucalyptus, fennel, helichrysum, jasmine, juniper, lavender, peppermint, pine, rose, rosemary, St. John's wort, spruce, thyme, valerian, vetiver, and ylang ylang.

Apply TMJ Massage Oil on the joint several times daily, especially before performing acupressure, massage, or tapping

on the area. Borage, calophyllum inophyllum, evening primrose, flaxseed, and hemp oils are carrier oils that can relieve inflammation and swelling associated with TMJ syndrome.

AROMATHERAPY BLENDS

You can prepare the aromatherapy blend below using pure essential oils. For a more detailed explanation of how to put together and use this blend, see Part Three: Ways to Use Aromatherapy. To review general guidelines for using essential oils, see page 142.

TMJ MASSAGE OIL

1 ounce flaxseed oil
½ ounce borage oil
½ ounce hemp oil
4 drops helichrysum oil
3 drops spruce oil
2 drops vetiver oil
1 drop valerian oil

In a clean container, add the essential oils to the carrier oil and blend. Massage into the muscles around the TMJ joint as needed.

TOOTHACHE

A toothache usually results when the pulp, the innermost layer of the tooth and the part that contains the blood and nerve supply, becomes irritated and inflamed. The ache may be a persistent dull, throbbing pain or a sharp, stabbing one, or it may hurt only when you chew or bite down on the tooth. Your tooth may be sensitive to heat or cold.

Toothaches commonly occur when decay erodes the tooth enamel (the outer covering of the tooth) and the dentin (the body of the tooth), the two layers that surround the pulp. Gum disease, poor dental work, infection or inflammation of the pulp, death of the tooth's nerve, injury to a tooth, a loose tooth, loss of a filling or crown, or receding gums can also cause a toothache. A sinus infection sometimes causes pain that mimics a toothache.

HELPFUL TREATMENTS

If you develop a toothache, you should consult your dentist immediately. Failure to treat the underlying cause of a toothache could result in the loss of the tooth.

Aromatherapy can provide temporary relief until you visit your dentist. Essential oils that help ease toothache pain include chamomile, coriander, ginger, lavender, myrrh, niaouli, oregano, peppermint, rosemary, and tea tree. Apply a drop of Toothache Oil to the tooth and the surrounding area to ease the pain. Holding a clove bud in the mouth next to the offending tooth or chewing on fresh oregano leaves can help numb the pain. For additional relief, apply a Toothache Compress on your face near the aching tooth. To soothe teething pain in babies, chamomile oil provides a safe and effective remedy.

Massage Baby's Teething Blend into the affected gums.

AROMATHERAPY BLENDS

You can prepare the aromatherapy blends below using pure essential oils. For a more detailed explanation of how to put together and use these blends, see Part Three: Ways to Use Aromatherapy. To review general guidelines for using essential oils, see page 142.

TOOTHACHE OIL

⅛ ounce carrier oil
3 drops tea tree oil
2 drops chamomile oil
1 drop oregano oil
1 drop peppermint oil

Place the carrier oil in a clean container and add the essential oils. Gently turn the container upside down several times or roll it between your hands to blend. Apply 1 drop on the aching tooth and the surrounding gum as needed.

TOOTHACHE COMPRESS

1 quart hot water
2 drops peppermint oil

Pour the water into a 2-quart glass bowl and disperse the peppermint oil in the water. Saturate a clean cloth in the water and apply the compress to your face near the aching tooth. Repeat as often as necessary.

BABY'S TEETHING BLEND
½ ounce sunflower oil
1 drop chamomile oil

Add the chamomile oil to the sunflower oil and blend. Massage a drop into your baby's gums as needed.

VAGINITIS

Vaginitis is a general term for an inflammation or infection of the vagina. Numerous microorganisms commonly cause vaginitis, including bacteria *(Gardnerella),* protozoa *(Trichomona),* and *Candida albicans,* which causes the type of vaginitis known as a yeast infection.

Symptoms of vaginitis can include a burning sensation, discharge or dryness, itching, painful and frequent urination, and an unpleasant odor. Poor hygiene, sexually transmitted diseases or infections, and the use of products such as artificially fragranced bath oils or bubble baths, commercial douches, birth control devices (especially diaphragms), spermicides, tampons, and vaginal deodorant sprays all are factors that can lead to or promote the development of vaginitis. Hormonal imbalances, certain drugs, notably antibiotics, and poor nutrition are often contributing factors.

A yeast infection occurs when *Candida albicans,* a fungus commonly referred to as yeast, multiplies uncontrollably in the vagina. This often happens as a result of a change in the normal acidity of the vaginal environment. Symptoms of a yeast infection include leukorrhea (a thick, white, even cheesy-looking, vaginal discharge), a burning sensation, irritation, severe itching, and sometimes pain or discomfort during intercourse or urination.

Antibiotics; birth control pills; diabetes; pregnancy; excessive douching; steroids; and a diet high in alcohol, dairy products, refined carbohydrates, sugar, and yeast or fermented products can create or contribute to the development of a highly acid internal environment where yeast organisms flourish. Nutritional deficiencies, particularly deficiencies of the B vitamins, can also be a factor.

Any substance—douches, sexual aids or preparations, semen, and condoms treated with dyes, fragrances, or lubricants—that enters your vagina can contribute to vaginitis. Traces of anything your partner consumes—sugars, yeast-containing foods, alcohol, cigarette residues, and drugs—can concentrate in his semen and alter the environment of your vagina. His personal hygiene is another factor since bacteria, yeast, and other microbes can thrive on his penis, hiding in its skin creases and folds. Even the soap he washes with can alter the environment in your vagina.

HELPFUL TREATMENTS

Many doctors treat vaginitis with antibiotics (for bacterial vaginitis) or fungicidal preparations (for yeast infections). Unfortunately, when you take an antibiotic for bacterial vaginitis, you actually increase the likelihood that you will then develop a yeast infection, because antibiotics destroy the beneficial bacteria that keep *Candida albicans* under control.

You can take numerous precautions to prevent vaginitis. Always wash yourself thoroughly with a mild, unscented body soap and gently pat yourself dry. Wear cotton underwear. Avoid using fragranced bubble baths and bath oils, colored or scented condoms, commercial douches, fragranced detergents and fabric softeners, deodorant tampons or sanitary pads, scented toilet paper, and vaginal deodorant sprays. Do not allow any product that contains synthetic fragrance, scent, or perfume; coloring or dyes; artificial or synthetic ingredients; or preservatives to come into contact with the delicate skin in and around your vagina.

Reduce the amount of sugar, cheese, dairy products, and foods containing yeast in your diet. If you already have a yeast infection, or are prone to recurring yeast infections, eliminate these foods entirely. Wipe from front to back following bowel movements. Always urinate before and after intercourse and after bathing.

Recurring yeast infections may indicate a systemic candida infection, which may require more than a localized approach. (*See* CANDIDIASIS.) Sexual partners may pass infections back and forth. Therefore, your partner also may need treatment to completely clear up an infection. Since diet is a major contributing factor in *Candida albicans* or yeast infection, until both you and your partner modify your diets, you may continue to suffer from recurring yeast infections. Insist on immaculate hygiene from your partner.

Aromatherapy can relieve some of the discomforts of vaginitis. Some essential oils that are useful for vaginitis are benzoin, chamomile, juniper, laurel, lavender, myrrh, niaouli, oregano, palmarosa, patchouli, and tea tree. If you begin treating vaginitis when the symptoms first appear, you may halt the infection, or at least minimize the severity, the discomfort, and the duration of the symptoms.

Take a Vaginitis Sitz Bath at the first sign of symptoms and repeat once or twice daily thereafter, as needed. You can use a Vaginitis Douche either alone or in conjunction with the baths. A douche of 3 drops of lavender, niaouli, or tea tree oil in 1 quart of warm water can relieve the discomforts of a yeast infection. You can also apply several drops of lavender, niaouli, or tea tree oil to a clean cotton ball and insert it into the opening of the vagina (but no further), as a tampon. The cotton ball makes an economical substitute for this purpose; to saturate a tampon requires a lot of essential oil. If the area surrounding the vagina is tender or raw, apply Vaginitis Soothing Oil. If symptoms persist for more than one or two weeks, consult your health-care professional.

AROMATHERAPY BLENDS

You can prepare the aromatherapy blends below using pure essential oils. For a more detailed explanation of how to put together and use these blends, see Part Three: Ways to Use Aromatherapy. To review general guidelines for using essential oils, see page 142.

VAGINITIS SITZ BATH

2 drops niaouli oil

2 drops tea tree oil

1 drop lavender oil

Add the oils to a shallow tub filled with warm water. Sit hip-deep in the water for fifteen minutes. Repeat once or twice daily, as needed.

VAGINITIS DOUCHE

1 quart warm water

1 tablespoon apple cider vinegar

2 drops lavender oil

2 drops tea tree oil

Add the vinegar, lavender oil, and tea tree oil to the warm water and mix well. Fill a douche bag or syringe with the mixture and douche. Repeat one to three times weekly, as necessary.

VAGINITIS SOOTHING OIL

1 ounce jojoba or sunflower oil

2 drops laurel oil

2 drops lavender oil

2 drops tea tree oil

1 drop chamomile oil

In a clean container, add the essential oils to the jojoba or sunflower oil and blend. Apply the oil externally to irritated areas several times daily, as needed.

VARICOSE VEINS

Varicose veins occur when veins lose their tone and elasticity. They can appear anywhere in the body, but they are most common in the ankles, calves, and thighs. Varicose veins develop when the little valves in the veins that normally propel blood throughout the circulatory system cannot close properly and no longer push the blood upward toward the heart. Blood flow slows, and blood cannot move properly through the veins. Instead, it seeps into smaller superficial capillaries where it stagnates. Legs become congested, swollen, and inflamed. This prevents the delivery of adequate nutrients and oxygen to the tissues of the legs and inhibits the removal of wastes from the legs. The veins turn purple, cranberry, or dark blue in color and begin to bulge. The legs may feel hot and heavy and become sensitive to pressure.

Heredity is usually a primary factor in the development of varicose veins. Hormones also play a role. Varicose veins rarely appear before puberty, and women are more prone to develop varicose veins than men. Many women develop them during pregnancy due to the extra pressure on their blood vessels, particularly those in the legs. The increase in blood flow during pregnancy also places a bigger burden on a woman's veins.

Other factors in the development of varicose veins include age, muscular atrophy, chronic constipation, excess weight or obesity, extremes of temperature, insufficient exercise, poor circulation, prolonged bed rest, the consumption of alcohol or spicy foods, and the wearing of constrictive clothing or hosiery, high heels, or other unsuitable shoes. Sitting or standing in the same position for long periods of time can restrict proper blood flow into and out of the legs. Strenuous physical exertion or injury can damage a valve in a vein or form blood clots that permanently destroy the valve and impair circulation. In some cases, varicose veins can signal other health problems.

HELPFUL TREATMENTS

Walking helps pump blood through the veins, making it perhaps the best preventive measure, as well as the best treatment, for varicose veins. Exercises that elevate the legs are especially beneficial. Exercise improves lymphatic drainage, improves muscle tone, and increases muscle size. Larger, more developed muscles exert more pressure on the veins, encouraging the flow of blood toward the heart. Compression, such as that provided by athletic bandaging, support hose, or stockings, helps the veins thrust the blood supply upward from the legs to the heart.

Regular massage of the feet and legs can improve or prevent varicose veins. Deep-breathing exercises increase circulation, aiding the delivery of nutrients and oxygen to the affected areas. A person with varicose veins should avoid standing or sitting in one position for a prolonged period of time. When varicose veins are painful, elevating the legs often affords some relief; relax with your legs elevated whenever possible. Severe cases require medical treatment such as injection sclerotherapy, which permanently closes off the varicose veins, or surgery to remove all or some portion of the affected veins.

Used by itself or in conjunction with medical treatments, aromatherapy can diminish the discomfort and improve the appearance of varicose veins. Essential oils such as cypress, geranium, ginger, juniper, lemon, neroli, patchouli, peppermint, rosemary, and St. John's wort are especially effective in restoring good circulation to the areas with varicose veins. Use alternating applications of Warm Compress for Varicose Veins with Cool Stimulating Compress for Varicose Veins to stimulate circulation, relieve inflammation and swelling, and ease pain. Cold constricts blood vessels, while heat dilates them; alternating the temperatures of the compresses exercises the veins. Apply Varicose Vein Massage Oil to the affected areas twice daily and gently massage the skin above the varicose veins upward toward the heart. Elevate your feet during these treatments. Bathe in a Bath for Varicose Veins once a day to promote circulation to the legs and ease discomfort. Foot baths can also provide relief.

AROMATHERAPY BLENDS

You can prepare the aromatherapy blends below using pure essential oils. For a more detailed explanation of how to put together and use these blends, see Part Three: Ways to Use Aromatherapy. To review general guidelines for using essential oils, see page 142.

WARM COMPRESS FOR
VARICOSE VEINS

1 quart warm water
2 drops geranium oil
1 drop lemon oil
1 drop rosemary oil

Pour the water into a 2-quart glass bowl and add the essential oils. Blend well. Soak a clean cloth in the water and apply the compress to the affected areas. Elevate your legs for fifteen minutes. Follow with a Cool Stimulating Compress for Varicose Veins. Do this as needed.

COOL STIMULATING
COMPRESS FOR VARICOSE VEINS

1 quart cool water
2 drops cypress oil
1 drop ginger oil
1 drop peppermint oil

Pour the water into a 2-quart glass bowl and disperse the essential oils in the water. Soak a clean cloth in the water and apply it to your legs. Elevate your legs for fifteen minutes. Follow with Varicose Vein Massage Oil. Do this daily or as needed.

VARICOSE VEIN MASSAGE OIL

1 ounce carrier oil
3 drops cypress oil
2 drops patchouli oil
2 drops rosemary oil
1 drop juniper oil

Place the carrier oil in a clean container and add the essential oils. Gently turn the container upside down several times or roll it between your hands to blend. Beginning directly above the varicose veins, massage your legs with the oil, using strokes directed upward toward the heart. Repeat once or twice daily.

BATH FOR VARICOSE VEINS

2 drops cypress oil
2 drops lemon oil
1 drop geranium oil
1 drop juniper oil

Disperse the oils in a bathtub filled with warm water. Soak in the bath for fifteen to twenty minutes daily or as needed.

WEAKENED IMMUNE SYSTEM

Your immune system is a complex mechanism that works to protect and heal your body from infection and injury by foreign matter that could compromise health. It involves the blood, bone marrow, lymphatic system, skin, spleen, thymus, and special immune cells. These special cells patrol your body to locate, identify, and destroy any foreign substances that threaten your health. They differentiate between cells and molecules that are "self" and those that are "non-self." When anything is identified as "non-self," the immune cells take action to eliminate it. They do this by stimulating the production of antibodies to protect you against foreign substances, or antigens, that can attack healthy tissues, upset your body's balance, and cause illness. A weakened immune system cannot respond adequately to the presence of antigens, rendering the body even more susceptible to all sorts of illnesses.

Poor nutrition and nutritional deficiencies are common contributors to low immunity. High cholesterol levels, stress, and sugar consumption also weaken immunity. Other factors that can weaken immunity include chemotherapy treatment for cancer; the consumption of alcohol; exposure to environmental pollutants, pesticides, radiation, food additives, food colorings, and preservatives; food allergies; heavy metal poisoning; hormonal imbalances; obesity; vaccines; the prolonged use of antibiotics, cortisone, steroids, and over-the-counter, prescription, or recreational drugs; and sunburn and sun exposure.

Signs that you may be suffering from lowered immunity include allergies, candidiasis, chemical sensitivities, chronic fatigue, chronic infections, colds, recurring asthma or bronchitis, and slower-than-usual healing from illness or injury.

Certain medical conditions, including acquired immune deficiency syndrome (AIDS), AIDS-related complex (ARC), and certain types of cancer, can severely depress the immune system. Although these serious illnesses are beyond the scope of this book, people who suffer from them may still derive benefit from using essential oils. Even in cases where it cannot address an underlying physical problem, aromatherapy can often successfully combat stress and address emotional issues. (*See also* EMOTIONAL ISSUES *and* STRESS.) However, if you have an illness that seriously impairs your immunity, you should consult with your health-care provider before using any essential oils.

HELPFUL TREATMENTS

There are a number of nutrients that can help restore and revitalize your immune system. These include antioxidants such as beta-carotene, selenium, zinc, and vitamins A, C, and E. Other important nutrients are iron and vitamin B_6. The herbs echinacea, goldenseal, and licorice root have immune-stimulating properties as well. Digestive enzymes are helpful in supporting the immune system; they improve the digestion, absorption, and assimilation of foods and nutritional supplements you consume.

Modify your diet, if necessary, to focus on fresh vegetables and fruits, whole grains, and legumes; avoid any foods that trigger allergies. You may wish to consult a nutritionist to determine if you have any food allergies or nutritional deficiencies and to set up an immune-boosting program. Stress management and regular exercise will also strengthen immunity.

Aromatherapy can boost immunity by prompting your body to heal itself. Essential oils that improve immunity are bergamot, chamomile, clary sage, elemi, eucalyptus, geranium, ginger, laurel, lavender, lemon, myrrh, niaouli, orange, oregano, rosemary, rosewood, sandalwood, spruce, tea tree, thyme, and vetiver. These oils promote the production of white blood cells, increase immune response, and fight bacteria, fungi, and viruses.

Aromatherapy can also reduce stress and help stabilize emotions. Long-term emotional upset and stress can compromise the immune system, preventing it from performing properly. Essential oils can help you to bring your body and mind back into balance. Take a Morning Immunity Bath or an Evening Immunity Bath or both, each day. Apply Immune-Boosting Massage Oil over your body once or twice daily. Carrier oils that promote immunity include borage, calophyllum inophyllum, coconut, and flaxseed.

AROMATHERAPY BLENDS

You can prepare the aromatherapy blends below using pure essential oils. For a more detailed explanation of how to put together and use these blends, see Part Three: Ways to Use Aromatherapy. To review general guidelines for using essential oils, see page 142.

MORNING IMMUNITY BATH

3 drops tea tree oil
2 drops rosemary oil
1 drop ginger oil
1 drop lemon oil

Disperse the essential oils in a bathtub filled with warm water. Soak in the bath for fifteen to twenty minutes.

EVENING IMMUNITY BATH

2 drops rosewood oil
2 drops thyme oil
1 drop elemi oil
1 drop oregano oil

Disperse the essential oils in a bathtub filled with warm water. Soak in the bath for fifteen to twenty minutes.

IMMUNE-BOOSTING MASSAGE OIL

2 ounces coconut oil
4 drops geranium oil
4 drops niaouli oil
2 drops lemon oil
2 drops spruce oil
1 drop elemi oil
1 drop myrrh oil

Place the carrier oil in a clean container, add the essential oils, and blend gently. Massage the mixture over your body once or twice daily.

YEAST INFECTION

See VAGINITIS.

APPENDIX

Aromatherapy Resource Guide

✳

RECOMMENDED SUPPLIERS

Omega Nutrition
6514 Aldrich Road
Bellingham, WA 98226
800–661–3529 or 604–253–4223
www.omeganutrition.com
Organic carrier oils.

Original Swiss Aromatics
P.O. Box 6842
San Rafael, CA 94903
415–479–4120
Pure essential oils, essential oil blends.

Redmond Minerals
P.O. Box 219
6005 North 100 West
Redmond, UT 84652
435–529–7402
www.realsalt.com
Clay, earth salt, sea salt.

Roberta Wilson Aromatherapy
P.O. Box 1717
Elephant Butte, NM 87935
www.robertawilsonaromatherapy.com
Pure essential oils, organic carrier oils, ready-to-use aromatherapy blends, aromatherapy skin-care

products, aromatherapy body-care products, aromatherapy bath products, Dead Sea salts, clay products, and fragrances made from pure essential oils.

PUBLICATIONS

Aromatherapy Today
P.O. Box 211
Kellyville, NSW 2155
Australia
011–61–2–9894–9933
www.aromatherapytoday.com

e-scentual news
P.O. Box 1717
Elephant Butte, NM 87935
www.oneminutearomatherapy.com

Inside Aromatherapy
P.O. Box 6723
San Rafael, CA 94903
415–479–9120
www.pacificinstituteofaromatherapy.com

The International Journal of Aromatherapy
P.O. Box 156
Avenel, NJ 07001
877–839–7126
www.harcourt-international.com/journals/
    ijar

EDUCATION

Pacific Institute of Aromatherapy
P.O. Box 6723
San Rafael, CA 94903
415–479–9120
www.pacificinstituteofaromatherapy.com

ORGANIZATIONS

International Federation of Aromatherapists, Australia
P.O. Box 786
Templestowe, VIC 3106
Australia
011–61–1–902–240–125
www.ifa.org.au

International Federation of Aromatherapists, England
182 Chiswick High Road
London W4 1PP
England
011–44–0–20–8742–2605
www.int-fed-aromatherapy.co.uk

The National Association for Holistic Aromatherapy
4509 Interlake Avenue North, No. 233
Seattle, WA 98103-6773
888–ASK–NAHA or 206–547–2164
www.naha.org

RESEARCH

www.oneminutearomatherapy.com

A website that allows you to participate in research programs and studies that use simple procedures and essential oils to treat common physical and emotional conditions, and to share your aromatherapy adventures, experiences, and successes with others online.

Recommended Reading

Blevi, Viktor, and Gretchen Sween. *Aromatherapy*. New York, NY: Avon Books, 1993.

Catty, Suzanne. *Hydrosols: The Next Aromatherapy*. Rochester, VT: Healing Arts Press, 2001.

Davis, Patricia. *Aromatherapy: An A–Z*. Essex, England: C.W. Daniel, 1988.

Fischer-Rizzi, Suzanne. *Complete Aromatherapy Handbook*. New York, NY: Sterling Publishing, 1990.

Harvey, John, Lilias Folan, Annemarie Colbin, Roberta Wilson, Don Campbell, Kay Gardner, Shakti Gawain, Ohashi, Dan Millman, Michael Hutchison, and Terry Patten. *The Big Book of Relaxation*. Edited by Larry Blumenfeld. Roslyn, NY: The Relaxation Company, 1994.

Keville, Kathi, and Mindy Green. *Aromatherapy: A Complete Guide to the Healing Art*. Freedom, CA: The Crossing Press, 1995.

Lavabre, Marcel. *Aromatherapy Workbook.* Rochester, VT: Healing Arts Press, 1990.

Lawless, Julia. *The Encyclopaedia of Essential Oils.* Rockport, MA: Element, Inc., 1992.

Mojay, Gabriel. *Aromatherapy for Healing the Spirit.* Rochester, VT: Healing Arts Press, 1999.

Ryman, Danièle. *Aromatherapy: The Complete Guide to Plant and Flower Essences for Health and Beauty.* New York, NY: Bantam Books, 1993.

Schnaubelt, Kurt. *Advanced Aromatherapy: The Science of Essential Oil Therapy.* Rochester, VT: Healing Arts Press, 1998.

———. *Medical Aromatherapy.* Berkeley, CA: Frog, Ltd., 1999.

Sellar, Wanda. *The Directory of Essential Oils.* Essex, England: C.W. Daniel, 1992.

Worwood, Valerie Ann. *The Complete Book of Essential Oils and Aromatherapy.* San Rafael, CA: New World Library, 1991.

Bibliography

Arctancer, Steffen. *Perfume and Flavor Materials of Natural Origin*. Elizabeth, NJ: By the author, 1960.

Atkinson, Holly. *Women and Fatigue*. New York, NY: G.P. Putnam's Sons, 1985.

Baker, Don, and Emery Nester. *Depression*. Portland, OR: Multnomah Press, 1983.

Balch, James, and Phyllis Balch. *Prescription for Nutritional Healing*. Garden City Park, NY: Avery Publishing Group, 1990.

Balch, James F., and Phyllis A. Balch. *Prescription for Nutritional Healing,* 2nd ed. Garden City Park, NY: Avery Publishing Group, 1997.

Bell, Robert. *Dictionary of Classical Mythology*. Santa Barbara, CA: ABC Clio, 1982.

Benjamin, Ben, with Gale Borden. *Listen to Your Pain*. New York, NY: Viking Press, 1984.

Berger, Stuart. Dr. Berger's Immune Power Diet. New York, NY: New American Library, 1985.

Blevi, Viktor, and Gretchen Sween. *Aromatherapy.* New York, NY: Avon Books, 1993.

Bremness, Lesley. *The Complete Book of Herbs.* New York, NY: Viking Penguin, 1994.

Bricklin, Mark. *Rodale's Encyclopedia of Natural Home Remedies.* Emmaus, PA: Rodale Press, 1982.

Brooke, Elisabeth. *Herbal Therapy for Women.* London, England: Thorsons Publishing, 1992.

The Burton Goldberg Group, ed. *Alternative Medicine: The Definitive Guide.* Fife, WA: Future Medicine Publishing, Inc., 1995.

Catty, Suzanne. *Hydrosols: The Next Aromatherapy.* Rochester, VT: Healing Arts Press, 2001.

Cooley, Donald G., ed. *Family Medical Guide,* 5th ed. New York, NY: Better Homes and Gardens Books, 1976.

Cunningham, Scott. *Magical Aromatherapy.* St. Paul, MN: Llewellyn Publications, 1989.

Davidson, Paul. *Chronic Muscle Pain Syndrome.* New York, NY: Villard Books, 1989.

Davis, Patricia. *Aromatherapy: An A–Z.* Essex, England: C.W. Daniel, 1988.

———. *Subtle Aromatherapy.* Essex, England: C.W. Daniel, 1991.

Dobelis, Inge, ed. *Magic and Medicine of Plants.* Pleasantville, NY: Reader's Digest Association, 1986.

Dodt, Colleen K. *The Essential Oils Book.* Pownal, VT: Storey Publishing, 1996.

Dorland, W.A. Newman. *Dorland's Illustrated Medical Dictionary,* 27th ed. Edited by Elizabeth J. Taylor, Douglas M. Anderson, Joseph M. Patwell, Katharine Plaut, and Kathleen McCullough. Philadelphia: W.B. Saunders Co., 1988.

Drury, Susan. *Tea Tree Oil: Nature's Miracle Healer.* Lindfield, Australia: Unity Press, 1989.

Egide, Stacey, ed. *A Guide to the Art of Aromatherapy.* Petaluma, CA: Tisserand Aromatherapy USA, 1993.

Ehrmantraut, Harry. *Headaches: The Drugless Way to Lasting Relief.* Berkeley, CA: Celestial Arts, 1987.

Fife, Bruce. *The Miracles of Coconut Oil Healing.* Colorado Springs, CO: Health Wise Publications, 2000.

Finnegan, John. *The Facts About Fats.* Berkeley, CA: Celestial Arts, 1993.

Fischer-Rizzi, Suzanne. *Complete Aromatherapy Handbook.* New York, NY: Sterling Publishing, 1990.

Foster, Steven. *Herbal Renaissance.* Layton, UT: Gibbs Smith Publishers, 1997.

Garrison, Robert, Jr., and Elizabeth Somer. *The Nutrition Desk Reference.* New Canaan, CT: Keats Publishing, 1990.

Gattefossé, René-Maurice. *Gattefossé's Aromatherapy.* Essex, England: C. W. Daniel, 1937; reprint, 1993.

Genders, Roy. *A History of Scent.* London, England: Hamish Hamilton, 1972.

Gerson, Joel. *Standard Textbook for Professional Estheticians.* Bronx, NY: Milady Publishing, 1986.

Grieve, M. *A Modern Herbal,* Vol. 1. New York, NY: Dover Publications, 1971.

———. *A Modern Herbal,* Vol. 2. New York, NY: Dover Publications, 1971.

Groom, Nigel. *The Perfume Book.* New York, NY: Chapman & Hall, 1992.

Guiness, Alma, ed. *Family Guide to Natural Medicine.* Pleasantville, NY: Reader's Digest Association, 1993.

Hoffman, David. *The Herbal Handbook.* Rochester, VT: Healing Arts Press, 1988.

Hogan, Elizabeth, ed. *Sunset Western Garden Book.* Menlo Park, CA: Lane Publishing, 1988.

Junemann, Monika. *Enchanting Scents.* Wilmot, WI: Lotus Light, 1988.

Keville, Kathi, and Mindy Green. *Aromatherapy: A Complete Guide to the Healing Art.* Freedom, CA: The Crossing Press, 1995.

Kowalchik, Claire, and William Hylton, eds. *Rodale's Illustrated Encyclopedia of Herbs.* Emmaus, PA: Rodale Press, 1987.

Lanctôt, Guylaine. *How to Have Great Legs at Any Age.* New York, NY: New Chapter Press, 1988.

Lautié, Raymond, and André Passebecq. *Aromatherapy: The Use of Plant Essences in Healing.* Wellingborough, England: Thorsons Publishing Group, 1979.

Lavabre, Marcel. *Aromatherapy Workbook.* Rochester, VT: Healing Arts Press, 1990.

———. "Essential Oil Distillation." *Beyond Scents Newsletter,* Vol. 1, No. 3, Summer 1993.

———. "Essential Oil Production: Traditional Versus Modern Distillation." *Beyond Scents Newsletter,* Vol. 1, No. 2, Spring 1993.

Lavabre, Michael, and Michael Scholes. Aromatherapy Seminars Advanced Certification Course. Los Angeles: Aromatherapy Seminars, 1992.

Lawless, Julia. *The Encyclopaedia of Essential Oils.* Rockport, MA: Element, Inc., 1992.

Lee, William, and Lynn Lee. *The Book of Practical Aromatherapy.* New Canaan, CT: Keats Publishing, 1992.

Livingston, Lida, and Constance Schrader. *Wrinkles.* Englewood Cliffs, NJ: Prentice-Hall, 1978.

Maple, Eric. *The Magic of Perfume.* New York, NY: Samuel Weiser, 1973.

McArdle, William, Frank Katch, and Victor Katch. *Exercise Physiology: Energy, Nutrition, and Human Performance.* Philadelphia: Lea & Febiger, 1986.

Mee, Charles L., Jr., ed. *Massage: Total Relaxation.* Alexandria, VA: Time-Life Books, 1987.

Mojay, Gabriel. *Aromatherapy for Healing the Spirit.* Rochester, VT: Healing Arts Press, 1999.

Morris, Edwin. *Fragrance.* Greenwich, CT: E.T. Morris & Co., 1984.

Murray, Michael, and Joseph Pizzorno. *Encyclopedia of Natural Medicine.* Rocklin, CA: Prima Publishing, 1991.

National Academy Press. *Jojoba.* Washington, D.C.: National Academy Press, 1985.

Novick, Nelson Lee. *Super Skin.* New York, NY: Clarkson N. Potter, Inc., 1988.

Olsen, Cynthia. *Australian Tea Tree Oil Guide.* Pagosa Springs, CO: Kali Press, 1992.

Pearsall, Paul. *SuperImmunity.* New York, NY: McGraw-Hill Book Company, 1987.

Pugliese, Peter. *Advanced Professional Skin Care.* Bernville, PA: APSC Publishing, 1991.

Quirin, K.W., and D. Gerard. "Supercritical CO_2 Extraction of Natural Products Used in Cosmetics and Perfumery." *Zeitschrift für die Chemisch-Technische Industrie, die Technische Chemie und Spezialchemikalien,* 24 October 1991.

Rector-Page, Linda. *Healthy Healing,* rev. ed. Privately printed, 1990.

Reynolds, James E.F., ed. *Martindale: The Extra Pharmacopoeia,* 30th ed. London, England: Pharmaceutical Press, 1993.

Richard, David. *Anoint Yourself with Oil for Radiant Health.* Bloomingdale, IL: Vital Health Publishing, 1997.

Rimmel, Eugene. *The Book of Perfumes.* Philadelphia, PA: J.B. Lippincott, 1866.

Ronsard, Nicole. *Beyond Cellulite.* New York, NY: Villard Books, 1992.

————. *Cellulite.* New York, NY: Bantam Books, 1975.

Rose, Jeanne. *The Aromatherapy Book.* Berkeley, CA: North Atlantic Books, 1992.

Ryman, Danièle. *Aromatherapy: The Complete Guide to Plant and Flower Essences for Health and Beauty.* New York, NY: Bantam Books, 1993.

Sagarin, Edward. *The Science and Art of Perfumery.* New York, NY: McGraw-Hill Book Company, 1945.

Schnaubelt, Kurt. *Advanced Aromatherapy.* Rochester, VT: Healing Arts Press, 1998.

————. *Aromatherapy Course.* San Rafael, CA: Pacific Institute of Aromatherapy, 1985.

————. *Medical Aromatherapy.* Berkeley, CA: Frog, Ltd., 1999.

————. *Science and Emotion.* San Rafael, CA: Pacific Institute of Aromatherapy, 1998.

————. *Wholistic Aromatherapy.* San Rafael, CA: Pacific Institute of Aromatherapy, 1995.

————. ed. *Essential Oils and Cancer.* San Rafael, CA: Terra Linda Scent and Image, 2000.

Scholes, Michael. *Beyond Scents Home Study Course.* Los Angeles: Aromatherapy Seminars, 1991.

Sellar, Wanda. *The Directory of Essential Oils.* Essex, England: C.W. Daniel, 1992.

Serrentino, Jo. *How Natural Remedies Work.* Point Robert, WA: Hartley & Marks, 1991.

Shayevitz, Myra, and Berton Shayevitz. *Living Well with Emphysema and Bronchitis.* Garden City, NY: Doubleday & Company, 1985.

Soltanoff, Jack. *Natural Healing.* New York, NY: Warner Books, 1988.

Thompson, C.J.S. *The Mystery and Lure of Perfume.* London, England: John Lane The Bodley Head Limited, 1927.

Tisserand, Maggie. *Aromatherapy for Women*. New York, NY: Thorsons Publishers, 1985.

Tisserand, Robert. *The Art of Aromatherapy*. Rochester, VT: Inner Traditions, 1979.

————. *The Essential Oil Safety Data Manual*. East Sussex, England: The Tisserand Aromatherapy Institute, 1988.

Todd, Pamela. *Forget-Me-Not: A Floral Treasury*. Boston: Bulfinch Press, 1993.

Trueman, John. *The Romantic Story of Scent*. London, England: Aldus Books Limited, 1975.

Turin, Alan C. *No More Headaches!* Boston: Houghton Mifflin Company, 1981.

Valnet, Jean. *The Practice of Aromatherapy*. New York, NY: Destiny Books, 1980.

Van De Graaff, Kent M., and Stuart Ira Fox. *Concepts of Human Anatomy and Physiology*. Dubuque, IA: William C. Brown Publishers, 1986.

Verrill, A. Hyatt. *Perfumes and Spices*. Boston: L.C. Page & Company, 1940.

Vogel, Virgil. *American Indian Medicine*. Norman, OK: University of Oklahoma Press, 1970.

Wall, Carly. *Naturally Healing Herbs*. New York, NY: Sterling Publishing Company, 1996.

Weinstein, Alan. *Asthma*. New York, NY: McGraw-Hill Book Company, 1987.

Wellness Encyclopedia, The. Boston: Houghton Mifflin Company, 1991.

Wildwood, Chrissie. *The Encyclopedia of Aromatherapy*. Rochester, VT: Healing Arts Press, 1996.

Wilson, Roberta. *The Cellulite Control Guide*. Albuquerque, NM: By the author, 1994.

————. *The Cellulite Control System*. Los Angeles, CA: By the author, 1988.

————. *The Facial Rejuvenation Program*. Santa Monica, CA: By the author, 1984.

Worwood, Valerie Ann. *Aromantics*. London, England: Pan Books, 1987.

————. *The Complete Book of Essential Oils and Aromatherapy*. San Rafael, CA: New World Library, 1991.

Zohary, Michael. *Plants of the Bible*. Cambridge, MA: Cambridge University Press, 1982.

Index